Innovation in community care and primary health

Patrick C Pietroni
MB BS MRCP FRCGP DCH
Director of the Centre for Community Care and
Primary Health, University of Westminster, London, UK

Professor Patrick Pietroni is married with three children
and has practised acupuncture and homoeopathy
for over 15 years. He has taught yoga and lectured
widely on the topic of complementary medicine. He is
an associate regional adviser with the British
Postgraduate Medical Federation, and was formerly
Council member of the Royal College of General
Practitioners, a member of the Medicines
Commission, and also, Senior Lecturer in General
Practice at St. Mary's Hospital Medical School. He is a
founder member and past-Chairman of the British
Holistic Medical Association set up in 1983, and is a
practising Jungian analyst. Professor Pietroni is the
principal of a National Health Service health centre
which, as part of a research project, incorporates
complementary therapies, audit, community outreach,
and education and self-help programmes. As a result
of this research work, the Marylebone Centre Trust
was set up in 1988 to both promote and develop the
experimental work of the health centre, with education
and training programmes, the aim being to encourage
similar models of health care within the NHS. In
August 1993, the Centre for Community Care and
Primary Health, based at the Trust offices, was established within the Faculty of Business Management
and Social Studies at the University of Westminster
with the validation of a Masters in Community and
Primary Health Care, and in January 1994, a Masters
in Therapeutic Bodywork. Other programmes in the
process of being validated include an MSc in General
Practice and Primary Health, an MA, Diploma and
Certificate in Community Development, and an MA
and Diploma in Community Observation.

For Churchill Livingstone:

Commissioning editor: Inta Ozols
Project development editor: Valerie Bain
Project manager: Valerie Burgess
Project controller: Pat Miller
Design direction: Judith Wright
Copy editor: Anita Hible
Indexer: Tarrant Ranger Indexing Agency
Sales promotion executive: Maria O'Connor

Community Care and Primary Health

Innovation in community care and primary health

The Marylebone experiment

Edited by

Professor Patrick C Pietroni FRCGP MRCP DCH
Director of the Centre for Community Care and Primary Health, University of Westminster, London, UK

Christopher Pietroni BA (Oxon)

Foreword by

Kenneth Calman MD PhD FRCS FRCP FRCGP FRCR FFPHM FRSE
Chief Medical Officer, Department of Health, London, UK

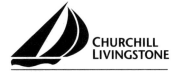

CHURCHILL LIVINGSTONE

NEW YORK EDINBURGH LONDON MADRID MELBOURNE SAN FRANCISCO AND TOKYO 1996

CHURCHILL LIVINGSTONE
Medical Division of Pearson Professional Limited

Distributed in the United States of America by Churchill
Livingstone Inc., 650 Avenue of the Americas, New York,
N.Y. 10011, and by associated companies, branches and
representatives throughout the world.

First published 1996

ISBN 0 443 05296 4

British Library of Cataloguing in Publication Data
A catalogue record for this book is available from the British
Library.

Library of Congress Cataloging in Publication Data
A catalogue record for this book is available from the Library
of Congress.

The
publisher's
policy is to use
**paper manufactured
from sustainable forests**

Produced by Saxon Graphics Ltd, Derby
Printed in Singapore

Contents

Contributors

David Aldridge PhD
Researcher, Marylebone Health Centre, London, UK

Veronica Barry
Community Service Volunteer, Marylebone Health Centre, London, UK

Pauline Benson BSc
Research Officer, Academic Department of Psychiatry, St. Mary's Hospital, London, UK

Linda Bridge BSc
Research Officer, Academic Department of Psychiatry, St. Mary's Medical Hospital, London, UK

Derek Chase MA MBBChir MRCGP DRCOG
Lecturer, Department of General Practice, St. Mary's Hospital Medical School, London, UK

Sybilla de Uray-Ura
Patient Liaison Worker, Marylebone Health Centre, London, UK

Peter Davies PhD
Director of Research (Clinical Audit), Marylebone Centre Trust, London, UK

Arnold Desser BA (Hons) CAc MRTCM
City Health Centre Acupuncturist, Marylebone Health Centre, Senior Lecturer, London School of Acupuncture and Traditional Chinese Medicine, London, UK

J Fleming HNC
Researcher, Marylebone Health Centre, London, UK

Clare Harrison BA (Hons) DTM
Research Assistant, Marylebone Centre Trust, London, UK

Jenny Hewison MSc PhD
Researcher, Marylebone Centre Trust, London, UK

Anthea Hey
Senior Research Fellow and Postqualifying Tutor, Brunel University, Middlesex, UK

Anne Kilcoyne BA DCP CertEd TQAP
Clinical Psychologist & Psychotherapist, Arts Health Research, Totnes, Devon, UK

Michael H Kottow MA(Soc) MD
Professor of Ophthalmology, University of Chile, Chile

Julienne McLean
Department of General Practice, St. Mary's Hospital Medical School, London, UK

Claire McCormack
Massage Therapist, Marylebone Health Centre, London, UK

Helen Martyn
University of London Goldsmith's College, London, UK

Harriet Meek
Researcher/Social Worker, Chicago, USA

Chrissie Melhuish RSCN ITEC
Marylebone Health Centre, London, UK

Brian Minty
Lecturer in Social Work, Manchester University,
Manchester, UK

Sue Morrison MBBS MRCGP
Marylebone Health Centre, London, UK

David Peters MB MFHom MLCOM MRO
Medical Osteopath, Marylebone Centre Trust,
London, UK

Christopher Pietroni BA (Oxon)
Research Assistant, Marylebone Centre Trust,
London, UK

Marilyn Pietroni MA
Principal Lecturer in Community Care and
Primary Health, University of Westminster,
London, UK

Robert G Priest FRCPsych
Professor of Psychiatry, Academic Department of
Psychiatry, St. Mary's Hospital, London, UK

Peter Reason PhD
Centre for the Study of Organisational Change
and Development, University of Bath, Bath, UK

Alan Rushton
The Maudsley Hospital, Institute of Psychiatry,
London, UK

Alan Shuttleworth
Tavistock Clinic, Polytechnic of East London,
London, UK

Jill Spratley BSc DipEd Res
Independent Consultant, Devon, UK

Judith Trowell MBBS DCH TPM FRCPsych
Consultant Child Psychoanalyst, Tavistock
Clinic, London, UK

Dorothy Wallstein RSHom
Northern College of Homoeopathic Medicine,
Newcastle, UK

Vivien Webber BSc ALCP
Social Worker/Psychoanalytic Psychotherapist,
Marylebone Health Centre, London, UK

Foreword

For many reasons it could be said that there has never been a better time to be in primary care. It forms the basis of our health services and provides high quality care for the population, close to where they live. Improvements in primary care have been continuous over the last 30 years, in clinical practice, education and in practice management. The context in which primary care operates has also been changing, in social, demographic and political terms and by the way in which advances in medical practice have provided new opportunities for delivering effective care in the community setting.

Primary care has always had a strong educational base, and has developed a tradition of innovation and research. It has, from the beginning, recognized the importance of involving the patient and the public in decision making about the quality of care provided and of making available information from which choices can be made. The team approach has been central to this with a recognition of the roles and responsibilities of each member, and of the wide range of skills required. It has been concerned with the whole patient, and has extended the range of treatment options available to ensure that the needs of all patients can be met.

This book provides the reader with both breadth and depth, and encourages a reflective approach to primary care. It sets out some new directions and in the spirit of the title considers creativity and innovation as part of practice philosophy. It sets out a particular view of primary care which will be readily recognized by those who wish to see primary care at the heart of the process of health care and is very much in tune with a primary care led health service.

Learning is central to the process of improvement, both for the individual and the organisation. Education is as important as training, and the distinction between the two words is important. To be trained is to have arrived, to be educated is to continue to travel, the essence of professionalism. We need skilled and highly trained primary care teams. But we also need them to have an educated view of clinical practice and be able to respond to change and to have the motivation to continue to learn and grow in experience and knowledge. There is an important ethical element in continuing education as patients expect that the doctor and other members of the team will be well informed and able to provide them with high quality care.

Those at a leading edge of any specialty recognize that there may be few sign posts ahead, and that the road is not well trodden. It is for this reason that to innovate and change can be difficult. The words of an Aboriginal saying, 'there are no paths, paths are made by walking' will strike a chord with many who will read this book. But we do need to see change and to take primary care forward with continual improvements in quality. That is the challenge for all who believe that the community is the place to deliver care, and that the patient is the central focus of the primary care team.

Kenneth Calman

Preface to the series

The combination of academic rigour and clinical practice has been a difficult one to achieve in secondary care. To attempt this fusion in Community Care and Primary Health is a challenge not yet attempted. This series will endeavour to record the work undertaken by the Centre of Community Care & Primary Health at the University of Westminster. There are currently eight separate Masters programmes:

- MA in Community & Primary Health Care: towards reflective practice

- MA in Community Development: towards reflective practice

- MA in Community Observation: towards reflective practice

- MSc in General Practice & Primary Health

- MSc in Evaluation of Clinical Practice: audit and quality improvement

- MA in Continuing Professional Education

- MSc in Complementary Therapy Studies

- MA in Therapeutic Bodywork

and an undergraduate degree in Therapeutic Massage.

Each book will serve to capture both the relevance of the clinical encounter as well as the rigour of the academic enquiry. The separate volumes will be a combination of already existing work as well as additional material written specifically for the area of exploration. Health and Social Care is rapidly evolving under the pressure of recent reforms. Complementary therapy, once excluded from mainstream enquiry, is receiving serious academic attention. It is vitally important that this transitional stage in the evolution of the new structures is recorded and critiqued. We welcome this new series and look forward to the forthcoming issues.

1996   P.P

Preface

I am very grateful for the opportunity to read again this comprehensive collection of papers describing experiments in community and primary health care which have developed in and around the Marylebone Health Centre since 1987. These experiments are combined in a way which I believe to be unique. Some – perhaps the smaller ones – are completed. There are also more ambitious ones which could not possibly be completed in 7 years; they are continuing and will be worth watching after this introductory volume is published.

A principal aim of the whole project is to study how far social isolation can be reduced and physical and psychological well-being can be enhanced in an inner city, by encouraging patients to accept more responsiblity for their own health, by involving them in their own care when in trouble and by inviting as many as possible to play an active part in the practice. Both the practice and the Trust which grew out of it have become increasingly concerned with interprofessional collaboration and the interprofessional education. Collaboration has been with those professions which are now working together in many other primary care teams, but also with several complementary therapists who use their particular theories about the cause of illnesses and their particular methods of treatment within the Centre. The problems of exposing and understanding fundamental assumptions and identifying different meanings attached to the same familiar words is not confined to cooperation between orthodox and complementary practitioners, although it may be most obvious and difficult there.

An overall characteristic of the practice, the Trust and of this collection of papers is breadth. This is a strength. Other strengths are in the basic setting – a National Health Service general practice; in the continuous monitoring of what is done, through the constant presence of a social scientist; and in the association with a university, which ensures the integration of teaching and research with the practice, and increases the likelihood of further development.

June 1995
John Horder
Past President of the Royal College of General Practitioners
President, The National Centre for the Advancement of Interprofessional education in Primary Health and Community Care (CAIPE), London, UK

Acknowledgements

The following studies were funded by the Wates Foundation and the authors acknowledge the Foundation's generous and continuing support:

- Calculation of the underprivileged area score for a practice in inner London
- The impact of a volunteer community care project in a primary health care setting
- Disabilities issues in the provision of health care: an initial investigation
- Informal complaints procedures in general practice—a one year audit
- Self-care—who does best?
- A controlled trial of self-care classes in general practice, taught by staff members with a short training, to long-term users of anxiolytic, hypnotic and anti-depressant drugs
- Counselling in an inner city general practice: analysis of its use and uptake
- The musculoskeletal clinic in a general practice: a study of one year's referrals
- Towards a clinical framework for collaboration between general practice and complementary practitioners: discussion paper
- Power and conflict in multidisciplinary collaboration
- Traditional Chinese medicine in general practice: an analysis of one year's referrals

Grateful acknowledgement is given to sources, as indicated in footnotes to articles, for permission to reproduce copyright material.

Introduction

The Marylebone Centre Trust is a charity dedicated to the promotion of a new, integrated and exploratory approach to community and primary health care. It is based on the experimental work of the Marylebone Health Centre, which is an NHS general practice incorporating:

- community care and outreach programmes
- patient participation and education schemes
- clinical research and audit
- complementary therapy such as counselling, osteopathy, homoeopathy, traditional Chinese medicine and massage therapy.

The Marylebone Health Centre was itself a continuation of a small pilot study undertaken by Dr Patrick Pietroni at the Department of General Practice, Lisson Grove Health Centre in 1984/85. The study resulted in a 5-year grant from the Wates Foundation, accompanied by great support and encouragement from Neil Wates, the Chairman, to establish a new general practice in Marylebone to continue the work. This marked the beginning of a long and fruitful association with the Wates Foundation, which generously funded much of the work of the Marylebone Health Centre and Marylebone Centre Trust over a period of years. The overall objective for the new practice was 'to explore and evaluate ways in which primary health care can be delivered to an inner city area in addition to the general practice component. The approaches used would include an holistic component comprising an educational self-help model, as well as a complementary medicine component'.

This project, while unique at the time, was in many ways a revival of the approach to health care undertaken by Dr George Scott Williamson and Dr Inness Pearse in the 'Peckham Experiment' of the 1920s. The health centre run by these doctors was designed to investigate the hypothesis that 'health is more infectious than disease'. Their focus on health promotion and self-care—notions that are now taken for granted—was in the climate of their times a revolutionary step. While it was hoped that the success of the Peckham Experiment would inform the design of the NHS, this was not to be. Indeed, the service that emerged after 1945 was one based on a model of disease which was reactive rather than proactive. With the deaths of Scott Williamson and Pearse, in 1953 and 1979 respectively, the impetus for the development of their health care approach was lost.

In Spring 1987 the Marylebone Health Centre project was undertaken by Dr Patrick Pietroni and Dr Derek Chase who combined their NHS practices and moved into the Crypt of St Marylebone Church. The Marylebone Health Centre was an autonomous but philosophically linked part of the Healing and Counselling Centre then being developed by the Church. Christopher Hamel-Cooke, then Rector of St Marylebone, had long been interested in the practical links between religion and medicine and had exploited these links as a central part of his ministry. In terms of the Marylebone Health Centre research project, being situated in the Church alongside the healing and counselling ministry fitted exactly with the belief in the need for inner city 'care agencies' to develop new ways of working together. The Crypt Centre was seen as a unique opportunity for exploring effective cooperation between all the caring professions.

The work of the Marylebone Health Centre was in many ways prescient, focusing as it did on asking new questions about the delivery of primary health care. Challenging the traditional forms of delivery and involving patients in decisions about the nature and form of their health care are increasingly the stuff of primary health. Moreover, an understanding of the importance of evaluating the quality and cost of primary health care services has been placed at the centre of government policy on the NHS. When the Department of Health specifically asked practitioners to consider the prevention of ill-health and the promotion of good health in The Health of the Nation (Department of Health 1990), the Marylebone Health Centre had been looking at these precise questions for the previous 5 years. Furthermore, the interprofessional approach of the Marylebone Health Centre, together with its clear objective to involve the local community in the work of the health centre, foreshadowed the move to 'community care'.

At the heart of the Marylebone Health Centre lies a firm belief in empowering the people using its services and encouraging them to become responsible for and to take control of their own health whenever possible. Indeed, a principal aim of the project is to explore the possible impact that patient participation might have on reducing social isolation and enhancing patients' physical and psychological well-being. The Marylebone Health Centre also sets out to explore collaborative working within the community and primary health care settings with GPs, complementary therapists and other health centre staff. From the outset the Marylebone Health Centre team were committed to an on-going programme of rigorous and innovative research into the numerous fields within their remit. The 'Marylebone Model' of community and primary care is best summarised by the 'flower diagram' developed by the Health Centre (Fig. I.1).

The Marylebone Centre Trust, founded in 1988, developed with the Health Centre and was established to further the work, research and philosophy of the Health Centre. As part of this general aim the Trust has become increasingly involved in interprofessional education and training. In association with the University of Westminster, the Marylebone Centre Trust has helped to establish a new Centre for Community Care and Primary Health. This centre aims to provide the kind of training needed by health and community care practitioners in the 1990s and onwards and is informed by the work of the Marylebone Health Centre and the Marylebone Centre Trust. The first course, an MA entitled Community and Primary Health—Towards Reflective Practice, began in 1993, and in 1994 it was joined by an MA in Therapeutic Bodywork. It is estimated that by 1997, 300 professionals will be studying at the joint Centre for Community Care and Primary Health in a range of innovative courses.

This collection of papers is a résumé of the work of the Marylebone Health Centre and the Marylebone Centre Trust from their inception to the present day. It aims to reflect the developing interests and concerns of those involved with the Marylebone projects, as well as acting as an authoritative source for those with interests in one or more of the varied, though related, fields in which the Health Centre and the Trust operate. As such, its chapters range from the philosophy of holism and medical ethics to the clinical trials of complementary therapies in a primary health care setting and the increasingly important area of interprofessional collaboration. The very nature of the interdisciplinary approach adopted by the Marylebone Health Centre and Trust has meant that the research projects and papers generated are themselves multifaceted, multidisciplinary and interprofessional. For this reason many of them have areas of overlap. Yet it is important to realise that overlap does not mean repetition; similar areas of inquiry can be valuably, and indeed necessarily, investigated from different perspectives. Consequently, the articles included in this reader have been reproduced in their original form. No attempt has been made to

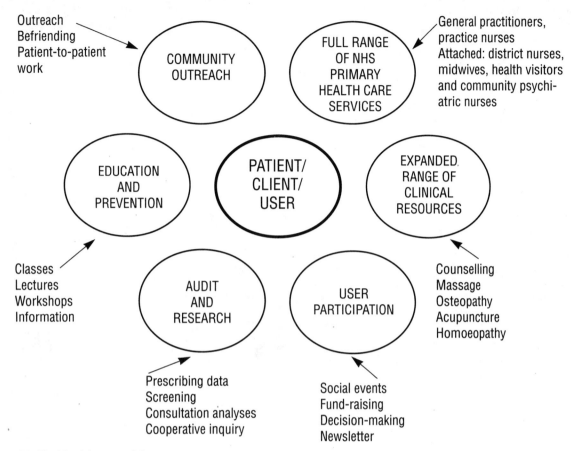

Outreach
Befriending
Patient-to-patient
work

COMMUNITY
OUTREACH

FULL RANGE
OF NHS
PRIMARY
HEALTH CARE
SERVICES

General practitioners,
practice nurses
Attached: district nurses,
midwives, health visitors
and community psychi-
atric nurses

EDUCATION
AND
PREVENTION

PATIENT/
CLIENT/
USER

EXPANDED
RANGE OF
CLINICAL
RESOURCES

Classes
Lectures
Workshops
Information

AUDIT
AND
RESEARCH

USER
PARTICIPATION

Counselling
Massage
Osteopathy
Acupuncture
Homoeopathy

Prescribing data
Screening
Consultation analyses
Cooperative inquiry

Social events
Fund-raising
Decision-making
Newsletter

Figure I.1 The Marylebone model.

place a false homogeneity onto this work. Rather, the natural links and connections between the different aspects of the work undertaken have been allowed to emerge naturally. The papers look forward as well as back and taken as a whole might be seen as a series of investigations into and suggestions for the development of community and primary health care.

REFERENCE

Department of Health 1990 The health of the nation. HMSO, London

1

The philosophical context of the Marylebone Model

INTRODUCTION

The work of the Marylebone Centre Trust and the Marylebone Health Centre is, above all, concerned with putting certain ideas about health into practice. Finding practical ways of dealing with the provision of innovative and flexible forms of health care is what the Trust exists to examine, and the Health Centre to provide. However, neither the Trust nor the Health Centre would exist at all were it not for the ideas from which they gain their inspiration.

The Marylebone model derives its intellectual and philosophical base from a belief in an holistic approach to health care. This term, as Pietroni points out in 'Holistic medicine—new map, old territory' (pp. 4–14), is a mixed blessing since it has come to be so widely used (or misused) that it is now almost meaningless. In terms of its application to the work of the Marylebone Centre Trust and the Marylebone Health Centre holism means treating the 'whole patient' but also treating the patient as part of a 'whole': a member of a family, a community, a society, etc. Holism is concerned with contextualising existence and hence its application to health and social care is concerned with treating the patient/client in context. The expansion of the Trust and Health Centre's work into issues concerning the nature and meaning of community and primary care was, therefore, a natural development of the original interest in holism (see Ch. 2).

More than this, however, holism also means

discovering and maintaining a certain awe and wonder at the interconnectedness of all nature, all people, all places and all times. In his paper, Dr Pietroni shows the vitality of an holistic approach to health care (and indeed to life) by demonstrating that it is a way of bringing together in harmony some of the latest ideas and discoveries to have emerged from modern science and some of the oldest ideas of philosophers and thinkers down the ages. That Einstein may give an insight into the functioning of traditional Chinese medicine, for example, is proof in action of the principle of holism. With an holistic eye, the complexities and subtleties of man and his place in his macrocosm may be teased out, and the insights thus gained can be put to use when treating individuals. Indeed, the holistic approach would suggest that unless this perspective were adopted when caring for individuals their care would always be limited.

The development in the public interest in holism is clearly linked to a growing awareness of how humankind relates to its wider environment. Politics, economics, social theory and medicine have all come under the influence of the 'green' movement. In 'The greening of medicine' (pp. 15–18), Dr Pietroni identifies five major areas of change associated with the 'greening process' and shows the effect that these have had on the ideas and practice of medicine. Far from being concerned only with the natural environment, the 'green revolution' has altered the ways in which men and women think about themselves and the services which they receive. All too often holism and 'green' issues are confused and considered to be one and the same thing. While this is certainly not the case, Dr Pietroni demonstrates how it would be foolish not to recognise the ways in which each of these ideologies has affected the other.

The idea that an holistic approach to man's health is the most beneficial and productive is not new. Nevertheless, a willingness to accept and implement this idea has waxed and waned with changing fashions. These changes have had a determining effect on the practice and nature of health care. By charting the changes

and the development in the way Europeans have thought about and conceived of the doctor/patient relationship (see 'Alternative medicine', pp. 19–31), Dr Pietroni illustrates this point in the context of the history of ideas. He demonstrates how it was that Western cultures, in their haste to free their 'rational' faculties from the thrall of the 'irrational' Christian Church, succeeded in also separating their understanding of the body from their understanding of the mind and spirit. Arguably, the medieval Christian Church had already done the same thing in reverse by insisting that attention to the cure of souls must come before attention to the ills of the body. Where modern cultures neglected the whole by putting the emphasis on the physical body, medieval cultures neglected the whole by putting the emphasis on the spirit. Both approaches, it is argued, were equally flawed.

It had not always been thus: primitive societies had made use of shamans who had acted as intermediaries between humans and gods (body and spirit) to heal and cure them. The Greeks too were acutely aware of the interrelatedness of the many aspects of humankind and the world in which it lived. The notion of health applied by Hippocratic doctors incorporated moral and spiritual, as well as physical, considerations. Indeed, Hippocratic doctors were so aware of the unity of humankind that they would not treat patients whom they believed to be 'leading improper lives'. What would be the point in easing physical symptoms if the mind and spirit remained in ill-health?

As Dr Pietroni shows, this understanding of the unity of humankind has parallels in the subjective approach to patient care developed in the late nineteenth century. The most complete articulation of this approach can be found in the psychoanalytic techniques of Freud. Freud raised the importance of subjective data to a new level and suggested that it could be used to help discover the very nature of a malady. The birth of the idea of psychosomatic illness was a further elucidation of the principle of holism although, if taken as a closed approach to ill-health, it is clearly as limited as any other.

Dr Pietroni demonstrates that what is now termed 'holism' has had many different incarnations and has been understood in varying degrees and in different ways by different people at different times. Holism as defined by Dr Pietroni contends that an approach to man, to life and to nature which insists on splitting up these three elements is fatally flawed. Yet this is no esoteric philosophy. On the contrary, it is a system of thought which is fundamentally rooted in daily action. As such it has a direct and practical applicability, both to the issues facing community and primary health care now, and to those which will become more central in the future.

One critical aspect of this applicability is investigated by Dr Pietroni in 'Towards reflective practice—the languages of health and social care' (pp. 32–41). Here he shows that the many ways in which health and social care have been thought about historically have a legacy in the many different languages which are used to talk about health and social care today. Dr Pietroni identifies 11 different languages used by health and social care professionals and suggests that these languages constrain and determine the ways in which these people think about themselves, their work and their colleagues. He points to a crisis in interprofessional communication arising from the professionals' inability to really understand what their colleagues mean. They are neither 'multilingual' not do they speak a 'common language' and as a result confusion, hostilities and resentments can develop. In the context of a health service which aims increasingly to provide integrated health and social care in one 'care package', rather than as a series of disconnected services, this is clearly a concern. It is especially so given it is the patient who is most likely to suffer from a breakdown in communication. This is reflected not only in major and well documented disasters, such as the Cleveland episode, but also in the daily experience of both service providers and consumers. Dr Pietroni implies that the fracturing of the health professions, and thus the health care professionals, and the resulting difficulties in communication have arisen because of the absence of an holistic approach to health and health care. The way out of the impasse, he argues, lies in encouraging professionals to develop into what Schön has called 'reflective practitioners' (Schön 1983). The approach to health care suggested by this term means not only treating a patient as a whole but also recognising that each practitioner is himself only one part of a whole nexus of healing potentialities. These will range from a series of therapeutic interventions, be they 'orthodox' or 'complementary', to the love and care given to an individual by his family, friends and care workers. The reflective practitioner acknowledges this and seeks to discover what it is that he can learn from all those involved in and concerned with the health of the individual patient. Each interaction with a colleague thus becomes a potential opportunity for broadening understanding and, in Dr Pietroni's terms, learning a new language. It is only through this kind of holistic approach that the changes now necessary in the interactions between health care professionals can be effected.

The notion of holism then, far from being a collection of abstract ideas, is a doorway to a whole approach to life which is fiercely and avowedly practical. Exploring the nature and range of these practicalities forms the basis for all the work of the Marylebone Centre Trust and the Marylebone Health Centre. It is the golden thread that links what at first sight may seem to be a series of unrelated activities.

REFERENCE

Schön D 1983 The reflective practitioner. Temple Smith, London

HOLISTIC MEDICINE—NEW MAP, OLD TERRITORY

Patrick Pietroni

The basic philosophical and scientific assumptions that have guided our thinking over the last 300 years have been largely *dualistic, mechanistic* and *reductionistic*. This has resulted in tremendous advances for medicine and mankind but these advances have produced a structure much like the leaning tower of Pisa—if we pursue in building higher, we are in danger of toppling over. The time has come to balance the dualistic approach with a *monistic* one, to replace our attempts at objectivity in the quest for further knowledge with one where the emphasis is not on subjectivity but on *authenticity*. We should replace our mechanistic approach to the study of health and disease with a *humanistic* one where aspects of human nature such as caring, sharing, loving, touching, hoping and hugging play as important a part in our endeavours to help the sick as the study of alpha feto-protein and T-suppressor cells. We should replace the reductionistic approach to the care of the sick with a *holistic* one, where the transplant surgeon will be as concerned about his patient's life-style, and will recognise its relevance to the outcome of his skilled interventions, as he is about the level of the patient's lymphocytes.

HOLISTIC MEDICINE

Holistic medicine is the label applied to a collection of different trends current in health care today. Like the word 'stress' it is fast becoming over-used, carrying different meanings for each person. This article is an attempt to map out my own personal understanding of the label and to describe those trends in science and medicine which have led to its current usage.

First, the argument concerning its spelling. The term 'holism' was first introduced by Jan Christian Smuts (1926). As used by Smuts, the term 'holism' described the study of whole organisms and systems. The English spelling with a 'w' is a relatively recent innovation, a fourteenth century addition. Our words 'hail', 'hello', 'health' and 'hi' are derived from the

Reprinted with permission from the British Journal of Holistic Medicine: 1(1)pp. 1–13 April 1984.

original spelling 'w(hole)', meaning complete.

Secondly, holistic medicine is not just about alternative or complementary medicine, nor should it be seen as an attack on current medical practice. It certainly incorporates some of the alternative therapies into its practice. Nevertheless, I have met many alternative practitioners who are not in the least holistic, treating their clients as objects to whom 'things are done'. Similarly, I have met many surgeons who I believe practise whole-person medicine.

Thirdly, whole-person medicine is a concept we are all relatively familiar with, and indeed good clinical care requires us to approach the patient as a whole. But the 'whole' we choose to recognise is determined by the prevalent scientific–medical model used to describe and understand that whole. It is a great advance that in general practice we are encouraged to make diagnoses in physical, psychological and social terms, and we owe a great debt to those courageous physicians who helped resuscitate general practice in the 1950s and 1960s and who have brought about such a tremendous change within general practice.

Holistic medicine is indeed about whole-person medicine, but its strength and vitality lie in the fact that it incorporates into its map of a 'whole-person' some of the more recent scientific discoveries that enhance our understanding of how we function as human beings. Up till now, these discoveries have not been included in the undergraduate curriculum.

These discoveries include:
1. The psycho-physio-neuro-immunological mechanisms of stress (Solomon et al 1974, Stein et al 1976, Pelletier 1978).
2. The insights of modern physics (Capra 1975, 1982).
3. The concept of field force in human functioning (Sheldrake 1981).
4. Systems theory and its implication for treating the individual patient (Miller 1965, von Bertalanffy 1968).
5. The holographic theory of brain storage mechanisms (Bohm 1980, Wilber 1981).
6. The nature of healing and healing energies (Meek 1977, Krippner & Vollobolo 1976).

At the same time as drawing on up-to-date science, many of the concepts and principles in holistic medicine have roots that go a long way back, and indeed, some of these roots precede the onset of the scientific method as we have known it. But the exciting and inspiring paradox is that these very basic concepts and principles are now being supported by discoveries rooted in science itself.

Some of these basic, universal, fundamental principles include:

1. The human organism is a multidimensional being, possessing body, mind and spirit, all inextricably connected, each part affecting the whole and the whole being greater than the sum of parts.
2. There is an interconnectedness between human beings and their environment which includes other human beings. This inter-con-nectedness acts as a force on the functioning of the individual isolated human being.
3. Disease or ill-health arises as a result of a state of imbalance, either from within the human being or because of some external force in the environment, and by environment I include the family.
4. We each possess a powerful and innate capac-ity for healing ourselves, or bringing our-selves back into a state of balance.
5. One of the primary tasks of someone entrust-ed to heal, be he doctor, priest or acupunctur-ist, is to encourage the self-innate capacity for healing of the individual in distress.
6. This primary task can often be better accom-plished through education than through direct intervention, whether the intervention be penicillin, surgery or a homoeopathic pre-scription.
7. To enable him to accomplish his task effective-ly the healer needs to be aware of his own multidimensional levels of existence and have some expertise and ability in achieving a state of balance and harmony within himself— 'physician heal thyself'.

Rather than attempt to describe the underly-ing scientific concepts in detail, a task that would take far too long and is beyond the scope of this article, I would like to highlight some of the important steps which have led us to review our current assumptions and beliefs.

For the last 300 years our reality has been shaped by the Newtonian view of the universe as a solid body where all events took place in a three-dimensional sphere governed by the laws of Euclidean geometry. Before Newton, Copernicus had bravely published his life work and put the sun at the centre of the universe, thus displacing the earth from its central posi-tion. Galileo, who followed him, set about prov-ing the brilliance of Copernicus' deductions and did so with the development of the telescope. He himself was arrested, put on trial and eventually recanted.

Nevertheless, the advancement of knowledge that occurred during the Renaissance was unstoppable and the separation of religion from science had begun. These new discoveries received the support from another great man, René Descartes, who brought together and refined the principles which have guided the subsequent 300 years of philosophical and scientific thought. Descartes' first major contribution was to free man from the domination that had up till then prevailed, whereby all events were determined by some form of divine intervention. He affirmed the concept of dualism and helped bring about the separation of body from mind. In his famous dictum 'I think therefore I am', he helped establish the primacy of logical, rational thought, separate from and independent of external influences.

His second major contribution was to see the body as a system of mechanisms much like a clock and he writes:

I consider the human body as a machine. My thought compares a sick man and an ill-made clock with my idea of a healthy man and a well-made clock . . . I desire I say that you consider that these functions occur naturally in this machine solely by the disposi-tion of its organs; not less than the movements of a clock (Vrooman 1970).

Since then we have largely viewed the body as a machine separate from the mind.

Descartes' third major contribution was the

statement concerning how we should set about studying the workings of this machine, called the body. He writes of the need 'to divide each of the difficulties into as many parts as possible and as might be necessary for its adequate solution' (Vrooman, 1970).

Here we have the reductionist statement of belief which has influenced most of our research and much of our clinical work. It is the combination of Descartes' philosophical statements expressing the dualistic, mechanistic and reductionistic viewpoint and Newton's brilliant discoveries that still largely govern our approach to the study of our external and internal worlds.

Before proceeding, let me say that a genius other than Newton and Descartes foresaw the limitation of these revolutionary ideas which nevertheless, for those times, were immensely liberating. Although man was being liberated from the belief in one true religion, he unknowingly was being delivered into the grasp of the 'one true science'. William Blake, a visionary hundreds of years ahead of his time, parodied this new scientific method (*ration* as it was labelled), best encapsulated in the paintings of God and then Newton measuring the universe with a compass. Blake's meaning must be seen in the context of his own writings:

And who shall bind the infinite with an external hand
To compass it with swaddling band (Blake 1958a).
May God keep us from single vision and Newton's
sleep (Blake 1958b).

Blake also foresaw the emergence of holism and holographic paradigm when he wrote those beautiful words:

To see a world in a grain of sand and a heaven in a
wild flower
Hold infinitely in the palm of your hand
And eternity in an hour (Blake 1958c).

Nevertheless, for the next 300 or 400 years man benefited from the liberation of science and religion. In medicine the Church kept to the cure of the souls and we were given the body, and mind. The body and its component parts became the true study of medicine and when Darwin helped free man from yet another of the Church's dogmas we were well on the road to our supposed goal of

understanding the human condition. With the advent of Freud and his descriptions of unconscious processes, a further chapter was added, although his discoveries are still not fully integrated within our medical framework because the progress of the study of the body and the material world seemed to be producing such good results.

With Pasteur, Koch, Ehrlich and Fleming, the search for the 'magic bullet' had begun and the age of modern pharmacology spread into the area of mental diseases as well as physical ones. In passing, let me say it is not often known that Pasteur on his death bed uttered the heretical words 'The bacteria is nothing, the terrain is everything', or as Thomas McKeown (1979) has shown, that 90% of the total decline in mortality from such diseases as scarlet fever, cholera and tuberculosis occurred before immunisation and antibiotics.

Nevertheless, we were patiently saving people's lives that could never have been saved before and progress in medicine was apparent everywhere. Sepsis had all but disappeared from the operating room, modern safe anaesthetics were developed and we were moving on from a bacterial and vitamin-deficiency based concept of disease to a biochemical and molecular based one. The search for the 'magic bullet' had become the search for the 'twisted molecule'.

Let us go back to the turn of the present century and see what was going on in other areas of man's incessant search for knowledge. With the discovery of the atom in 1805 by Dalton it was thought we had at last found the smallest unit of matter. In 1897 J J Thompson discovered the electron and in 1911 Rutherford described the atom as we best understand it, with a central nucleus and orbiting electrons. At the same time as Rutherford was working on the atom, Max Plank was studying energy in the form of electromagnetic radiation. He showed how energy not only came in the form of waves but also in lumps which he termed *quanta*. It was the putting together of these various strands of discovery and adding their own by Einstein, Neils Bohr and Heisenberg that finally resulted in a clearer appreciation of the basic building blocks of nature, which has required us to look again at our understanding of causality and the relationship between matter and energy.

What the insights from the new physics show us is that matter and energy are interchangeable and that the idea of an indivisible, indestructable unit of matter is not supportable by the evidence. It is the relationships between the particles that help to determine the shape, structure and form these particles take, not the particles themselves. The relationship of the particles is in turn influenced by a field force, much like the iron filings that are displaced around a magnet, and it is more accurate to describe matter as a concentration of field force or energy, or as Einstein (1952) wrote 'We may therefore regard matter as being constituted by the regions of space in which the field is extremely intense. There is no place in this new kind of physics both for field and matter for field is the only reality.'

At one level of our being we are a bio-energetic organism, and with these discoveries it has at last been possible to explore and gain some preliminary glimpses into the nature of such diverse healing traditions as acupuncture, homoeopathy, spiritual healing and many other alternative forms of therapy that have remained outside our generally accepted view of the biochemical and molecular theory of disease (Motoyama 1978, Vithoulkas 1980).

The body can no longer be regarded as a separate individual entity surrounded by empty space. We ourselves are largely empty space in an even emptier space, and as has been described by Capra and others, there is a non-ending stream and flow of energy between bodies, that he has labelled 'the bio-dance of the universe'.

T S Eliot (1963) expressed it more poetically when he wrote:

At the still point of the turning world.
Neither flesh nor fleshless;
Neither from nor towards; at the still point, there the dance is,
But neither arrest nor movement. And do not call it fixity,
Where past and future are gathered. Neither movement from nor towards,

Neither ascent nor decline. Except for the point, the still point,
There would be no dance, and there is only the dance.

What is exciting about the early part of this century is not only that discoveries were being made in science which are only now beginning to have their impact, but that similar stirrings were happening in literature, art and music. The basic form and structure were being challenged by many of the greats of that time. In art the classical representation of reality was giving way to the cubist, dadaist and surrealist movements. Picasso's *Demoiselles D'Avignon* was and is seen as as great a departure from classical art and as shattering to old concepts as Einstein's and Bohr's works were to prove to be to the scientific world.

James Joyce's *Ulysses* was a crack in the form of the written word, and the very units of language, like the atom before, became no longer the stable elements we knew. In music, the public were woken to a new sound as the old classical form began to give way. Stravinsky's *Rite of Spring* created an uproar when first performed. He, together with Ives and Schonberg, were experimenting with the basic building blocks of their chosen field and in their own way were making the same fundamental observations and discoveries as their scientific colleagues.

Medicine was also progressing in many different directions and it seemed as if treating the body as a machine was paying great dividends to the progress of curing man's ills. However in 1925 a recently qualified medical student was not too happy with the answers he was getting from his teachers, especially as they did not seem to fit the clinical observations he was making.

Hans Selye (1978) the father of modern stress work, or as he first called it 'the syndrome of just being sick', began the difficult and painstaking job of putting body and mind back together again. I met him twice in his last year of life and he had by then incorporated spirit as well into his understanding of the syndrome of just being sick. We now have a fairly good understanding of the neurological, biochemical, hormonal, immunological, psychological and environmental aspects of stress; and even though we may as scientists disagree as to what the term means, most of us as individuals have a personal experience of what it does mean to us. Hans Selye helped to put the parts together and as a result of his work, stress was reintegrated into clinical medicine.

Once the realisation occurred that stress underlay much of what we considered as individual separate illnesses, with individual separate causes, a spate of stress clinics were developed. This coincided with the invasion of the West by the East, which had begun after Sir John Woodroffe translated the Upanashads in the nineteenth century, and we now need to introduce this thread into our canvas.

Schopenhauer was the first Western philosopher to comment on Eastern texts. He wrote 'compared to these ancient rishis, we philosophers in the West are still in the kindergarten' (Worthington 1982). In 1893, Vivekenanda, a disciple of Ramakrishna, was the first of the great yogis to visit the West and attend the Parliament of religions in Chicago. It may well be that the greatest benefit that occurred as a result of the British occupation of India is not that we brought our culture and language to the Indian, but that the rich world of Vedas' Upanashads and yoga was brought to the attention of the West. Jung was heavily influenced by Eastern writers, and the emergence of the Theosophical Society in the 1920s was a major factor in spreading the richness and depth of Eastern philosophy and science to this country. A third wave of influence occurred in the late 1950s and 1960s with the popularisation of transcendental meditation by Mahrishi Yogi and the publicity given to the Beatles' visit to India. Several yogis were being investigated in biofeedback laboratories in the United States, and their claims to be able to alter heart rate, blood pressure, skin temperatures and brainwave activities were being verified to the astonishment of many scientists (Green & Green 1977).

Other clinicians, including Luthe, Benson, Ballantyne and Green were exploring whether any of these approaches were relevant to the 'syndrome of just being sick' and were repeatedly finding that without recourse to drugs, many of the symptoms and signs of just being sick could be reversed using approaches to healing many thousands of years old (Luthe 1969, Benson 1977, Green & Green 1977, Ballantyne 1978).

The latest chapter in the integration of body, mind and spirit was occurring as a result of the coming together of a mathematician, a new form of photography, a physicist and a neuroscientist.

Ever since Penfield in the 1940s did his classical experiments using microelectrodes to pinpoint the topographical representation of brain function, from which he developed the sensory homunculus we all learned about at medical school, the question that puzzled neurosurgeons and neurophysiologists was: 'Where is memory stored, and how is it stored?' Aristotle had described memory as resulting from a physical impression on the surface of the brain much as a printer makes an impression on the surface of a wax tablet. Penfield thought he located memory in the temporal lobes, but this was soon to be disproved by Karl Lashley (1950), a neurosurgeon who removed more and more bits of cerebral tissue from animals only to find that they still retained the memory of the task learnt before the operation. He is said to have despaired at ever localising memory in the brain and to have said 'I sometimes feel . . . that the necessary conclusion is learning just is not possible.'

In the 1950s and 1960s Sperry did his classical split brain experiments and it seemed as if we were at last beginning to get nearer to an understanding of brain topography. The importance of the right hemisphere was discovered and the intuitive, spatial, non-verbal, imagery functions were recognised as counterparts to the rational, verbal, linear modes being governed by the left hemisphere (Sperry 1970). Memory though, still eluded the experimenters. At about the same time as Penfield was working on his experiments, in the 1940s, Dennis Gabor, a mathematician, had worked out the formulae (for which he won a Nobel Prize) for describing a form of wave pattern storage system which he called a *hologram*. It was not until the development of the laser beam (a beam of pure light) that his discovery could be made concrete, and this new form of photography could be demonstrated. Lyall Watson, the biologist, has produced the best and most succinct description

I have read:

If you drop a pebble into a pond, it will produce a series of regular waves that travel outward in concentric circles. Drop two identical pebbles into the pond at different points and you will get two sets of similar waves that move towards each other. Where the waves meet, they will interfere. If the crest of one hits the crest of the other, they will work together and produce a reinforced wave of twice the normal height. If the crest of one coincides with the trough of another, they will cancel each other out and produce an isolated patch of calm water. In fact, all possible combinations of the two occur, and the final result is a complex arrangement of ripples known as an interference pattern.

Light waves behave in exactly the same way. The purest kind of light available to us is that produced by a laser, which sends out a beam in which all the waves are of one frequency, like those made by an ideal pebble in a perfect pond. When two laser beams touch, they produce an interference pattern of light and dark ripples that can be recorded on a photographic plate. And if one of the beams, instead of coming directly from the laser, is reflected first off an object such as a human face, the resulting pattern will be very complex indeed, but it can still be recorded. The record will be a hologram of the face.

The two aspects that differentiate a hologram from an ordinary photograph are:

1. It is three dimensional, like the stereo effect one achieves standing between two balanced speakers.
2. If the hologram is broken, a part of it will reconstruct the whole, i.e. the information of the whole picture is contained in each part, unlike the pinpoint representation of a normal photograph.

It was this revolutionary discovery in photography that provided the clue to memory storage in the brain, and Karl Pribram, the neuroscientist at Stanford, had the courage to make the imaginative leap, develop the theory and subsequently produce evidence that the brain, as far as memory is concerned, functions like a holgram. In other words memory is not located in any one area but is spread throughout the brain. There has been much criticism of Karl Pribram's work and his evidence is still relatively scanty. Nevertheless it does appear as if science has come close to demonstrating one of the fundamental principles that the monist philosophers and writers from Plutonius, Leibnitz Bergson and Koestler had always maintained. The whole is contained in the smallest part—or recalling Blake's words 'To see the world in a grain of sand . . .'.

It has been Karl Pribram and David Bohm (1980), Professor of Physics at Birkbeck College in London, who have done most to explore and develop this apparent paradox, and their writings make exciting and inspiring reading. The discoveries and insights that are being put forward as a result of the understanding of the nature of holography, together with those I have briefly outlined, have brought science and religion closer than they have ever been for over 300 years, when Descartes and Newton helped to separate them. Hans Kung remarked that the standard answer to 'Do you believe in spirit?' used to be 'Of course not, I am a scientist', but it might very soon become 'Of course I believe in spirit, I am a scientist.'

I will outline very briefly some of the conclusions that I believe can be drawn from this fundamental paradigm shift in the areas of clinical medicine, patient care, medical education and research.

CLINICAL MEDICINE

The therapeutic interventions that will be used increasingly are those where:

1. The patient actively participates.
2. There is a re-ordering of the patient's experience.
3. The therapies are not therapist-dependent.
4. The therapies increase the patients' wisdom of their own nature.

I will describe three of the most commonly used holistic therapies.

Meditation

There must be over 500 papers on the psychophysiological responses during meditation, and its clinical uses. We now know that during meditation there is a fall in pulse rate, blood pressure and oxygen requirements and an increase in alpha wave brain rhythm activity. We also know that people who meditate regularly have a fall in their cholesterol, an increase in the high density lipoprotein and a decrease in their free fatty acids. There is a carry-over effect, and by all of the known parameters, people who meditate regularly experience less anxiety; their requirement for sleep diminishes; they describe a greater locus of control within themselves, and feel less at the mercy of the outside world (Kasamatsu & Hirai 1966, Wallace 1970, Soloman & Schwartz 1976, Wallace & Garrett 1971, Wallace & Benson 1972). The work with meditation in clinical conditions is equally encouraging and its use in hypertension has been well documented (Patel 1973, Benson et al 1974).

Exercise

Exercise as a form of self-therapy is something most people have at one time engaged in, for both physical and psychological benefit. Wilhelm Reich drew attention to the link between physical posture, body movements and emotional and psychic conflict. Bio-energetics, the Alexander technique and massage are all approaches to healing the mind through the body. Lately, jogging has been shown to be as effective as short-term psychotherapy and drugs in the treatment of non-psychotic depression (Griest et al 1978). At the same time, exercise programmes have been fashioned for a number of different physical disorders, particularly cardiovascular disease and asthma. It has been suggested that some of the beneficial effects of exercise therapy on cardiovascular function include (Fuller et al 1974):

1. Decreased myocardial oxygen requirement.
2. Decreased infarction rate and sudden death.
3. Decreased risk factors, including cholesterol, blood sugar, and triglycerides.
4. Increased myocardial collateral circulation.
5. Increased cardiac reserve.

More work is required to develop this fascinating and neglected approach to healing, for like all approaches, it has its indications and con-

traditions. My own approach to exercise with patients is to help them explore the four categories of exercise that appear to have separate characteristics:

1. Intensive, very active, intermittent form, where you achieve a varying pulse rate, e.g. football, tennis, squash.
2. Sustained continuous moderate form, where a more regular pulse rate can be achieved, e.g. running, cycling, swimming, walking.
3. Non-aerobic form, isotonic or isometric, e.g. Hatha yoga, Canadian airforce exercises, simple stretches, tai chi or weightlifting.
4. Breathing exercises, varying from simple diaphragmatic breathing to complex forms described in the classical texts of Ayurvedic medicine.

All these exercises can be indulged in competitively or non-competitively, although it is more common for competition to occur in the first group than the last. Nevertheless, we have seen how jogging, which was hailed as the solitary healthy pursuit of physical, mental and spiritual oneness, has developed into a multi-million pound activity with goals, programmes, times and marathons. It is a sad fact that our cultural heritage will prevail in most of us and we will try to turn every approach to wholeness into a method with *dos* and *don'ts* and *shoulds* and *musts*.

Lawrence Durrell wrote 'To realise the importance of pleasure and get contemplative enough to really enjoy it is something achieved.' I would change the word 'pleasure' for 'exercise' and use it as a guide. To realise the importance of exercise and get contemplative enough to really enjoy it is something achieved.

Breathing and relaxation

Our medical education has focused solely on breathing as a physiological fact. It nevertheless has an important symbolic meaning reflected in our language. We talk of being 'inspired' and of the 'the breath of life'. Similarly, we are aware of how breathing and emotional states are closely linked. Anxious people breathe rapidly and talk on the height of inspiration and depressed people sigh, have long pauses and talk on the depth of expiration. The hyperventilation syndrome is well documented as an accompaniment to many psychophysiological conditions, and effective therapeutic retraining has been well described (Innocenti 1983).

What is not so well known is the importance of diaphragmatic breathing as opposed to thoracic breathing, and the significance of mouth breathing, snoring, and sleep apnoea, especially its relationship to heart disease. The link between the breath cycle and the functioning of the sympathetic/parasymphathetic neuronal discharge has been recently outlined (Clark 1981). Because it is possible consciously to alter our breathing patterns through retraining, it has been possible to reverse some of the chronic autonomic imbalance that is a feature of many clinical disorders.

Positive results following respiratory retraining have been described in such varied clinical conditions as:

1. Hyperventilation syndrome (Lum 1975).
2. Hypertension (Patel & North 1973).
3. Post-operative analgesic requirements (Hymes 1980).
4. Migraine (Sargent, Green & Walters 1972).

Muscle relaxation accompanies diaphragmatic breathing and it is this fact that has resulted in its use in many chronic stress disorders, from mild anxiety neurosis to insomnia.

PATIENT CARE

The concept of holism as it applies to patient care implies a shift from the disease/medical model to a health/whole-person model. It involves adopting an educational approach with patients and seeing every encounter as an opportunity for increasing the patient's wisdom in looking after himself. The word *doctor* means teacher and it is necessary for this aspect of the doctor's work to be reincorporated into the overall framework. The very individualised basis of the delivery of health care needs to be re-evaluated.

An individual diseased organ needs to be examined in the context of an individual human being who inhabits a family unit. The explosion of self-help and patient participation groups suggests that patients are aware of the importance of such support—and seek it out.

As the importance and fundamental value of the educational model is appreciated, then certain basic changes in patterns of work will alter. Patients will be seen together in a 'classroom' setting. The architecture of our health centres and hospitals will alter to allow for these activities, including the provision for a meditation or quiet room.

It will not be possible for doctors to address the health problems of the twenty-first century unless we learn how to share our power, not only amongst our colleagues in the health team but also with our patients. Without being cruel, and whilst recognising that there will always be a place for the totally active doctor and the totally passive patient, there is a very great need for the power equation present in the majority of doctor–patient interactions to be redressed.

MEDICAL EDUCATION

There are hundreds of papers on the need to humanise medical education and suggestions on how to go about achieving this. Let me quote from one:

When a patient enters a hospital one of the first things that commonly happens to him is that he loses his personal identity. He is generally referred to not as Henry Jones, but as 'that case of mitral stenosis in the second bed on the left'. [There are plenty of reasons why this is so, and the point is relatively unimportant—but the trouble is that it leads more or less directly to the patient being treated as a case of mitral stenosis and not as a sick man. The disease is treated but Henry Jones lying awake nights while he worries about his wife and children represents a problem that is much more complex than the pathological physiology of mitral stenosis and he is apt to improve very slowly unless a discerning houseman discovers why it is that even large doses of digitalis fail to slow his heart rate.] Henry happens to have heart disease, but he is not disturbed so much by dyspnoea as he is by anxiety for the future and a talk with an understanding physician who tries to make the situation clear to him, does more to straighten him out than a book full of drugs. Henry has an excellent example of a certain type of heart disease, and he is glad that all the staff find him interesting, for it makes him feel that they will do the best they can to cure him, but just because he is an interesting case, he does not cease to be a human being with very human hopes and fears.

That was written in 1927. I know it still occurred when I went to medical school and I know it still occurs now. There are still some medical schools in this country that have no departments of general practice and several that have them in name only. Few, if any, medical schools provide any instruction or guidance on interviewing skills to their students. Our medical educational system has not adapted fast enough to the changes that occur in society. When I was at medical school, if you wanted to enter general practice, you were considered a failed hospital doctor. Your consultants would shake their heads in sorrow and pity. Even though over 50% of our graduates now enter general practice, they still experience this particular subtle form of pressure, despite the fact that in any group of 1000 adults, 750 in any one month will develop a symptom, 250 will go to their general practitioner, 10 will go to hospital and only one will be admitted to a teaching hospital. Medical students therefore get a very biased and incomplete picture of diseases and you will hear comments like 'Well, he had no decent pathology' or 'nothing I could really get my teeth into'.

We are moving from a time when we looked to curing the patient to a time when often the most we can do is 'care for the patient'. This requires a different outlook on the part of the students, but more importantly, a different sort of medical education. The medical school years are divided into pre-clinical and clinical years. They unfortunately also become the pre-cynical and cynical years. Medical students arrive at medical schools with some sense of hope, concern, compassion and idealism as befits many 19-year-olds. As they struggle with the enormous amount of information required to pass exams, they begin to have some of their idealism blunted by the many hours of hard work required. When they eventually go on the wards, they meet patients who are ill, but also who are anxious, frightened, depressed, angry and at times, rude and difficult. They see patients in pain, in tears and witness the last breath of a human being as he struggles for his life.

The instruction and guidance they get is not on how to handle these difficult human situations. Rather, they are asked about the state of the patient's liver or the latest blood test. They are expected to know when the last article on some new investigation was written. There is no doubt that this sort of instruction is essential the high technical competence of our doctors is proof enough of that—but at what cost?

As the students struggle, not only with having to amass a new set of knowledge, they are overwhelmed with feelings they do not understand. Even worse, they may stop feeling altogether, as a protection from these difficulties. The high rate of depression, alcoholism, divorce and suicide amongst our profession is a glaring illustration of what lies ahead for those students who succumb to the extraordinarily difficult task of caring for a human being, as opposed to curing a disease.

Oliver Cape said 'the practice of medicine today reflects the education of yesterday'. If we are to provide our students with the education they deserve, then we need to complement our medical education with activities that will allow them an opportunity to explore and understand these aspects of our work.

Such activities might include a comprehensive interviewing course; small group discussions and seminars on human sexuality, death and dying, human awareness and the value of healing.

RESEARCH

I believe that we have too much and not too little research. If we were only to implement a tenth of what we know already, we would have made great progress.

Secondly, research and the publication of papers have for too long been accorded an importance they do not deserve. Promotion and preferment have been dictated by the length of the curriculum vitae over and above the human qualities of the registrar or houseman. We do not reward compassion, sensitivity and humaneness and it is time we did.

Thirdly, there is a need to explore what sort of research and what methodology is needed to explore these new and not so new approaches to healing. As has been indicated earlier, science, at least in the new physics, has realised and come to terms with the impossibility of achieving 'objectivity'. Rather than sanitise research procedures to the point of the 'double-blind controlled crossover trial', it is important to accept that the subjectivity of the researcher and the patient being researched is an inherent, important and often crucial factor in the efficacy of the method of therapy under examination. It is not possible to study fish out of water any more than it is possible to divorce the effect of the healer from the treatment under study.

CONCLUSION

These are difficult, perplexing and immensely challenging concepts and I would like to conclude with a story which describes why I believe our current research approach has to be challenged.

This is the story about Nasrudin—a sufi—who is variously referred to as 'very stupid, improbably clever or the possessor of mystical secrets'. Someone saw Nasrudin searching for something on the ground. 'What have you lost Mulla?', he asked. 'My key', said the Mulla. So they both went down on their knees and looked for it. After a time, the other man asked 'Where exactly did you drop it?' 'In my house.' 'Then why are you looking here?' 'There is more light here than inside my own house.' We have unfortunately looked for the answer to our question where our measuring instruments have taken us, not in the dark areas where I suspect the answer may lie.

REFERENCES

Ballantyne R 1978 Diet and nutrition: a holistic approach. Honesdale, Pennsylvania, Himalayan Institute.

Benson H 1977 The relaxation response. London, Fontana.

Benson H, Marzetta B R, Rosner B A 1974 Decreased blood pressure associated with the regular elicitation of the relaxation response: a study of hypertensive subjects. In: Eliot R (ed) Stress and the heart. Mount Kisko, New York, Futura.

Blake W 1958a Europe. In: Keynes G (ed) The complete writings of William Blake. London.

Blake W 1958b To Butts—second letter. 22 November 1802 Ibid.

Blake W 1958c Auguries of innocence. Dream, mirage or nemesis. Ibid.

Bohm D 1980 Wholeness and the implicate order. London, Routledge & Kegan Paul.

Capra F 1975 The Tao of physics. Berkeley, Shambhala.

Capra 1982 The turning point. London, Wildwood House.

Clark J 1981 Respiration, heartrate and the autonomic nervous system. Himalayan Institute Research Bulletin, 3, 4-6.

Einstein A 1952 The principle of relativity. New York, Dover.

Eliot, T S 1963 Burnt Norton. The four quartets. Collected Poems 1909–1962. London, Faber & Faber.

Fuller E 1974 The role of exercise in the relief of stress. In: Eliot R (ed) Stress and the heart. Mount Kisko, New York, Futura

Green E, Green A 1977 Beyond biofeedback. San Francisco, Delacorte Press.

Griest J H, Klein M H, Eischens R R, Faris J W 1978 Running as a treatment for non-psychotic depression. Behavioural Medicine, 6, 19–24.

Hymes A 1980 Diaphragmatic breath control and post surgical care. Himalayan Institute Research Bulletin. Winter, 9–10.

Innocenti D K 1983 Chronic hyperventilation syndrome. In: Downie P A (ed) Cash's textbook of chest, heart and vascular disorders. London, Faber & Faber.

Kasamatsu A, Hirai T 1966 Studies of EEG's of expert zen meditators. Folia Psychiatrica Neurologica Japonica, 28, 315.

Krippner S, Vollobolo A 1976 The realms of healing. Millbrae, California, Celestial Arts.

Lashley K 1950 In search of the engram. Society for Experimental Biology Systems Symposium No 4, 454–482.

Lum L C 1975 Are breathing exercises of benefit to the chest patient? Health, 8, 1–4.

Luthe W (ed) 1969 Autogenic therapy. Vols 1 and 3. New York, Grune and Stratton.

McKeown T 1979 The role of medicine. Oxford, Blackwell.

Meek G W 1977 Healers and the healing process. Quest. Wheaton, Illinois, Theosophical Publishing House.

Miller J G 1965 Living systems: basic concepts. Behavioural Science, 10, 193.

Motoyama H 1978 Science and the evolution of consciousness. Autumn Press.

Patel C 1973 Yoga and biofeedback in the management of hypertension. Lancet, 2, 1053–1055.

Patel C, North W R S 1973 Randomised controlled trial of yoga and biofeedback in the management of hypertension. Lancet, 2, 93–95.

Pelletier K 1978 Mind as healer, mind as slayer. A holistic approach to preventing stress disorders. London, Allen & Unwin.

Sargent J, Green E, Walters E 1972 The use of autogenic feedback training in a pilot study of migraine and tension headaches. Headache, 12, 120–125.

Selye H 1978 The stress of life. New York, McGraw-Hill.

Sheldrake R 1981 A new science of life. Paladin, Boulder,

Colorado and London.

Smuts J C 1926 Holism and evolution. New York, Macmillan.

Soloman D, Schwartz G E 1976 Meditation as an intervention in stress reactivity. Journal of Consulting and Clinical Psychology, 44, 456–466.

Soloman G F, Amkraut A A, Kasper P 1974 Immunity, emotions and disease. Psychotherapy and Psychosomatics, 23, 209–217.

Sperry R 1970 Perception in the absence of neocortical commissures. Research Publication of The Association for Research in Nervous and Mental Diseases No 48.

Stein M, Schiavi P, Camerino M 1976 The influence of brain and behaviour on the immune system. Science, 191, 435–440.

Vithoulkas G 1980 The science of homoeopathy, New York, Grove.

von Bertalanffy L 1968 General systems theory. New York, Braziller.

Vrooman J R 1970 René Descartes. New York, Putnam.

Wallace R 1970 Physiological effects of transcendental meditation. Science, 167, 1751–1754.

Wallace R, Benson H 1972 The physiology of meditation. Scientific American, 226, 84–90

Wallace R, Garrett M D 1971 Decreased blood lactate during transcendental mediation. Federation Proceedings, 30, 376.

Wilber K (ed) 1981 The holographic paradigm. Berkeley, Shambhal.

Worthington V 1982 A history of yoga. London, Routledge & Kegan Paul.

THE GREENING OF MEDICINE

Patrick Pietroni

> Originally the Green revolution was a phrase used to describe new high-yield wheat strains that had been developed in Mexico and were subsequently exported to India to help solve the sub-continent's chronic food shortages. Since then, the 'greening process' has affected many of our social organisations as well as our individual beliefs and has come to mean much more. We can identify five major areas where change has taken place and the ways in which this has or has not affected the practice of medicine.

THE CONSUMERIST ELEMENT

The consumer movement is second only to the concern for the environment as a principal feature of the greening process. It can be understood in terms of power-relationships between consumer and supplier or in medicine, between patient and doctor. We now see evidence of this in changing attitudes amongst both doctor and patient. The 'doctor knows best' approach has had to alter as it has become clear to some patients that we don't always know best. Questions which we must now ask ourselves and indeed have a legal obligation to do so include:

- How much to tell a patient about his diagnosis and/or prognosis.
- How much to involve a patient in the decision-making regarding treatment.

The vexed question of informed consent in complex operations and research studies will not go away.

The growth of the self-care movement—and alternative medicine—are probably the two most obvious examples of the consumer/patient wanting more power. In the first group the patient wants to be an active participant in both

Reprinted from Health and Disease: a reader, with permission from the Open University Press

the treatment and prevention of his condition (the explosion in health clubs, jogging, yoga groups, keep-fit, etc, are an expression of that), and the alternative medicine movement is in part an expression of the consumer/patient voting with his feet. The consumerist element in health care is seen in the various campaigns often mounted successfully by patients themselves, either against a particular medical attitude, e.g. the natural birth movement or for 'breast is best'.

THE ENVIRONMENTAL ELEMENT

The need to care for the environment is the one overriding and unifying belief that binds the Green movement together. Petitioning for the abolition of a planned by-pass or the preservation of a wildlife sanctuary are quintessential Green issues. Concern over the pollution of rivers, the ozone layer, the emission of CFCs, the dumping of nuclear waste, etc, is now at the forefront of public debate and is no longer merely a fringe or counter-culture activity. How can we live on our planet and not destroy it or so affect the quality of our lives that we do not make ourselves sick?

The major area for concern has been over food and water. Interest in nutrition is one of the hallmarks of Green medicine—the level of additives, the question of preservation and irradiation, the use of antibiotics and hormones in meat production, the question of salmonella in eggs and the purification of water are only some recent glaring examples of how all of a sudden doctors have had to wake up to the real concern there is amongst patients regarding these aspects of our environment.

The concern for the environment is linked to the 'back to nature' movement. For a section of the population the doctors' insistence on drugs as the only intervention for treatment is unacceptable.

It is increasingly clear that if we are to understand the relationship between ill-health and ecological destabilisation, the medical profession will need to involve itself more directly in matters regarding the environment. Not only are many of the modern epidemics (heart disease, arthritis, cancer) partly related to environmental factors but also political reactions stimulated by the rise of the Green movement will ensure that no government will be able to ignore the validity of public concern. The specialties of community health, environmental health and occupational health have all been relegated to Cinderella status in the medical profession. The next two decades may see these areas of medicine requiring more government research than the 'high status' specialties of heart surgery, transplantation and genetic engineering.

THE INTERPERSONAL ELEMENT

Like the consumer movement and the environmental movement, the feminist movement has been one of those broad sea-changes against which we can both understand and make sense of many of the changes we see in our society and in the practice of medicine. The emergence of the feminist movement has not only had profound changes on, say, the number of women who now become doctors, but it has also increased our understanding of the psychological processes of diseases and treatments that heretofore have been described through masculine eyes using masculine language.

Notwithstanding the presence of white witches, midwives and nurses, healing and health care has always been a masculine-dominated preserve. The gods of medicine, Apollo, Aesculapius and Chiron, were all male and equally important were warrior gods. We still talk of 'fighting the disease','the war against cancer','the magic bullet' and 'stamping out infection'.

Menopause is described as a 'process of failure', the 'ovaries are shrunken','breasts and genitals atrophy', and it is not too difficult to comprehend why there is a widely accepted view that the menopause is a pathological process. It is in highlighting the words and phrases found in medical text-books both past and present that the male bias towards women can be identified. This bias ensured that women's role in medicine was limited to that of the *comforting healer*. Female practitioners were few and far between and almost always attracted the opprobrium and disapproval of their male colleagues.

We can see more clearly the masculine bias in medicine when we look at those conditions and disorders which affect women in particular— child birth, menstruation, menopause, breast feeding, contraception, cervical smear, breast cancer, obesity, anorexia and bulimia, sexual dysfunction. One does not have to be an ardent feminist to recognise that much of medicine, with its male bias, has ensured that the exchange between a male doctor and a female patient results in women feeling less in control and more at the mercy of the doctor.

Another feature of the greening process is the move towards more gentle nurturing interventions and therapies. If we categorise drugs, surgery and radiotherapy as the active, interventionist, masculine therapies, then we can see the emergence of listening, counselling, massage, relaxation and meditation as more nurturing, containing, feminine therapies.

THE SPIRITUAL ELEMENT

Until very recently, scientific Western medicine has been content to view man and his diseases from a perspective which is primarily a form of mechanistic materialism. Since the Renaissance and Descartes, we have separated the physical from the metaphysical. Descartes saw the body as a clock. The pursuit of reason and reductionist science enabled us, as Francis Bacon said, to put the body on the rack and make it reveal its secrets. Nowhere is this move away from the spiritual to the material more evident than in our approach to terminal illness and death. There is no greater factor which determines the nature of our health care systems than our attitudes towards death. Much of medicine is organised and devoted to do battle with death. This has now been extended to the ageing process as well. We have developed an impressive array of procedures, clinical agents, multivitamins, mineral preparations and reconstructive surgical procedures, transplants, etc, whose aim is to prolong life. There is clearly a legitimate task for medicine, but we need to begin to ask ourselves the question 'why?' What is it that we are afraid of and is this attitude towards ageing and death healthy? Certainly within ecological texts the relationship between life and death and the survival of one species at the expense of another form a very central part of their study.

Once we begin to ask questions about death, we inevitably have to ponder on the question of the spirit/soul. Following the Age of Reason, the cure of the soul was given to the priests, whilst medicine concentrated on the body and, latterly, on the mind. This, of course, is a fairly recent separation for medicine has always been closely linked to the spirits and the gods. Many of the earliest healers were indeed priests. Jesus was known as the great healer. Plato, the father of Western philosophy wrote:

The cure of the part should not be attempted without treatment of the whole. No attempt should be made to cure the body without the soul and if the head and body are to be healthy you must begin by curing the mind, for this is the greatest error of our day in the treatment of the human body that physicians first separate the soul from the body.

What we are now witnessing in our society and what forms an essential part of many Green groups is the return of the spirit—the recognition that man cannot live by bread alone, that to be whole and healthy implies an integration of that part of ourselves that medical science discarded 300 years ago. Its modern expression in health care takes several forms. First, the vast majority of alternative practitioners are spiritual healers. Over 40 000 are registered with one or other organisation in this country—more than the number of GPs. The number of patients seeking 'laying on of hands' or some spiritual intervention, grows each month. Another manifestation of the return of the spirit has been in the use of the concepts of energy or life-force that underpins many of the alternative therapies. Patients seek these practitioners because they will be asked about their energy flow, their sense of harmony and balance. Acupuncture, homoeopathy, reflexology, spiritual healing, all operate on the understanding that ill-health occurs as the result of some 'energy block'. Many patients understand this language and respond to it. It is the language of the spirit. Science has rejected this model and regards it as an outdated concept.

THE SUSTAINABLE ELEMENT

The final characteristic of the greening process in society is the most difficult to describe but is probably the most important to grasp. It is much less tangible than the other four so far outlined. For Greens, one of the factors that causes many of the problems they describe—pollution, over-population, resource scarcity—is over-consumption or the pursuit of growth (in the economic sense) that typifies many Western economies. In the 1960s, when concern regarding the world's resources seemed to reach a peak, many of the prophecies outlined in the books, reports and conferences were doom-laden, and the solutions proposed had a 'hair shirt' air about them. No growth and negative growth were phrases that were often used. Today, the accepted wisdom is that to address many of the problems that beset us, we need to adopt a policy of *sustainable* growth. If it is to be pursued, how then does this principle apply to medicine and health care?

The pursuit of health and positive health has become a major industry, much of it taking place within the alternative health movement. The health food industry and the 'look good–feel well' approach has overwhelmed the public and the medical profession alike. It is in danger of creating a tyranny of its own in the same way as we have created an expectation that all disease would eventually be eradicated if we were given enough research grants, developed the proper instrumentation and discovered the appropriate drugs. Gene therapy is now held up as the latest saviour in the way antibiotics were in the 1950s, steroids in the 1960s and interferon in the 1970s. At the other end of the pole, the public is told 'if you eat the right lentils, meditate in the right way and exercise, you will be healthy'. Both of these approaches, in my view, are misguided. We can no more eradicate disease than we can rid the sea of storms.

If we are to develop the notion of sustainable health, we need first to acknowledge the limitations of what is possible, recognise that ageing and death are normal and moderate our drive for perfection with a pursuit of the ordinary.

CONCLUSION

What impact, if any, have these 'green' ideas had on the practice of medicine today? The Government reforms in the UK-NHS and Community Care Act 1990 (DOH 1990), appear to address the need to 'put the patient first'. The rhetoric underpinning the reforms—'the user-centred seamless service'—suggests that the power relationship between patient and doctor is being addressed at policy level. It is still unclear whether this will provide for a better service or whether the adversarial relationship between patient and doctor will result in a deterioration of care at all levels.

With regard to health, the environmental concerns have, as yet, to influence the training of doctors in any substantial way and medicine remains a personal service profession, where the community and global issues are rarely addressed. We may need to develop and train a new form of 'planetary doctor' if the issues are to be tackled with any seriousness. The feminist influence on medical care is making inroads, not only into research areas, but also into the training of future doctors. Many of the more feminine modes of healing—counselling, massage, hydrotherapy—are beginning to find a legiti-mate place within many general practices and hospital out-patient departments.

The hospice movement and the debates around euthanasia suggest that the taboo regarding our approach to death and dying is gradually being eroded. Many more people are making living wills and doctors are more openly discussing the conflict they encounter when caring for someone who is terminally ill.

It would appear from the above conclusions that one could be reasonably optimistic regarding the future in health care. Unfortunately it is the case that most Western economies and cultures have not addressed the last of the 'green ideas'—that of sustainability. Medicine is still striving to find the 'magic bullet' for cancer. Gene therapy, embryo research and transplant surgery are all seen as the next phase in medical care. No doubt miracle cures will occur but these approaches to health care are not sustainable and we continue to neglect the 'simple needs of the many in order to concentrate on the complex and costly conditions of the few' (De Kadt 1975).

REFERENCES

Department of Health 1990 UK-NHS and Community Care Act 1990
De Kadt E 1975 Inequality and health. University of Sussex. London, HMSO

ALTERNATIVE MEDICINE

Patrick Pietroni

Chairman, British Holistic Medical Association and Senior Lecturer in General Practice, St Mary's Hospital Medical School

Delivered to the Society on Wednesday 1 June 1988, with Sir Peter Baldwin, KCB, a Vice-President of the Society, in the Chair

The Chairman: Our subject tonight has some natural affinity with this Society, because the RSA is interested in noticing improvements in health as in other fields. We talk about a health service and then do anything but look after health; we look after ill-health.

Dr Pietroni is Senior Lecturer in General Practice at St Mary's Hospital Medical School, with responsibility for student education. He is also Senior Tutor and Associate Regional Adviser with the British Postgraduate Medical Federation. In 1983 he helped set up the British Holistic Medical Association, of which he is now Chairman. This year he established the Marylebone Health Centre in the converted crypt of Marylebone Parish Church, in the heart of the community. As part of a research project, several complementary therapies have been introduced into that centre in the hope that such methods will eventually be incorporated into all National Health Service centres.

INTRODUCTION

The last 5–10 years have witnessed a major interest in what has been called alternative medicine. One can trace a number of critical steps that have led to this development, not least of which was Prince Charles' valedictory address as President of the BMA in 1983. Since then, numerous reports, surveys, public hearings, seminars and parliamentary debates have all taken place, and tonight it is my task to try and present to you a brief survey of this topic. I have chosen to divide my talk into four sections. The first will be an historical sketch on the growth of medicine, with specific relevance to the philosophy of ideas that

Reprinted with permission from the RSA Journal: Vol. CXXXVI, No. 5387, October 1988 and delivered to the RSA on 1 June 1988.

underpins the relationship between a health care practitioner, be he a doctor or an acupuncturist, and his patient. The second will be an outline of what is understood by the term 'alternative medicine'. The third will be a description of the current status in the UK and the fourth will be a tentative offering as to how some of these models of health care could be integrated within both the NHS and scientific medicine.

Throughout the history of medicine, certain individuals have either propelled themselves, or been propelled by society, to perform the functions of a 'doctor'. The nature and roles of doctors have changed and continue to change. Different influences are brought to bear on this task. Some are to do with changes in society and the expectation of patients, some to do with advances in health care and therapeutic discoveries. Pathology also changes: the diseases doctors deal with now are fundamentally different from those experienced in the nineteenth century. In addition, patient's responses to their diseases change—social pressure on such things as abortion, terminal care and sexual promiscuity all affect not only the nature of the disease but the nature of the illness as well. With so many changes affecting both doctor and patient, it is not surprising that the nature of the relationship between them changes. Yet as we shall see, although these changes are there to be observed, the fundamental nature of the relationship has not altered very much and we can trace some basic elements that were present in primitive societies, ancient Greece, medieval Britain, post-industrial Europe and modern-day practice.

THE PRIMITIVE ATTITUDE

Primitive here refers to the fact that this is the earliest form of healing known to man. It still exists as the strongest force in many cultures and has not been totally supplanted by later attitudes. The 'primitive' practitioner was the witch-doctor, tribal religious leader or shaman. The shaman (Tunguistic word) is found in almost all cultures. His place amongst the tribal group was of great importance. The shaman was not always male, and on occasions was an ex-patient, yet was equally likely to be the son of the previous shaman. He was often selected as a result of some social occurrence at birth, either breech delivery or propitious astrological confluence. He learnt his 'art' through an apprenticeship which at times was exceedingly hazardous. The role of shaman was not taken up lightly, for it often involved a 'descent into the underworld'. The shaman acted as a mediator between mortal man and the supernatural. He lived in both worlds and, like Mercury, adopted the role of fool or trickster. The religious nature of the healing ceremony involved him in combining the roles of priest and doctor. The separation of these roles did not occur until well into the seventeenth century.

The shaman's relationship to the 'patient' was complex and took several forms. More often than not, the treatment was not individualised but directed towards the patient's home, family or tribe. Healing ceremonies were common, their purpose often to encourage a transformation of consciousness. The shaman would enter into a trance induced through the drinking of some hallucinatory drug or as a result of repetitive chanting or dancing. Whilst in a trance, he would engage with the evil spirits that had invaded the patient and transform them, thus ridding the patient of his illness. The magical element of the ritual was often accompanied by more empiric interventions—drugs, herbs, poultices, enemata and physical manipulations. Study of the details of these empiric interventions suggests that the shamans were astute physicians as well as magicians. Distance healing was practised using effigies, spells and masks.

Primitive man dealt kindly with patients and people who were handicapped. Euthanasia was often practised, but the nature of the relationship between the shaman and his patient involved a certain distance. He was held in awe and maintained his power by surrounding himself with acolytes and accessories (drums, sticks, feathers, etc). This attitude towards healing might be contrasted with our present-day ward round, with the white-coated consultant surrounded by students and expensive pieces of equipment, talking in a language that the patient cannot understand. However, the shaman had additional tasks in relation to the tribe. He was involved in weather forecasting, the collection of the harvest and the warding off of natural disasters. He acquired his skills through an elaborate training, and his methods were often passed on by word of mouth. Payment was often in kind, and shamans would refuse to treat someone when they did not feel they would be successful. Shamans were often made ill by their treatments—occasionally they died—and if unsuccessful, ran the risk of shame, punishment and death. The shamans form the primogenitor from whom all healers are descended.

THE ANCIENT GREEK ATTITUDE

Hippocrates is seen as having laid the foundations for much Western medicine, and some medical schools ask their students to read the Hippocratic Oath on completion of their studies. No one is quite sure who wrote the body of works that come under the name of Hippocrates, but they were clearly written by several different physicians.

The three great philosophers who followed each other, Socrates, Plato and Aristotle, all involved themselves in matters medical and taught on the appropriate nature of the relationship between doctor and patient. The Greek notion 'philia' enthused this relationship. Philia, or 'friendship', took on several forms leading to agape or eros. Much of the early discourses of Plato and Aristotle describe and delineate the difference. In a medical relationship, philia on the part of the doctor implied either a philia for the patient (philanthropy) or a philia for the art of doctoring (philiotechnia). For the Greeks, these two forms of philia blended together within the one doctor, and we can see the progress and development of these strands today. The technique (not technology) or art of medicine involved both empiric, reasoned, imitative and creative acts, and it was Aristotle who outlined the nature of these tasks as they related to medicine. So for the Greek doctor, influenced by the philosophers, his relationship with his patient was influenced by his love for man and by his love for his art. One of the crucial differences, however, was that the philanthropy was related to man and nature as a concept, and not man, the person, the patient. The patient was the individualised form of nature, and it was not until the late nineteenth and twentieth centuries that the patient as a subject in his own right began to be entertained in any major way.

One feature that does seem to remain constant throughout history, however, is the differential treatment of the 'rich', 'poor but free' and 'slaves'. Strict guidelines ensured that 'slaves' were generally treated by the doctor's assistant, communication was kept to a minimum and individualised treatment was unusual. The free but poor visited the doctor's place of work and a fee structure was negotiated. Nevertheless, the need for the patient to work and earn his living necessitated that he be returned to health as quickly as possible. This relationship did not include a discussion on prevention or causation of his illness, as is so well outlined by Plato, reporting on one of Socrates' dialogues (Lovelock 1988):

When a carpenter is ill he asks the physician for a rough and ready cure, an emetic or a purge or cautery or the knife—these are his remedies. And if someone prescribes for him a course of dietetics (diet) and exercise and that he must swathe and swaddle his head, and all that sort of thing, he replies at once that he has not time to be ill and that he sees no good of a life which is spent in nursing his disease to the neglect of his customary employment.

Although health education and preventative health care were seen as important by ancient Greeks, their understanding was that neither the slaves nor the artisans could profit from such a model. The 'discourse' into causes and life-style only took place between the doctor and his 'rich patient', usually in the latter's home, for only the rich had the time and the money to pursue the doctor's instructions. The Greeks were also careful as to the ethics of medical care, and the fundamental difference was that, as has been stated, the philanthropy related to 'man in nature' and not 'man in man'. Thus it was unethical for a doctor to treat a patient who was in the grip of a deadly disease, for to do so the doctor pitted himself against Nature and ran the risk of that fateful hubris that waited those mortals who challenged the gods. Aesculapius, himself the son of Apollo and the father of medicine, was slain by Zeus for raising the dead—only gods had that power. The Hippocratic doctor knew his limitations and refrained from treating the incurably sick or terminally ill. Moreover, it was felt that 'persons who were leading improper lives—no wise physician would wish to heal'.

We see similar debates nowadays in relation to what are thought of as self-inflicted conditions—smoking and lung cancer, alcohol and cirrhosis, food indulgence and obesity, sexual promiscuity and AIDS. It seems clear that for the Greeks there was no normal imperative for the doctor to concern himself with these ailments.

THE CHRISTIAN ATTITUDE

Jesus personified 'the great healer', and under the influence and writing of his Apostles and St Paul, the nature of the relationship between doctor and patient was transformed. The philia of the Greeks became centred around the 'anthropos' as opposed to the 'technie', and the quality of this friendship was also affected. The parable of the good Samaritan is held to indicate the substance of this change. The love for 'man in nature' became 'love thy neighbour', and the doctor could or could not be your 'friend' but a neighbour he had to be. As we shall see, a gradual division between love for the body of man and love for the soul of man often dictated the medieval doctor's relationship with his patient, but the general admonition was that the physician should practise an active effusion of the soul towards other people and their needs.

Under the Christian influence, therefore, we begin to see an attempt to shift the three-tier nature of medical care towards a more egalitarian one: the doctor responds to his patients in a similar manner, irrespective of their class, status or ability to pay. In addition, Christian ethics implied that medical care should go beyond the possible and that the priest/doctor's task did involve the care of the dying and the consolidation of the sick and terminally ill. The latter existed alongside the belief, still strongly held today, that there was some form of therapeutic moral value in the endurance of pain and hardship. This of course reached its most obvious expression in the medieval 'trial by ordeal'; for example, if your soul was pure, no harm would be done to your body if it were dunked in hot oil or in a burning brazier. The medieval medical development occurred under the Church's domain, and although we see how the Christian ethic influenced the nature of the relationship, we can also see how the Church began to exercise its powers over doctors. Initially they were priest/doctors and the early monasteries were places of healing, where the monks practised Christian charity and religious observances. The practice of empiric medicine or Hippocratean medicine began to lose its influence, and instructions such as these were not uncommon:

The sick man must think of his soul before medicine for his body, and what punishment is deserved by a physician who treats him any other way.
When a doctor visits a sick man his first duty is to make him think of his soul and confess—and if the physician does otherwise Holy Church would think fit to cast him out for having acted against her laws.

That some doctors were a little more psychologically attuned is noted by this additional comment:

Before going to a sick man's house ask whether he has confessed to the priest—and if he has not done so let him do so or promise to do so, for if this is spoken after seeing the sick man and considering his symptoms it will be thought that the time has come to despair of a cure, since you despair of it yourself.

With the advent of the medieval universities, we begin to see the return of medicine as an 'art' to be studied, but the Church forbade the dissection of the body and it is not until the seventeenth century that we begin to see the re-emergence of secular medicine. Nevertheless, the Christian influence added to the notion of the doctor–patient relationship elements which we still value today: an egalitarian model of the doctor–patient relationship and the element of caritas towards the incurable and dying. The Church introduced the notion of the 'office of

healing', or ritual as it relates to healing, but this latter element was minimised and secularised by the rationalists and scientists who emerged in the seventeenth century. Towards the end of the medieval period, we see the re-emergence of the three-tier structure of health care. The poor were seen in the monasteries/hospitals, the artisan visited the precursor of the family doctor, and the rich were seen in their own homes usually by their private and exclusive doctor.

THE RATIONALIST ATTITUDE

The explosion of the Renaissance heralded a major shift in medicine, as in all other areas. The process of secularisation led to a division of the patient. The care of his soul became the sole task of the Church and priests, and medicine developed into the study of the body. It was not until the late nineteenth century that attempts to study the mind were made with any earnestness. Descartes and Newton heralded the age of reason. Descartes, in his discourse, laid down the foundation of the future direction of enquiry. The dualistic nature of the human experience, as expressed in the dictum 'I think therefore I am', was followed by the 'mechanistic' description of the body as if it were a clock. He writes: 'I consider the human body as a machine. My thought compares a sick man and an ill-made clock with my idea of a healthy man and a well-made clock.' Descartes' third major contribution was to espouse the cause of reductionism. To study the body, Descartes wrote of the need 'to divide each of the difficulties into as many parts as possible and as might be necessary for its adequate solution'.

Like Bacon before him, who wrote, 'We must put the body on the rack and make it reveal its secrets', the rationalist doctor became the objective, scientific doctor. The wish to help was overwhelmed by the wish to know, and we begin to see a return to the Greek 'philotechnie'. The philotechnie of the past, however, was different from that outlined by Socrates, who emphasised that the love of the art arose out of the initial love of man. Art for art's sake, or more accurately, knowledge for knowledge's sake, determined the nature of the doctor's task. The doctor's task is not to obey or love nature, but to penetrate it and control it. The patient is almost an uncomfortable appendage to this pursuit. The notion that incurable diseases are part of 'nature' and should be tolerated is an unacceptable ethos for the nineteenth and twentieth century doctor. For him, his knowledge tells him that no disease is incurable or that if it is, then the relentless pursuit of knowledge will eventually overcome ignorance. Not only is no disease incurable, but no disease is necessary, so that the notion of morality and punishment as evidenced in the medieval approach to disease is banished under the advances of the microscope, the surgical operating theatre and the magic bullet.

In addition, we have seen how this thrust and acquisition of knowledge has allowed the doctor to imitate nature and surpass the gods—test-tube babies, genetic engineering, etc. The doctor as scientist and the instruction to medical students 'not to get involved or be affected by your patient' are a far cry from the Greek notion of philia-anthropy, let alone the Christian concept of neighbourliness. Nevertheless, the successes resulting from this approach to medicine have become evident, and it has become the dominant form of medical practice, certainly in the Western world. The industrial revolution heralded the growth of hospitals, and a new form of doctor arose, one who was employed by the institution to provide medical services. His relationship with his patient was no longer governed by a financial transaction, in the sense that he neither asked for a fee from the patient directly, nor, if he chose, could he donate his services free to the patient.

The structure of health care practice, however, remained much the same: the poor received free hospital care, the artisan and worker paid for his health care in kind, and the rich were visited at home. The nineteenth century, with its passion for facts and knowledge, allowed for the emergence of the doctor as a sociologist. Armed with accurate figures, it was possible to demonstrate the effect of social class, unemployment, poverty and poor housing on health status, and the beginning of the influence of central government on

doctors and patients. Until then, the major legal and governmental decrees involved the education of doctors and the granting of licences to practise. Now government, like the Church before it, became involved in controlling the tasks that doctors could or could not perform. Legislation concerning the spread of infection, clean air and drainage formed the basis of the public health and hygiene movement. Individual doctors were at the forefront of these campaigns, but by and large the duty of the individual doctor remained the same to his patient. More importantly, however, his duty to the pursuit of the art of medicine, which now was labelled a science, remained paramount. The definition of science as being concerned with the objective and the measurable further distanced the doctor from his patient. Instrumentation introduced the required element of objectivity, and the old skills of taking the pulse, conducting a verbal dialogue, observing the tongue and examining the urine all began to fall into disrepute.

THE SUBJECTIVE ATTITUDE

The philosophers of the late eighteenth and nineteenth centuries, Rousseau, Voltaire, Kant, Nietzche, laid the groundwork for the emergence of the subject. The crisis point in medicine is nowhere better seen than in the differing attitudes to 'hysteria' as evidenced by Charcot, the great French neurologist, and Freud, the rising star of Vienna. Freud followed Charcot on his rounds at the Salpêtrière Hospital in Paris, where the latter demonstrated the nature of 'hysteria' as it affected mostly young women patients. Autopsies failed to reveal any abnormalities, and Freud's notion of the subject's mind scarred not by organic lesions but by unconscious forces, eventually necessitated his return to Vienna and the emergence of psychoanalysis.

There then followed a full-scale return to the study of the patient not as an object but as a subject. Feelings, thoughts, dreams, fantasies, slips of the tongue, all became the data for the diagnosis and the treatment of the patient's ailment. The patient was encouraged to talk and the doctor sat and listened. This, probably more than anything else, is the lasting influence of psychoanalysis on the doctor and his patient. The notion that somehow the subjective responses of the patient were an important ingredient not only in arriving at a diagnosis but in deciding on treatment were, of course, not new. Hippocrates and others all stressed the importance of listening and observing, watching the demeanour and noting the state of clothing. Freud of course took the nature of the subject's remarks much further and endeavoured to demonstrate how they indicated the nature of the malady. With the re-introduction of the subject came the notion of patients' rights. The patient no longer was prepared to hand over his body to the doctor to do with it what he will.

Medical care began to involve not just the serious diseases and surgical operations but the response to disorders of mood or desire. Psychosomatic medicine was born in the early part of the twentieth century, and the doctors who were still practising the objective medicine found that their methods and interventions proved unequal to the task of treating the great epidemic of functional disorders which was soon to develop. We are still witnessing the results of this conflict, and we are a long way from the notion of friendship, neighbourliness or love when we observe the increasing dissatisfaction amongst both doctor and patient in the nature of their relationship. Sociologists, who took up the study of this relationship, began to map out the particular problem.

I have taken the trouble to give this brief historical outline because I feel it is only possible to understand the growth of alternative medicine against the background of these rather large historical sweeps. There has always been and there will always be some form of alternative medicine. What constitutes it will change, depending on the dominant ideology of the time. The rationalist or scientific growth of modern Western medicine arose in the seventeenth century—it was the alternative medicine of its day. We must not forget how the greats of that time, Copernicus, Galileo, Descartes and Newton allowed man to free himself from the dogma of the Church. The Church and its servants were the keepers of all knowledge. Galileo was tried

and had to recant, dissection of the body was forbidden, Darwin was desecrated, Freud was reviled. Man's progress has always been the result of a dominant ideology withstanding the forces of an alternative ideology. Sometimes this alternative ideology is a cry to 'go back to the good old days' or a call to scale the next peak of understanding. The holders of the dominant ideology will respond in a number of ways, either by denigrating, proscribing or ridiculing the upstart, or by incorporating, taking over and integrating. What we are now witnessing in the debate in medicine is a challenge to the dominant ideology, which we could label rationalist, scientific and objective, by a whole host of alternatives that are united only by being outside this dominant ideology. Some of these alternatives wish to incorporate the primitive and magical attitude, some the Christian one emphasising caring and love, some the subjective one with its emphasis on self-care and self-responsibility, and some wish to be accepted within the dominant ideology and see themselves as practising rational, scientific and objective modes of healing. In a hundred years' time there will still be an alternative medicine—its shape, however, will be different. Who knows, it may actually be a scientific doctor suggesting that we should go back to the good old days of penicillin and valium.

THE STATE OF ALTERNATIVE MEDICINE

Let us now look at the current status of alternative medicine. As I have indicated, the term 'alternative medicine' is used to describe those therapies and approaches to healing that are not covered by the traditional, Western, undergraduate medical curriculum. The word 'complementary' is finding more favour and is used by some as a way of avoiding the confrontational stance towards traditional medicine that the word 'alternative' implies. I find that my own understanding of what goes under the umbrella title of 'alternative medicine' is helped by the following model, which embraces four groups:

Group 1:   Complete systems of healing
Group 2:   Diagnostic methods
Group 3:   Therapeutic modalities
Group 4:   Self-help measures

I will now look at each of these in turn.

Complete systems of healing

These are systems of healing which have a theoretical base as to the causation of disease. They have a diagnostic, investigative and therapeutic understanding which shares some similarities with orthodox medicine. Some of these systems have been around for many thousands of years, others are relatively new. The major categories that are found in this country to any great degree are:

1. Acupuncture or traditional Chinese medicine
2. Herbal medicine
3. Osteopathy
4. Chiropractic
5. Homoeopathy.

Most of these systems of healing have an educational framework, publish ethical guidelines and attempt to regulate their practitioners in the same way as the General Medical Council might regulate doctors. They consider themselves, by and large, to be competent enough to deal with most of the problems that come their way, although the more sensible ones tend to suggest that most acute and life-threatening problems are better dealt with by orthodox medicine. Other systems of healing not included in this list are Naturopathy or Ayurvedic Medicine—the traditional healing model in India.

Diagnostic methods

These are ways of determining the presence or absence of disease using methods not normally linked with traditional medicine and include:

1. Kinesiology: as a test for allergies
2. Iridology: as a test for hidden disease
3. Hair analysis: as a test for nutritional defects
4. Aura diagnosis: as a test for levels of well-being.

There are many such methods, some not requiring the presence of the patient, such as intuitive diagnosis; some that claim to be 'scientific' and use many splendid-looking machines; others that claim to call on powers 'unknown to science'. I cannot say, nor do I know, whether there is any truth in these claims. Anecdotal evidence is easy to find, but any substantial body of evidence is absent.

Therapeutic modalities

These treatments again are not found in traditional medicine, and the list is endless. Most practitioners of these therapies do not claim any diagnostic skill but they do claim (and I would go along with some of their claims) that their treatments can and do work. It is probably within this group that the term 'complementary' is most suitable. The treatments complement or supplement what is already on offer. This group includes:

1. Massage—or therapeutic touch
2. Reflexology
3. Aromatherapy
4. Spiritual healing
5. Hydrotherapy.

Self-help measures

This group includes the package of self-help measures where patients are encouraged to undertake certain practices and exercises that will diminish their symptoms, improve their health or maintain their well-being. These self-help measures include:

1. Breathing and relaxation techniques
2. Meditation
3. Visualisation
4. Yoga and other exercise routines
5. Fasting or dieting, etc.

Again, the list is endless and I have mentioned only a few examples of such therapies.

So, the term 'alternative medicine' covers a pot-pourri of activities, some requiring a rigorous training akin to medicine, others faltering on the edge of deceit and charlatanism. There is no doubt of the increase in interest amongst both doctors and the public in many of these activities. Reilly (1983) found a positive attitude in 86 of 100 general practitioner trainees towards alternative medicine. Wharton & Lewith (1986), in their survey of 200 general practitioners in the Avon District, found that 38% had received some additional training in some of these activities, and 76% had referred patients to colleagues practising some form of alternative or complementary medicine. The last major survey in the UK, in 1982, identified a total of 30 000 practitioners of one sort or another. I suspect the figure to be much larger, although it should be pointed out that at least 20 000 of these were in fact spiritual healers. In what is considered the mainstream of alternative medicine (those that would like to be seen as 'scientific'), there are no more than about 3000–4000. We are talking about a small group, therefore, but one which is growing rapidly at a rate of 10% a year. As far as the public is concerned, the consumer magazine *Which* (1981), in its survey of almost 2000 readers, found that one in seven had visited a complementary/alternative practitioner in the previous year, 82% claiming to have been improved or cured. (These figures must be viewed with caution as the figures are highly selective.)

Why do people seek 'alternative medicine'? Information in this area is a little scanty but, as I suggested earlier, there always will be an 'alternative' to the dominant ideology that underpins medicine. This dominant ideology at the moment is the scientific rationalist one, so that one might assume that patients will seek alternatives when they perceive that their problems or difficulties are not being addressed by the group of practitioners trained in this dominant ideology. The survey undertaken by *Which* found that 81% of patients seeking complementary medicine identified dissatisfaction, due to poor symptom relief, as their reason. 71% sought help for joint or pain problems, 15% sought help for psychological problems, but I suspect that the majority of people seeking help, if the figure of 20 000 spiritual healers is correct, did so because scientific rational medicine does not address itself to problems of the spirit. Now spirit is a very difficult concept, and I do not want to get side-

tracked: suffice it to say that I suspect that many patients believe that powerful forces unknown to science still hold sway over our destiny, and like the patients in many so-called primitive cultures, their faith in the shaman is greater than their faith in the doctor.

The BMA (1986) Report on Alternative Therapy, which was produced almost certainly as a direct result of Prince Charles' intervention, was criticised, rightly I think, for being limited in its understanding and prejudiced in its approach. Nevertheless, it highlighted a number of common features in many of the techniques used, and suggested that the popularity of alternative medicine lay in the amount of time available to patients, the use of touch, the magical qualities surrounding alternative practitioners and the authoritative attitude and belief in their models and methods of healing.

THE MARYLEBONE HEALTH CENTRE

Finally, I should like to describe our own attempts to bring together some of these differing and at times conflicting developments in health care under one roof. If I can first remind you of the historical background that I outlined at the beginning of this talk: the primitive attitude with its focus on ritual and magic, the Hippocratean attitude with its emphasis on philotechne and philoanthropi, the Christian attitude with its emphasis on love and care, the scientific or rationalist attitude with its search for facts and knowledge, and the subjective attitude with the emergence of the person, self-responsibility and autonomy. I have described our own approach as the holistic attitude, one which draws on the understanding of the multifaceted nature of health and disease, that sees the importance of flexibility in therapy as well as the limitations of what is possible. I would say that the holistic attitude to health care eschews the dogma of the one true religion as much as it decries the tyranny of the one true science. We are body and mind enthused with spirit. We form only one species in this world and rely on plants, winds, the sea, the atmosphere, as well as the existence of other species to survive. Illness and disease are as much a part of our being human as health and vigour. To believe that we can create a model of health care which will banish all disease, get rid of all pain, cure sleepless nights, is a fantasy that is essentially inhuman. What we *can* do is draw on all the giants of yesteryear and retain some humility as to what we *can* achieve within our own spheres.

The Marylebone Health Centre was set up as an experimental project to explore whether it is possible to provide under one roof a holistic model. We were extremely fortunate to have the support of the Wates Foundation, which has underwritten the first 5 years. The project arose out of an initial research study we conducted at Lisson Grove Health Centre where I was a partner in General Practice. In my capacity as Senior Lecturer in General Practice at St Mary's Hospital Medical School, I set out to see whether some of these alternative methods could be incorporated within a normal NHS General Practice. Following the success of this initial project, we expanded our work and were again fortunate enough to find a new site for our team in the crypt of St Marylebone Parish Church. We now have under one roof a number of activities which I shall describe in turn.

Clinical programme

The National Health Service: General Practice is available, offering the range of normal GP services to the community, including all the necessary attached staff of health visitors, district nurses, etc.

The Complementary Therapy Unit: We undertake an outreach programme, identifying those of our patients who we know have a high requirement of health care but who may have difficulty obtaining it: the elderly, isolated patients, the homeless and unemployed, the ethnic minority groups and the single-parent families. We have organised a mutual support scheme whereby those of our patients who volunteer to give time with both practical or befriending tasks are matched with those of our patients who require extra help with baby-sitting, transport or loneliness.

The Joint Assessment Clinic: This facility allows patients to be examined by four different practitioners from different disciplines (medicine, acupuncture, homoeopathy, stress counselling), and a joint assessment is made as to the nature of their problem and a package of therapies is offered. Sometimes we may arrive at a decision that none of the therapies we have on offer may be of direct help, although we repeatedly find that listening to the patient is the best form of alternative medicine that is necessary.

Educational programme

Public programme: Lectures, seminars and skill-building activities occur throughout the week, and include stress reduction classes, yoga, meditation, relaxation, dietary counselling and all the other activities that are understood by the term 'self-help'. These courses are not the icing on the cake but form very much the substance of the cake. Patients are as likely to be asked to attend a class on diet or relaxation as they are to be offered massage or valium. My own view is that the educational, preventative and promotional nature of our task is vastly undervalued and underestimated.

Professional programme: Similar activities are offered to health-care professionals who wish to enlarge their therapeutic understanding. We provide both instruction and supervision for those practitioners who wish to undertake similar work.

Community/business programme: This is an outreach programme to our local school, youth hostels, community centres and businesses, to provide a focus of health education at the work or study site.

Research programme

Under this programme we attempt to evaluate in some detail both the clinical effectiveness of what we are doing and the cost effectiveness of this approach. Some of the studies are scientific controlled trials (e.g. the use of acupuncture in asthma), and some are to do with concepts of health and vigour and whether healthy people are also happy people. One study is looking at our prescribing patterns and whether we can demonstrate a cost saving on our drugs bill; another is looking at an holistic approach to cancer care, that is, one which draws on religious, scientific, subjective and alternative approaches to the management of cancer.

We are just finishing the second year of this project and it is too early to make any predictions. However, we all feel very privileged to have been given the opportunity to take part in this experiment.

DISCUSSION

Mr M H O Paterson (Community Programme Worker, Hospital Discharge Service, Winchmore Hill Neighbourhood Centre: The literature on this subject is not large, and I try to ensure that holistic publications are in some hospital libraries, but sadly they are not very obvious. I would commend *Caduceus,* and of course there is the *British Journal.* Can you mention any other publications?

The Lecturer: The growth of complementary medicine and interest in this area in the last 5 years has been parallelled by the growth of the number of organisations and publications. The British Holistic Medical Association (BHMA) was an attempt to bring together doctors, medical students and the public. We have expanded our constitution to include other practitioners, and have our own journal, newsletter and publications.

At the same time as the BHMA arose, the Research Council for Complementary Medicine (RCCM) was founded by Dr Richard Tompkin, who quite rightly realised that one of the ways in which we could convince our colleagues in scientific Western medicine that some of these therapies had a place was through appropriate research. It is very difficult to get funds for research studies outside the conventional medical domain. The RCCM has its own publication, in which many of the studies now being carried out are published.

One of the main criticisms levelled at complementary therapists is that they don't have a regulating body akin to the General Medical Council. A group of them set up a body called the Council for Complementary and Alternative Medicine (CCAM), which attempts to address the notion of educational standards and ethical guidelines, so that the public, quite rightly, can be protected against those practitioners of whom they should be wary. Many people who are not professionally trained have the capacity to heal. On the other hand, there are people with a host of letters after their names whom I would not think of approaching for medical help. So 'professionalisation' is no guarantee of healing, but nevertheless we have to address this problem and the CCAM has attempted to do so.

Mr W E Thompson FRCS, Edinburgh (retired Consultant Surgeon): I am an older practitioner and can remember many unfortunate legal cases 50 or more years ago which showed that the medical profession was not prepared to accept alternative medicine. Things have changed and now many are prepared to accept it, but you have to protect practitioners, because ethically the GMC would probably come down on doctors if they did certain things. Could you comment on the legal position?

The Lecturer: A lot of work has been done on the legal situation regarding doctors who refer their patients to complementary practitioners, both at the GMC and the BMA level as well as by the EEC. The whole issue is constantly under review. To the best of my knowledge, there is nothing to stop a general practitioner or a doctor referring a patient to a complementary practitioner, as long as he has made the necessary inquiries to ensure that that practitioner is competent and that he or she remains clinically responsible for that particular patient.

The major issue that patients take their doctors to court for (and there has been a 400% increase in the complaints procedures) is poor communication. What patients seem to prize most in their doctors is not necessarily their scientific skill and knowledge, but their compassion and awareness of the patient as another human being. It is not until we get this important part of health care into our medical system that we shall really begin to address some of the fundamental problems in our health service.

To my knowledge there is only one complementary practitioner who has been taken to court; he was actually a doctor, an acupuncturist, whose needles were not sterilised.

Mr Irving Osborne (Research Fellow, Centre for East London Studies, Queen Mary College, University of London): You have, quite rightly, concentrated on the British scene. Have you any comments on the global aspect? What are the attitudes of other countries?

The Lecturer: As far as Europe is concerned, a lot of legalisation is at present under review in Brussels. I sit on the DHSS Medicines Commission, and in the last 3 or 4 years we have been reviewing homoeopathic and herbal remedies, arising from a request from Brussels. The only country in Europe that has legislated for alternative and complementary practictioners is the Netherlands.

Anyone who has practised in Africa, as I did for 3 years, will have seen the tragedy of scarce resources spent on intensive care units, trying to emulate Western medicine because it was thought to be good. Now there is a great debate about intensive care wards in this country, let alone in the Third World. Our Western medicine is very good, but it is limited, not only for a particular group of diseases but for a group of cultures.

Dr Ian Lush (Senior Lecturer, University College London, Department of Genetics): I have listened to your holistic approach with great interest, but I still think you are trying to mix oil with water and getting a kind of emulsion which will eventually separate out. Let us suppose that you were able to arrange a properly controlled clinical trial of a basic tenet of one of these theories, homoeopathy, say, and let us suppose that the trial showed that the therapy did not work. Do you think that it would have any effect on the popularity of that particular form of health care?

The Lecturer: Let me turn the question around. Two years ago the *Lancet* published a trial using homoeopathic remedies for hay fever. It showed quite clearly, with statistical differences that you and I would accept in any scientific debate, that homoeopathy was superior to the use of antihistamines. Did that change anything amongst the scientific doctors? No. Research does not change

attitudes and practices very much. Our whole treatment is littered with conditions that we no longer use. We used to take the colon out for constipation; we used to do radical mastectomy for breast cancers (and some surgeons still do, which is an absolute tragedy). Research will not change doctors either. We identify with the mode, the language. We like to see ourselves as scientific and objective, or as intuitive and wise, or as alternative and anti-orthodox; all these stances which split, which say 'that is good and this is bad', will leave out the strengths of each. Research is required but it rarely changes attitudes.

Chandra Patel, a very eminent physician, did some wonderful trials in the mid-1970s, with long follow-ups, to show that up to 30% of patients with high blood pressure could come off their tablets if they used a simple breathing and relaxation technique. Yet hypertension is still treated solely by drugs: her research changed nothing. I do not want to be accused of saying that there is no place for drugs. We have to have flexibility.

So I would agree with you. If we could prove that homoeopathy does not work, I don't think it would stop being practised. But we are all very rigid, and the same thing would be likely to happen in orthodox medicine.

Mr Denis Haviland (Chairman, Confederation of Healing Organisations): The Confederation of Healing Organisations is an umbrella for 16 socially acceptable healing organisations in the country and 7500 healers. It is our policy and aim to establish healing as a standard therapy for the National Health Service, and we have two methods to achieve that. The first is by controlled trials. We are prepared to put to the test whether healing does or does not work, as measured by independent medical scientists. We are at the moment in the last stages of negotiating a series of controlled trials on arthritis, neuralgia and strain, on cancer, on pre-eclampsia in pregnant women, and on leg ulcers. We think it necessary to meet the scientists on their own terms before we can expect the medical profession to accept us.

The other method, which Dr Pietroni has touched on, is through cooperation with the National Health Service. So far we have offered a healing service and had it accepted in part by eight hospitals and 15 family practitioner committees, which is more than 10% of the whole. We want them to have experience of healing in advance of actually becoming responsible for it.

It seems to me that the division between alternative and complementary medicine is much too fuzzy at present. The Confederation is in favour of regulation of all therapies in order to keep the bad ones out. We have a policy which starts with the GMC rule that the doctor is in charge, the doctor prescribes, the doctor diagnoses and the healer is forbidden to interfere. The healer is there simply to help. Some therapists who are educated below the level of diagnosis nonetheless aspire to be alternative to medicine. I am inclined to share the view that many doctors have expressed to me that they are a danger to their patients. Do you agree?

The Lecturer: We live in a society regulated by laws. Professions are groups of people who come together to provide a particular service and they protect themselves through the existing legal framework; clearly that needs to be so in health care and medicine. I agree that the alternative and complementary practitioners are coming together to address that, and I also think there is a problem about the level of diagnostic skill in many of the complementary practitioners. There is, too, a concern about the level of diagnostic skill in doctors. Autopsy results show that we get it wrong 25% of the time. So we are not saints either; we need to approach this development towards bringing together complementary and orthodox under the one umbrella, and the legislative aspect will need to be considered too.

Mr S Lee (Member of British Tinnitus Association and Self-Help Group Organiser): Would doctors in areas where large numbers of sleeping pills and tranquillisers are being taken be concerned to find out the reason for it and get some action on a political basis? Would it not be beneficial for doctors and politicians to talk to each other more? And is there not a case for more preventive medicine?

The Lecturer: So far tonight we have not mentioned politics. The whole nature of health care is political, in terms of what we decide to treat and what we decide not to treat, and where the resources go. It is political in that we may have a campaign against drug abuse, yet allow or even increase time for drinking, and allow the use of tobacco. We talk about the drug epidemic. Yet one in ten of all patients in hospital is there because of some alcohol-related disease. We know tobacco causes lung cancer. What can we do about it at the preventive level? It is a political issue.

The time when this nation had its healthiest diet was during the Second World War, when the government legislated for the introduction of vitamin and mineral supplements in the bread. The decrease in infectious diseases is the result not of antibiotics, but of social changes, changes in housing and unemployment. Much of what we see in general practice, casualty and hospitals is the result of our social structure.

We are clearly in a very important phase in the development of the health service at the moment; change is in the air and we do not quite know which direction we should take. Prevention has always been the Cinderella of the health service. Until we establish a service where the preventive, promotional, health educational nature of our task is addressed, we shall continue to have an illness service, as was mentioned by the Chairman in his introduction. In traditional Chinese medicine there are three forms of doctors. The lowest is the doctor who treats you, who gives you your prescription. The second level is the doctor who diagnoses your condition. The top level is the doctor who tells you how to avoid the condition you contracted. Our system is slightly cock-eyed.

Mr Alfred Stern (Acupuncturist): Why do so many doctors view alternative medicine with such suspicion? Surely the main consideration is the patient's welfare. If the patient does not respond to conventional medicine, then why not try alternative medicine? But so many doctors refuse to countenance it. Are they afraid for their security? So often I come across patients who, not having responded to conventional medicine for arthritis, have tried alternative treatments. They have then returned to their doctor, stated that they have had relief, but the doctor does not want to know.

The Lecturer: I think things are changing. Some of the surveys, certainly within general practice, show that many of us are acknowledging that the skills we are given at medical school are not sufficient to deal with the problems we meet in general practice. Many of us have turned to alternative and complementary approaches because they are much more applicable to the problems we see. As far as hospital practice is concerned, the situation is not quite so gloomy. Two hospitals that I know of in London use acupuncturists in their anaesthetic departments. I don't want to perpetuate the conflict. We are moving towards an age where we have to have a greater dialogue with our colleagues from complementary medicine.

I should just add to my complementary colleagues that it is very important to try to address the doctors in language that they can understand. Doctors get terribly frightened when people talk about the chakras, the little bit to the left, the hair analysis of the selenium. This is not the language they have been brought up on.

Mr Gordon Wigglesworth: You used two terms, complementary medicine and alternative medicine, but there is another term which might be used: conviction medicine. In other words, people make their own diagnosis and may decide on one of the alternative medicines which you mentioned. People who are physically sound but may not be very happy can adopt certain disciplines which might give them some kind of comfort. They make their own diagnosis, and nothing on earth will shift them from it.

The Lecturer: I think you have made a very good point. Certainly in the sub-group of patients who seek out alternative and complementary medicine there is a group who wish to retain their sense of control over their own health care. Many of us who have to undergo medical treatment realise that part of being a patient is having to let go and lose that sense of control. An institutionalisation process robs the patient of his own particular prowess.

The metaphor of the wounded healer subserves the whole of the various attitudes and approaches to health care across cultures and across ages. The healer, to be able to heal, has to be aware of his wounds. In many of the shamanistic rituals, healers had to go through a process of acknowledging their wounds or indeed being wounded, in order to be aware of their limitations. In our culture that metaphor has been split; all the wounds have been put on the patient and all the healing potential supposedly put on the doctor. Many of us have the ability to heal ourselves, and what is required is a re-emergence or a marrying together of that split, both in patients and in doctors. For too long the passive patient has put the doctor on a pedestal. It is not just the doctor's fault; it is the patient's fault as well. If he accepts that passivity, then the split will continue. The patient must recognise his wounds but also his ability to heal himself. The doctor must recognise his healing potential but also his wounds and limitations. Only then will there be a true partnership between patient and doctor.

The Chairman: I am sure you will agree with me that those who are students of General Practice at St Mary's Hospital Medical School are extremely fortunate, and moreover that those who come within the postgraduate system over which Dr Pietroni presides are also very fortunate. I am very struck by Dr Pietroni's remark that the kind of diseases that had to be treated only recently, in the last century, are not the diseases to be treated now. Change is going on all the time, and education cannot keep up because not everyone can be educated all the time.

In the National Health Service, patients pass through our hands in some form or other. How little we know of them, or what they are inspired to make of their subsequent lives! But to have been treated as an entire person must be an enormous encouragement in itself, after leaving the hands of such a doctor as we have heard speak tonight. He spoke with extraordinary eloquence, and has given us an enthralling evening.

REFERENCES

BMA 1986 Report of the BMA Board of Science Working Party on Alternative Therapy, May
Lovelock J 1988 The ages of Govia. OUP, Oxford
Reilly D 1983 Young doctors' view on alternative medicine. BMJ, 287, 337–339
Wharton R W, Lewith G 1986 Complementary Medicine and the General Practitioner. BMJ, 292, 1498–1500
Which? 1981 Magic or medicine, August

TOWARDS REFLECTIVE PRACTICE— THE LANGUAGES OF HEALTH AND SOCIAL CARE

Patrick Pietroni

The complexity of interprofessional communication is illustrated by the description of 11 different language sub-sets in current use. The implications for collaborative work are explored and the emergence of the reflective practitioner is examined in the light of these different languages.

INTRODUCTION

If one surveys the ever-increasing literature on interprofessional work, one is faced with the 'litany of disappointment and frustration at the patchiness or absence of fruitful and democratic communication between professionals' (Kilcoyne 1991). This area of study, to paraphrase, is 'everybody's distant relative and nobody's baby' (Griffiths 1988).

In this paper I will put forward the view that the 'baby' of interprofessional work is at present separately represented by the different languages we use to describe our own individual work. I will describe how these languages perform the function of partial communication systems only. Each language and the associated professional way of thinking can be seen as representing the monosyllabic utterances found in the early communicative life of an infant. If this 'interprofessional' infant is to mature and develop a language that can be shared, then as collective godparents, we shall have to explore how these separate languages or 'word forms' can be strung together to form complete sentences. It is as yet unclear whether as collective godparents we shall need to become multilingual or develop a common language.

Jung, in the appendix to the Practice of Psychotherapy, describes the dreams of a patient who

Reprinted with permission from the Journal of Interprofessional Care: 6(1) pp. 7–16 1992.

'caused me no end of trouble' (Jung 1966). The dreams appeared incomprehensible and the patient, who had already left two analyses, was in despair. At about this time, Jung came across the book *The Serpent Power* by Sir John Woodroffe which is a treatise on Kundalini Yoga, and includes a description of the chakras. Jung (1966) writes 'to my astonishment I found in this book an explanation of all those things I had not understood in the patient's dreams and symptoms', and he adds that the difficulties encountered during an analysis 'may not always be in the analyst's evasion of his personal difficulties but in the lack of knowledge which has the same effect as unconsciousness'. In the same way, the difficulties we all encounter in interprofessional work may likewise be the result of the lack of knowledge of each other's language and not necessarily, as portrayed in much of the literature, as the result of personality clashes, power struggles and role confusions. By exploring the nature of these languages and the mode of thought made possible by them, it may be possible to bypass the often highly charged discussions that occur between health and social care professionals.

MEDICAL/MOLECULAR/MATERIAL

Box 1.1 The medical/molecular/material language

Key words: symptoms, signs, disease, aetiology, diagnosis, treatment, virus, genetic chromosome drugs, surgery, radiotherapy, specialist cure, science.
Key writers: Aristotle, Descartes, Newton, Hobbes, Bacon, Galileo, Osler, Fleming, Medawar, Kuhn, Popper.
Key concepts: Inductive reasoning, linear cause and effect, reduce to small bits, mind–body dualism, clinical trial, randomisation.

This is the language of classical science, as practised today, dominant for over 300 years after Copernicus, Galileo, Newton and Descartes freed man from over 1000 years of rigid adherence to ascribing all phenomena, including thought, to some form of divine intervention. It was Descartes' systematic method that gave rise to the mechanistic, reductionistic and dualistic concepts that have since become the hallmarks of rational, scientific enquiry. 'I consider the human body as a machine' he wrote, 'my thought compares a sick man and an ill-made clock with my idea of a healthy man and a well-made clock'. Just as Hobbes learned from Galileo's reconstruction of complex physical problems that even moral issues could be broken down to their constituent parts and then rebuilt to substantiate their logical meaning, so too did Descartes in his analysis of the relationship between mind and body.

There is always a need, he wrote, 'to divide each of the difficulties into as many parts as possible and as might be necessary for its adequate solution'. This is then the language of mainstream Western medicine and indeed Western science generally. Within this language, meaning is pursued usually in terms of causality; precision and measurement are the hallmarks of excellence. This language enables us to pursue a logical, rational and linear mode of thought. Practitioners familiar with this language will look for objectivity and 'hard evidence'. The nature of scientific knowledge acquired through modes of thought made possible by this language is considered to be impersonal, value-free, precise and reliable.

PSYCHOLOGICAL/PSYCHOSOMATIC/ PSYCHOANALYTICAL

> **Box 1.2**   The psychological/psychosomatic/psycho-analytical language
>
> **Key words:** Mind/brain consciousness, unconsciousness, neurosis, psychosis, symptom formation, psychosomatic, potential, growth, stimulus–response, desensitisation, psychoneuroimmunology.
> **Key writers:**
> *Analytical:* Freud, Jung, Klein, Bion, Winnicott, Lacan
> *Psychosomatic:* Groddeck, Balint, Levene, Engel
> *Behavioural:* Pavlov, Eysenk, Skinner, Marks, Ayer
> *Humanistic:* Perls, Maslow, Rogers.
> **Key concepts:** The unconscious, ego/superego/id, projection, splitting, defence mechanism, pleasure/reality principle, transference archetype.

This language is in part older than the first—both Hippocrates and Galen made observations on the mind–body link which are subject to research today—and in part more recent in that the study of the mind has been a relatively new study in health care. This language is also much less unified than the previous one. Nevertheless, within this language and mode of thought, attempts are made to link mind with body—there is a shared understanding that the meaning of an illness should be sought in the psyche as well as in the soma. Freud stood as the creative force behind the modern rebirth of the study of the mind but his approach was steeped in the language of reductionism as is the language of the organic psychiatrists. The behaviourists also pursued a linear cause and effect (stimulus–response) mode of study and it is from the Gestalt and humanistic psychologists that we observe a language that could be viewed as fundamentally different. Like Jung's idea of a causal connecting principle—later termed synchronistic principle—this mode of thought and language privileges 'the idea that correspondence has greater significance and replaces the idea of causality for things are connected and not caused'. In spite of this fundamental difference it is helpful to view these different sub-sets of psychological understanding within one framework. The psychosomatic school has made some attempt to integrate these different forms of psychological language and physicians, including Groddeck, Balint, Levene and Engel, have described models which allow for an integration and cross-over. Latterly the new specialty of psychoneuroimmunology has increased our understanding of 'mind–body' functions and has necessitated the creation of a new sub-set of words, thoughts and language so that it may now be possible to use language to describe how 'unhappiness enters a cell'.

SOCIAL/CULTURAL/EPIDEMIO-LOGICAL

> **Box 1.3**   The social/cultural/epidemiological language
>
> **Key words:** Class, ethnicity, culture, group, public health, privilege, disadvantage, poverty.
> **Key writers:** Parsons, Mechanic, Suchman, Illych, Black, Tudor-Hart, Jarman, Caplan, Cartwright.
> **Key concepts:** Health-beliefs, illness, behaviour, sick-role, knowledge/power, patriarchy/matriarchy, incidence, prevalence.

> **Box 1.4** Examples of the social/cultural/epidemiological language
>
> - An American opera singer in Vienna consulted an Austrian doctor who prescribed suppositories for her headache. Not used to receiving headache medication in this form, she ate one.
> - Pinto is a skin disease so prevalent amongst some South American tribes that not having it is considered an illness.
> - Asked to keep a calendar of symptoms over an 8-week time scale, 100% of social class I and II women mentioned the onset of periods and symptoms associated with them, whereas 78% of social class IV and V made no mention of periods. When asked why, their answers were invariably that for them, periods were part of being a woman, and were not therefore a symptom.
> - A child born into social class I can expect to live, on average, between 5 and 7 years longer than a child born into social class V.

Illnesses such as hiatus hernia, colonic cancer, hæmorrhoids, appendicitis, varicose veins and gallstones, are all diseases of the developed world and fairly uncommon in Third World countries. The link appears to be the low level of fibre in our Western refined diet. Cultural and epidemiological data on the incidence of such diseases as diabetes, atherosclerosis and multiple-sclerosis all suggest a meaning which cannot be derived from traditional biological or psychological studies. Writers in this field include Mechanic, Parsons, Suchman, Black, Illych. The importance of 'illness behaviour', sick-role and 'secondary gain' all help to enlighten the understanding of health care and allow us to debate how the concept of healthy behaviour is itself culture specific. Hallucinatory experiences are seen as totally acceptable and non-pathological in many traditional cultures, whereas in highly developed cultures, they are often the factor determining admission to mental hospital. As late as 1960, homosexuality was seen as an illness requiring treatment. Without the concepts and modes of thought made possible with this language, our health-care approaches would be impoverished, limited and unbalanced.

ANTHROPOLOGY/ETHOLOGY/ETHNOLOGY

> **Box 1.5** The anthropological/ethological/ethnological language
>
> **Key words:** culture, context, field-work, tribes, ritual.
> **Key writers:** Darwin, Lorenz, Levi-Strauss, Bowlby, Mead, Helman, Leach.
> **Key concepts:** Observation/participation, non-verbal behaviour, folk-care, folk-illness, health beliefs, rites of passage.

This language set draws on two previous 'languages' and has been described as a 'biocultural discipline concerned with both biological and sociocultural aspects of human behaviour, and particularly with the ways in which the two interact and have interacted throughout human history to influence health and disease' (Hehnan 1990). An anthropological study of healing practice will reveal systems of 'self-care', 'folk-care' and professional care present in all cultures. The 'health-belief' systems observed and described by medical anthropologists allow us to understand how the Western view of the 'body as a machine' contrasts with the humoral theories of illness and health and how, for some cultures, concepts of balance and harmony lead to health-care practices alien to traditional medicine as described by the first 'language' outlined. Anthropologists have described many 'folk-illnesses', e.g. amok in Malaysia, 'high-blood' in the USA and colds and chills in the UK. These 'folk-illnesses' will also have their 'folk-treatments' and health-care practitioners unfamiliar with this language will have great difficulty in responding to patients who present their problems in this way. The perception and response to the universal symptom of pain differs from culture to culture as different meanings are ascribed to what may objectively appear to be similar experiences. The response to the pain of childbirth may vary from the 'expected and accepted' to the request for spinal analgesia and cæsarian section.

The last 30 years have seen the emergence of the feminist movement which has challenged and changed actual word usage. The feminist perspective in health and social care has, in addition, made great in-roads to the accepted practices of child-birth, infant-feeding, contraception and hormone replacement therapy, etc. Medical textbooks that describe women's bodies through predominantly male doctors' eyes, have had to be rewritten and as a result, the traditional male/doctor and female/nurse relationship is being challenged and altered.

SYMBOLIC/METAPHORICAL/ ARCHETYPAL

Box 1.6 The symbolic/metaphorical/archetypal language

Key words: Ritual folk-lore, magic, image, gods, fairy stories, sacrifice, myths.
Key writers: Eliade, Zeigler, Hillman, Jung, Groddeck, Fowler, Louis von Franz, Fromm, Bettelheim.
Key concepts: The wounded-healer, healing ceremonies, archetypal patterning, connectedness.

This is the earliest language of health care—the language of the shaman. It still exists as the strongest force in many cultures including our own. The shaman acted as a mediator between mortal man and the immortal gods from whom it was thought all disease arose. Diseases were not seen as separate, distinct entities but carried messages to man from the gods.

Groddeck saw disease as a warning from what he labelled 'the it'—'Do not continue living as you do', says 'the it' to the individual. In this language, explanations are sought not from physiological, psychological or social texts but in fairy stories, myths and legends.

Nature's intention is to work towards continual prevention of one-sidedness. Thus the person with the 'A'-type personality structure—constantly active, striving, having little or no time for relaxation—meets his Nemesis through a coronary and like Icarus, who flew too close to the sun and plunged into the sea, is brought down in order to redress the balance of his nature. In archetypal medicine, the patient/client is encouraged to seek meaning, not through words and thought but through images, drawing, sculptures or music. The whole area of the creative arts is drawn upon both to provide meaning and to indicate possible treatment. The focus on the individual and his illness is reduced, and there is an emphasis on the family, the tribe and the collective experience. The shaman presides over the healing ceremony which is heavily ritualised. Shaman were often made ill by their treatments and it is within this language set that the concept of the wounded-healer can best be observed.

NATURAL/ENERGETIC/SPIRITUAL

Box 1.7 The natural/energetic/spiritual language

Key words: Natural balance, harmony, vital force, wholeness, Chi, healing.
Key writers: Dossey, Wilbur, Sheldrake, Pelletier, Capra, Ayurveda, Patanjali.
Key concepts: Field-force, participatory universe, homeostasis, holism, positive thinking, prayer.

This is the language of 'alternative' medicine and as such is directly opposed to the materialistic language of traditional Western medicine. Left alone, nature is considered to be beneficial and caring. The concepts of energy and life-force are central to the understanding of disease and health. Through all matter, both dead and living, 'energy flows'. Distress and disease(s) are the result of an imbalance in the flow of energy and the Eastern concepts of Chi, Yin and Yang are used to examine, explore and treat individual illnesses. More recently, this language sub-set has drawn upon the insights of modern physics to support its hypotheses. The human individual is seen as a 'bioenergetic organism', and the body is no longer regarded as a separate entity. Not only are our bodies largely 'empty space'—if we were able to reduce the 'space' between all the electrons and neutrons in all the atoms contained in the human body, the resulting matter would amount to no more than a grain of sand—but we are surrounded by a never-ending stream and flow of energy that has been labelled the 'bio-dance' of the universe. Therapeutic interventions such as homœopathy, acupuncture and the laying on of hands, all work through influencing the energy system and restoring a balance between positive and negative energies. 'Positive thinking', meditation and prayer are all felt to encourage healing energies, and bring about an increase in wholeness and harmony within both the individual and the universe. In this mode of thought 'illness' is seen as the result of a disturbance in the 'collective field force'. Like the previous sub-set, there is a greater emphasis on group activity, collective healing ceremonies and the acceptance of spiritual forces in human health and illness. The allegiance to 'natural' products and 'pure' foods has produced a culture which is anti-drug, anti-technology and anti-science. It is, nevertheless, finding increasing popularity amongst many patients. The miscommunication between doctors voiced in the first language described and patients who use this language to describe their illnesses has resulted in the increased popularity of alternative practitioners.

PREVENTION/PROMOTION/ EDUCATION

Box 1.8   The preventative/promotional/educational language

Key words: Self-help, risk factor, health-hazard appraisal, life-style, check-up.
Key writers: Selye, Cousins, Pietroni, Boston's Women's Handbook, Le Shan, Ballentyne.
Key concepts: Prevention is better than cure, empowerment, responsibility, positive health, knowledge=power, mind over matter, power=choice, choice=behavioural change.

This language stems from the belief that prevention is better than cure and that if one follows a particular set of life-style activities relating to food, exercise, sleep, stress reduction and simple mental exercises, one can not only prevent disease but one can also modulate the effects of a disease once it occurs. Health promotion clinics and life-style advice have now not only entered the language of health care but also heavily influenced the distribution of resources and monetary rewards, especially within General Practice. The epidemics of the latter half of this

century, epidemics of mood, desire and life-style (stress-related illnesses, the psycho-emotional disorders, cancer, arthritis, heart disease and, latterly, AIDS) are all thought to require a preventative approach rather than an interventionist approach favoured by the first two languages described. In the last 10 years there has been an explosion of self-help groups and jogging and aerobic classes, all aimed at giving consumers more knowledge and skills in taking an active responsibility for their own health care. The shelves of book stores are cluttered with '*How to*' books and many achieve best-seller status. Phrases like anticipatory care, risk-factor analysis and health-hazard appraisal have formed the basis of many official reports on health care. Illness is viewed as a consequence of a failure in teaching and learning preventative health, whether it be immunisation, adequate contraception, safe sex or dietary practices. Huge sums of money are expended in anti-smoking and other such campaigns and responsibility for these preventative measures is increasingly seen as one that is shared between health-care practitioners and the consumers. This language attempts to attribute meaning through the expression of individual choice, knowledge and the freedom to change.

ENVIRONMENTAL/ECOLOGICAL/ PLANETARY

Box 1.9   The environmental/ecological/planetary language

Key words: Green, pollution, acid rain, global warming, ozone layer, environment.
Key writers: Porritt, Lovelock, O'Riordan, Higgins, Hume-Hall, Dubos.
Key concepts: Ecological balance, environmental degradation, artificial additives, over-population.

This particular language arises out of the increasing concern for the degradation of the environment and the effect this has on health and disease. The advances and improvements brought about by technological developments are thought to have led to a disturbance in the ecological balance and led to many diseases and epidemics affecting us today. Man's concern with the environment is, of course, not new and many commentators argue that the improvements in health care that occurred at the beginning of the century are a direct result, not of advances in drugs or surgery, but of improvements in legislation regarding sewage control, clean air and housing. It is believed that we are now facing the consequences of a lack of control over pollution, food production and clean water management. There is a call for 'planetary doctors' to address the problem of acid rain, deforestation, the greenhouse effect, resource scarcity and over-population. All these aspects of modern industrial life are felt to have a much greater impact on individual health than the causative factors that form the basis for much medical research. This planetary language is relatively new and within the individual-based model of our health-care services, we are rarely able to find use for it. Nevertheless, more recently, there has been a clear and radical shift amongst establishment institutions, food manufacturers, multinational institutions and politicians from all parties, so that 'green' policies towards health care will inevitably form part of the language with which all of us will have to become familiar. New disease entities such as 'multiple allergy-syndrome', ME, food allergies and candidiasis are believed to have arisen because of environmental degradation and the new specialty of 'clinical ecology' addresses the consequences of this degradation on the individual.

LEGAL/MORAL/ETHICAL

Box 1.10 The legal/moral/ethical language

Key words: Rights, euthanasia, integrity, conscience, beneficence.
Key writers: Kennedy, Gillon, Vessey, Mills, Rawls.
Key concepts: Utilitarianism, deontology, quality of life, informed consent, medical paternalism, moral obligation, medical confidentiality.

As health care has become more complex, practitioners have had to embrace a level of practice which has involved them in both statutory responsibilities as well as issues of morality regarding experimentation, organ-transplant,

adoptions, foster care, in vitro fertilisation and euthanasia. Many of these issues have moral, legal and ethical implications. Practitioners could be helped to manage such dilemmas if they were more familiar with both deontological and utilitarian theories of philosophical ethics. Increasingly, legislation regarding experimentation, the prolongation of life, informed consent and the access to medical records will impinge on the individual practitioner's clinical task. Tragedies surrounding child-abuse and the management of terminal care inevitably highlight the practitioner's unfamiliarity and inability to make use of language and concepts that are derived from this body of work. The world of professional paternalism is gradually being eroded so that problem-solving is a far more difficult affair. It involves an ability to tolerate the confusion and uncertainty that is involved in these complex problems. The practitioner who is familiar only with the language of measurement and precision may be peculiarly unqualified in handling such problems, especially within the biomedical discipline.

Once the complexity of these judgements is appreciated and once their evaluative character is understood, it is impossible to hold that the doctor is in a better position to make judgements than the patient or his family. The failure to ask what sort of harm/benefit judgements may properly be made by the doctor in his capacity as a doctor is a fundamental failure of medical paternalism (Gillon 1985).

This failure applies to several of the other health-care disciplines and until the language of ethics is introduced into practice then the problems arising from this failure will inevitably occur.

RESEARCH/EVALUATION/AUDIT

Box 1.11 The language of research/evaluation and audit

Key words: Data computer, protocol, randomisation, co-operative enquiry, action-research.
Key writers: Medawar, Reason, Crombie, Howie, Metrof, Bradford-Hill.
Key concepts: Clinical trial, double-blind, long-term follow-up.

One of the phenomena of the latter half of the twentieth century has been the information explosion in almost all areas of academic and clinical work. To enable an individual to properly evaluate what information is valuable and indeed valid, systematic attempts at research now form the basis of thinking and progress. Within medicine, it is the clinical trial as a method of assessing and validating treatments that has largely governed the rules of research and has helped to determine progress in Western medicine. This model has been criticised as being too limited in assessing the outcome of clincial interventions. Other forms of research, including the sociological survey, participatory observation and cooperative inquiry now form the basis for studies in clinical outcome. Whichever method is adopted, there is nevertheless an increased awareness that the task of any professional, whatever his discipline, involves the ability to critically evaluate his work. How can one assess whether what one is doing is of value? Audit procedures have become the norm in many clinical settings and the desk-top computer, with its ability to provide immediate feedback on prescribing pattern, referral choices and consultation times is increasingly forming the basis of performance indicators. This is all language that was non-existent 10 years ago. Indeed, the willingness to subject one's work to these audit procedures as well as the undertaking of research studies will almost certainly become a factor in determining pay, status and promotion. This language, so closely linked with the first, can lead to an emphasis on measurement and on the need for distinct entities in disease labelling that is characteristic of the biomedical model. The psychosocial model of health care needs to develop its own sub-set of research and audit procedures which allows for the evaluation of the indeterminate and the imaginative qualities and intuitive perceptions that are associated with these disciplines.

ECONOMIC/ADMINISTRATIVE/POLITICAL

Medical bureaucracy began with the emergence

> **Box 1.12** The economic/administrative/political language
>
> **Key words:** Budgets, money management, committees, bureaucracy.
> **Key writers:** Maynard, Keynes, Bosanquet, Lethard, Tudor-Hart, Jarman, Hoggett.
> **Key concepts:** Resource-allocation, unit costs, internal and market, health-economics, indicative drug budgets, performance indicators.

of the hospitals and the need to develop a coherent management of bureaucratic institutions which possessed a dual system of authority. The administrative structure was managed separately from the professional task of caring for the patients. Doctors retained not only their administrative autonomy but were able to control the lay managers as well. Even with the emergence of the National Health Service in 1948, the medical profession retained both autonomy and control. The escalating costs of providing a 'free' health service forced politicians, both Labour and Conservative, to consider ways of controlling expenditure, and the appropriate allocation of resources. Government, which had so far restricted itself to matters of Public Health, began increasingly to get involved in planning and managing the health service. Professionals who had been used to total autonomy and control were having to recognise that not only was their administrative independence being challenged but their professional judgements as well. The pace of these changes has accelerated a great deal in the last decade and a completely new language set has emerged as all health-care professionals are subject to a managed health service. The development of information technology has ensured a massive increase in data collection and audit procedures. 'Independent hospitals', trusts and fund-holding practices have been introduced and have brought with them their own specialist language. Practitioners of all disciplines are now having to familiarise themselves with ways of thinking that have not formed part of their training.

IMPLICATIONS FOR THE PRACTICE

What conclusions can be drawn from this overview of health-care 'languages'? Is effective communication possible between professionals who speak different languages? For it is not only the language and words used that separate us, but the mode of thought that is made possible by the different languages. The use of language is a complex process whereby one's internal experiences, thoughts, fantasies and bodily sensations are transformed into words that are then used to reflect on and communicate these internal experiences. The context in which these internal experiences occur will influence the choice and formation of the words and the language construction arrived at. Language is never value-free and is contextual to a degree that may actually inhibit thought and imprison the imaginative growth of the individual.

The study of language and word construction has become a major academic discipline in its own right and has affected the nature of critical discourse profoundly. Structuralism and the theory and practice of deconstruction have been applied extensively to the study of literary texts and other cultural phenomena. The links between language, thought, ideology and culture, although firmly accepted within other disciplines have, as yet, to be made within our different health-care professions.

Attempts at solving the crisis in interprofessional work have centered around communication skills training, sensitivity groups and management training, but as Isabel Menzies (1988) points out:

It's money for old rope to make people sensitive, because they usually want to be more sensitive anyway. But then you send them back to where they came from and they're back in the old situation which does not allow them to deploy more sensitivity. All that happens is that they slip back or they get very disgruntled or discontented, or they leave or something.

A similar conclusion was noted in a recent survey on post-course experience amongst social workers: half said their experience was entirely disregarded and 65% changed their job within the first 2 years after completing a course (Rushton & Martin 1991).

If communication courses do not seem to provide the solution, what does? The Newcastle study, one of the most extensive in the field, suggested some practical steps to encourage collaboration:

1. The use of a common base record.
2. The development of medical, nursing and social work group practices with appropriate zoning of geographical catchment areas.
3. The encouragement of stable 'attachments' of district nurses, health visitors and social workers to group practices.
4. The development of joint educational sessions for interprofessional training. (University of Newcastle Health Care Research Unit 1985).

The recent Centre for the Advancement of Interprofessional Education (CAIPE) survey identified several such initiatives throughout the UK, but although the number of such courses was encouragingly high, the content and course membership seemed to suggest the majority did not address the issue of interprofessional work (CAIPE 1989).

Anthea Hey and colleagues, in their survey specifically addressing social workers, point out that 'team work', with its implied institutional base and high degree of collaboration, may be the wrong format for dealing with highly complex, anxiety-filled situations. She draws attention to the concept of networking and suggests that a finer discrimination is required before arriving at a generalised solution (Hey et al 1991).

Whether the containing concept is a network or a team, most workers in this field recognise the need for something additional in the training of health-care workers. Rosalie Kane has developed a framing series of knowledge skills and attitudes she believes are required for the future (Kane 1976), to enable, as Mary Kahn says, the practitioner to 'delight in another's work and in connecting their own to it' (Kahn 1977). Schön and his colleagues take a different perspective using a situation-specific model and describe four professional roles they perceive within health care.

1. The *practical*, professional is pragmatic, problem-solving, arrives at solutions by trial and error and is involved with the everyday clinical problems.
2. The *expert* professional claims expert knowledge which may result in being distanced from everyday problems. He calls on a body of expertise which he alone has and which can often be difficult to share with others.
3. The *managerial* professional is familiar from the field of social work and social services. This two-tier model applies where an experienced practitioner becomes a manager responsible for personnel, planning strategies and the management of resources. He may also provide a supervisory back-up to less experienced practitioners.
4. The *reflective* practitioner is an ideal that many of us may aim for. This practitioner recognises that others have important and relevant knowledge to contribute and that to allow this to emerge is a source of learning for everyone. Reflective practitioners look for a sense of freedom and real connection with, rather than distance from, clients (Schön 1983).

Schön, who has written most on the 'reflective practitioner' has also provided the drive for rethinking the basis to professional training. He calls for 'the liberation of the professions from the tyranny of the university-based professional schools'. He believes the latter have succumbed to the idea that rigorous professional practice is dependent on the use of 'describable, testable, replicable techniques derived from scientific research based on knowledge that is objective, consensual, cumulative and convergent'. He challenges this view of professional knowledge and puts forward an additional perspective that involves practitioners in 'making judgements of quality for which they cannot state adequate criteria and displaying skills for which they cannot describe procedures or rules'. These skills he believes form some of the most important aspects of competent practice. He contrasts these two aspects of the professional task as the dilemma of 'rigour or relevance'. He then explores how

training can be offered to professionals of whatever discipline to develop a 'reflection-in-action' as opposed to a knowing-in-action mode of practice (Schön 1987).

Schön's work has attracted much attention and he clearly has struck a chord for those involved in professional training. It is therefore critical that the idea of the reflective practitioner is itself reflected on before it becomes part of the accepted canon. A doctor who reflects on the problems of a patient with chronic rheumatoid arthritis may be familiar with only two or three of the language sub-sets described. He may lack the knowledge-base that will allow him to consider such possibilities as 'secondary-gain' or 'dietary-prevention', or the metaphorical-symbolism of the distribution of the arthritis. He may have no awareness of how a chronic, debilitating illness affects other family members and his 'reflection' may involve only the search for another effective drug, as opposed to considering acupuncture or spiritual healing.

Reflection which occurs within one language sub-set only runs the danger of repeating the same mistakes over and over again. For the reflective process to be truly creative, producing new solutions to old problems; the ingredients present need to be as diverse as possible. To exclude one of the language sub-sets from inter-disciplinary teamwork discussion may not be of great consequence, but to allow only two or three language sub-sets will almost certainly avoid the confusion, messiness and muddle that are inherent in the process of reflection.

To encourage such a wide-ranging reflective process amongst professionals is not at all an easy task. In another series of papers (see pp. 228, 235) we describe the outcomes of an attempt to explore these issues in depth during the life of a multidisciplinary clinic.

REFERENCES

CAIPE 1989 A report of a national survey on inter-professional education in primary health care
Gillon R 1985 Philosophical medical ethics. John Wiley, London
Griffiths R 1988 Community care agenda for action. HMSO, London

Helman C G 1990 Culture and health and illness. Butterworth-Heinemann, Oxford

Hey A, Minty B, Trowell J 1991 Interprofessional and inter-agency work: theory, practice and training for the 90s. In: Pietroni M (ed) CCETSW study 10. CCETSW, London

Jung C G 1966 The realities of practical psychotherapy. The Collected Works, 16 pp 327–338. Routledge & Kegan Paul, London

Kahn M 1977 Towards collaborative health practice: 9th annual meeting of the American Society of Allied Health Professionals, Journal of Allied Health Workers, USA

Kane R 1976 Paper to CSWE conference. Philadelphia, USA

Kilcoyne A 1991 Post-Griffiths: the art of collaboration in the primary health care team. Marylebone Monograph 1.

Marylebone Centre Trust, London

Menzies I 1988 Containing anxiety in institutions. Selected Essays Vol 1. Free Association Books, London

Rushton A, Martyn H 1991 Research findings from two post-qualifying courses. In: Pietroni M (ed) Right or privilege? CCETSW Study 10. CCETSW, London

Schön D 1983 The reflective practitioner. Jossey-Bass, London

Schön D 1987 Educating the reflective practitioner. Jossey-Bass, London

University of Newcastle Health Care Research Unit 1985 A study of interprofessional collaboration in primary health care organisations. University of Newcastle Health Care Research Unit 1 and 2

2

The community

INTRODUCTION

The 'community' is a term that has become one of the most important in late twentieth century health and social care. It is the place where people are increasingly expected and expect to receive health and social services and it is now widely agreed that, where possible, people should be cared for in their own homes, or home-like environments. People should be able to give birth, convalesce and die in the place where they are most comfortable and hospitals are increasingly becoming places where people go for short and discrete clinical interventions, rather than places to 'get well' per se. Yet despite this development in the thinking about the proper provision of care, there are still many unresolved issues concerning the meaning of community care in practice for both providers and consumers of care services. Indeed the very word 'community' is a loose one and not easily defined. Who makes up a community? How large is it? What makes one person a part of it and another excluded from it? How is it possible to integrate new and often different members into an already existing and perceived 'community'?

More than this, the delivery of community care is further complicated by the historical development of the idea of community care. In particular there have long been issues concerning the boundaries between community care, primary care and primary health care. The experiences of the Marylebone Health Centre and the Marylebone Centre Trust have not been exempt from these issues and conflicts. The Marylebone

Model of care (see Introduction, pp. 1–3) was developed from a notion of user-centredness but one which saw its task as providing a broad range of services in a primary care setting. The Health Centre never had a narrowly defined notion of 'primary health', and indeed its community outreach unit was crucial to the holistic approach adopted by the Centre. The emphasis was on enabling living connections to be made with the individual and between individuals and their environment.

However, the conceptual move towards providing community care at the Health Centre, while arising naturally out of the work already undertaken there, was given impetus by the Education and Training Unit of the Marylebone Centre Trust. The process of developing an MA in Community and Primary Health Care by the Education and Training Unit, which necessitated interprofessional and collaborative work by members of the Health Centre, the Trust and other professionals and organisations, helped to heighten the awareness of the issues at stake. For example, at the heart of the new framework for community and primary health care is user-centredness. Professional groups of all kinds and with widely differing training and backgrounds are expected to work together in a 'user-centered seamless service'. First hand experience, however, points to a divide between this service-led objective and the performance and cost-led framework for evaluation which now accompany it. Professional workers in community and primary health care, therefore, find themselves caught in a web of policy contradictions. The creative learning process that resulted in the MA in Community and Primary Health Care led not only to the decision to integrate community and primary health care in one Masters programme but also to a conceptual shift at the Health Centre. The Centre recognised that rather than providing primary care, an integral part of which was community outreach, it ought in fact to consider itself to be a provider of community care. Thus the services available at the Health Centre would be provided within a framework that recognised the difficulties, challenges and possibilities of care in the 1990s while staying close to, and indeed developing, the fundamental belief in an holistic approach to care.

The papers included in this chapter reflect the nature of this development and are drawn from its different stages. They fall mainly into two categories:

- The research and experimentation with various projects designed to meet the needs of the community served by the Marylebone Health Centre.
- The research that has been undertaken into the needs and issues of various minority groups represented within the Health Centre and indeed in almost every 'community' in the country.

Clearly the work undertaken in one area informs the work undertaken in the other and the papers included in this chapter reflect both these aspects.

The cost of serving different communities and the workload associated with serving them will vary. The debate over how these factors can best be measured has, however, been extensive. Chase & Davies (see p. 47) undertook a study designed to establish an accurate and useful profile of the patients registered with the Marylebone Health Centre and, in particular, to discover the underprivileged area score (UPA) for the Centre. Specifically, this study was designed to look at whether a UPA score for a given practice was better calculated on the basis of the UPA score of the wards in which the registered patients lived, as suggested by Jarman (1983, 1984), or on the basis of the patients actually registered and registering with that practice. In the course of their study Chase & Davies discovered that the UPA score calculated from the practice was consistently higher than might have been expected using the UPA score for the various wards. Moreover the research produced much additional information about the needs of the Health Centre's patients and suggested areas for development and improvement of services.

This type of research gives invaluable evidence which can be used effectively in the development of community care and primary health programmes. One such programme, which illustrates well the move towards providing community care, is described by Webber et al (see p. 53). The volunteer community care project which they initiated arose naturally from the Marylebone Health Centre's approach which contends that an integrated health care policy provides a wider range of services than simply the doctor–patient consultation. An additional aim of this outreach and patient participation project was to discover whether patient participation structures had a significant effect on the physical and psychological well-being of individual patients. That this is the case has been widely suggested, and may be borne out by anecdotal evidence, but the literature is still inconclusive on the matter. The difficulties associated with setting up such a scheme were varied and included the problems involved in both recruiting volunteers and recruiting people who were in need of and willing to accept the kind of volunteer services that the project could offer. Certain elements of the volunteer scheme, such as the befriending service, raised issues about confidentiality and professional/personal boundaries. It seems that both of these are natural areas to consider when this kind of volunteer patient participation is undertaken. However, in the context of a health service in which the neighbourhood is increasingly becoming the major unit of service management, these kinds of volunteer schemes clearly have a future and, as Webber et al suggest, they can be successful in improving the well-being of both the service consumers and the service providers—in this case the volunteers themselves.

Pietroni (see p. 60) reflects on these findings and suggests that they will prove to be extremely significant for the future development of all care services. In particular, he suggests that the ways in which the 'pastoral' function of health and social care are carried out will have to change and develop to meet new needs and new systems of care provision.

The successful provision of services to a community will necessarily involve providing services tailored to minorities within that community. These minority groups will have needs specific to their identity as a minority which will require to be identified and provided

for. One such group identified by the Health Centre was the homeless refugees whom they served. Specifically, the issues of racism which faced many of the homeless refugees with whom the Health Centre worked were of particular concern. These individuals often had particular problems integrating themselves into their community. In large part this was because they often spoke very little English and had come from cultures which functioned in very different ways from the one in which they now found themselves. More than this, however, many of the people with whom the Health Centre was working had undergone gross mistreatment before coming to England; not infrequently they had been tortured and beaten, and these experiences coloured the ways in which they responded to their new surroundings. If care is to be genuinely based in the community it must be flexible enough to respond to these kinds of challenges and must find ways of providing services tailored to the needs of these kinds of groups, many of which may be quite different from the kinds of services delivered ordinarily.

Pietroni & Pietroni (see p. 64) look at the needs of another minority group in their paper on access to health care services for people with physical disabilities. Here they show that it is in the long-term interests of both the provider and the disabled consumer of health services to make primary health care facilities as accessible as possible. The former will save money and the latter will be likely to have a higher all-round state of health as a direct result. Moreover, they demonstrate that improved access is not confined to putting ramps into buildings. On the contrary, it also means providing clear and, above all, accurate information about the provision and accessibility of facilities as well as developing a legislative framework which prevents the creation of a built environment which discriminates against people with physical disabilities. They go on to discuss the wider context of accessibility to health care with specific reference to transport to and from health care facilities.

A point which emerges strongly from all the work on the community and community care is that it is important for providers of health and social services to recognise the individual within the community. A community, after all, is made up from a series of individuals, each with individual needs. There may be identifiable groups within a given community and thus it may be possible to tailor services to groups. It should, however, be remembered that just as homeless refugees or physically disabled people may have specific needs, so there will be sub-groups of refugees and disabled people who have yet more specific needs. Ultimately, the level at which care will be provided will always be the individual, and it is

only as a way of providing better care to individual patients and clients that community care is valuable. Community care is a means to an end, not an end in itself.

REFERENCES

Jarman B 1983 Identification of underprivileged areas. British Medical Journal 286 pp 1705–1709
Jarman B 1984 Underprivileged areas: validation and distribution of scores. British Medical Journal 289 pp 1587–1592

THE CALCULATION OF A PRACTICE UNDERPRIVILEGED AREA (UPA) SCORE

Derek Chase
Peter Davies

A study was undertaken at a London inner city practice to determine an underprivileged area score (UPA) based on information derived from patient questionnaires. The practice studied was new, had a highly mobile population and operated an 'open door' policy to new registrations—factors which were all considered to be contributing to a high level of workload. This was confirmed by the practice UPA score which was found to be at variance with the Jarman score for the area. As such, the method used serves to highlight the differing workloads between practices and provides a means by which to make comparisons.

INTRODUCTION

Work by Jarman (1983, 1984) has shown that the socio-demographic characteristics of a population, as reflected in its UPA score, correlate with the level of workload as perceived by general practitioners serving that population. These perceptions have been supported by objective evidence showing that UPA scores correlate well with indices of need for general practitioner services, such as mortality (Charlton & Lakhani 1985) and infant mortality rates (Jarman B personal communication) and with actual general practitioner workload (Curtis 1990).

In April 1990, the Government introduced deprivation payments payable to general practitioners, for every patient living in a ward whose UPA score was greater than 30; larger payments being made for scores between 40–50 and 50 and above (Department of Health and the Welsh Office 1989).

However, since ward populations range between 56 to 41 875 people, the mean size being

Reprinted with permission from the British Journal of General Practice: 41 pp. 63–66 1991.

5237, Foy (Foy et al 1987) has pointed out that 'the aggregated socio-demographic data available from the census may hide large variations between smaller, more homogeneous groups.' A practice, therefore, may have a patient population which is unrepresentative of the ward in which it is located. This might be due to geographical reasons, for example if it were close to a large housing estate in a ward of relative affluence, or as a result of practice policy which limits registration to certain patient groups. Thus, whilst the Jarman score provides an indication of the expected workload for a ward, it may not reflect accurately workloads for individual practices within it.

The present study calculated a practice UPA score from information collected directly from the patient population of an inner city practice, the Marylebone Health Centre (MHC). The practice was new, having opened in February 1987, and was growing rapidly with an 'open door' policy towards registration of the local population. It is situated in an area of social extremes, being close to both Harley Street and a large number of bed and breakfast hotels for homeless families. These characteristics suggested that the practice and local ward scores might be different.

METHOD

800 new patients fully registering with the practice between 1 January 1988 and 30 November 1988 were each asked to complete a 'registration form'. This included questions relating to housing, ethnicity and other factors from which a UPA score could be calculated (See Table 2.1). Patients who did not complete the form at registration had their notes tagged and were asked to do so on their next attendance. Forms were completed usually unsupervised but with help from reception staff where patients had difficulty. These were then checked during the first consultation. At the end of the study, patients on whom information was still incomplete, (less than 5%), were followed up by telephone. No temporary residents were included in the study.

The definitions of the eight factors required to calculate a UPA score are listed in Table 2.1. These are slightly different from the definitions used

Table 2.1 The Jarman factor definitions compared with those used for the study

Factor 1 *Elderly living alone* — % of people of pensionable age living alone (males over 65, females over 60)
MHC: % of patients over 65 who state at registration that they are living alone

Factor 2 *Under 5* — % of children under 5 years old
MHC: % of children under 5

Factor 3 *One parent* — % of people in households of one person 16 yrs and over and one or more children under 16
MHC: Child under 16 in 'one parent' household
Adult over 16 and over in 'one parent' household

Factor 4 *Unskilled* — % of people in households headed by a person in socio-economic group 11
MHC: Child under 16 whose head of family is in group 11
Adult over 16 where the head of family is in group 11

Factor 5 *Unemployed* — % of people aged 16–64 seeking work or temporarily sick as a percentage of the economically active population
MHC: % people aged over 16 who state on registration that they are unemployed as a percentage of economically active patients aged 16–64 yrs

Factor 6 *Overcrowded* — % of people in households living in more than one person per room (excluding bathroom, toilet, kitchen and corridors)
MHC: Child under 16 yrs whose head of family states that he/she is living in such a household
Adult over 16 yrs who on registration states he/she is living in such a household

Factor 7 *Changed address* — % of people aged 1 or more with a usual address one year from the census different from their present address
MHC: Child over 1 and under 16 yrs who has moved in the last year
Adult over 16 yrs who has moved in the last year

Factor 8 *Ethnic minority* — people in households headed by person born in the New Commonwealth or in Pakistan as a percentage of all registered patients.
MHC: Child under 16 yrs whose head of family states he/she was born in the New Commonwealth or in Pakistan
Adult over 16 yrs who on registration states he/she was born in the New Commonwealth or in Pakistan

by Jarman (Irving & Rice 1984) because of the way the data was collected. The principal difference was the replacement of the term 'head of household' (defined in the 1981 census (OPCS 1981) as the 'person in the first column of the census form') by the term 'head of family' (defined in the 1981 census as the husband in a married couple family, or the lone mother, or lone father, or lone grandparent in a lone parent family). A second change was that all patients over 16 years of age were treated as individuals and not linked to their family head because of difficulties in doing this accurately. Children, though, remained linked to the head of family. A third change related to pensionable age. Although this is 60 years for women, it was taken as 65 years for both male and female patients.

A consequence of these changes meant that an English woman married to a Pakistani man, for instance, did not score positively for the 'ethnicity' factor (factor 8). Under the Jarman definition, assuming the husband was the head of the household, all family members would score. Applying a pensionable age of 65 years to both sexes, meant that factors 1 and 5 were slightly underestimated for the practice.

Individual codes were assigned to each factor and score so that these could be entered as part of a patient's records on the practice's computer system. Thus, a single parent who was unemployed and living in overcrowded accommodation had three codes recorded, one for each UPA factor, and a further code to indicate an individual score of three. This allowed an 'integrity' check to be made on the data—the sum of the factors being equal to the sum of the scores—and also meant that groups of patients with the same individual UPA score could be identified more easily.

Only when the information about all eight factors was known, was it recorded. Since factors 1, 2 and 5 ('elderly living alone', 'under 5' and 'unemployed') are mutually exclusive of one another, the maximum score a patient could have was six. Factors were derived from answers given on the registration forms for each patient (or in a few cases after follow-up by telephone) and were not updated during the 11-month period. The age of a patient was calculated from his/her date of birth at the time the information was entered on computer—usually within a week of the registration form being completed.

In order to obtain a comparative score from the 1981 census information, a listing of the patients' postcodes was given to a commercial mapping company (Pinpoint Analysis Ltd)

Table 2.2 Transformation procedure and the contribution of each factor to the final practice UPA score

Column	1	2	3	4	5	6	7
Factor %Contrib	%	%/100	Sq Rt	ARCSIN	Stand	Weighted	
	v*100	v	√v	(√v)	Value	Value	to UPA
1. Elderly living alone	3.62	0.0362	0.190	0.191	− 0.749	− 4.958	− 8.21
2. Child under 5	12.55	0.1255	0.354	0.362	3.726	17.287	28.63
3. Single parent	5.05	0.0505	0.225	0.226	2.585	7.782	12.89
4 Unskilled	6.21	0.0621	0.249	0.252	0.797	2.980	4.94
5. Unemployed	9.34	0.0934	0.306	0.310	0.292	0.977	1.62
6. Overcrowded	26.91	0.2691	0.519	0.545	3.885	11.188	18.53
7 Moved house	43.21	0.4321	0.657	0.717	7.238	19.399	32.13
8. Ethnic minority	14.75	0.1475	0.384	0.394	2.288	5.719	9.47

Practice UPA score (sum of weighted, standardised values) = 60.37 100.00%

which linked these to local electoral wards. By knowing the numbers of patients living in each ward, the Jarman score of which is known, an equivalent Jarman score was derived for the practice. This calculation is described in more detail below.

RESULTS

A total of 800 new patients registered at the Health Centre during the 11-month study period and the list size increased from 1210 to 2046. Information relating to all eight UPA factors was collected on 773 of these patients. Data on the remaining 27 patients was incomplete and therefore was not included.

Practice score

A UPA score was calculated following the transformation procedure defined by Jarman (1988) (see Table 2.2). The square root of each factor variable, expressed as a decimal (v), was:

- normalised using an 'ARCSIN' function (column 4)
- standardised using the means and standard deviations of the ward transformed values for England and Wales (column 5)
- weighted using the weightings from the national GP survey (column 6) (Jarman 1983, 1984)

The weighted values were then summed, resulting in a 'practice' UPA score of 60.37. In the case of factor 5, the percentage of patients unemployed (9.34%), was only of those patients who were economically active (n=557).

Score based on census information

The mapping company identified the total patient sample (n=773) as covering a total of 15 electoral wards (Table 2.3). Only in five of these wards was the number of sample patients more than 0.1% of the 1981 population (indicated by an asterisk). The numbers of patients expected to score for each factor were calculated by multiplying the census derived percentages (OPCS 1981) by the number of sample patients in each ward. Thus, in Baker Street ward with a sample population of 265, 28 were expected to score on factor 1 (elderly living alone). Summing those patients expected to score on factor 1 for all 15 wards gives a total of 79.6, or 10. 3% of the sample population (n=773). Applying the same procedure to the remaining factors and transforming these in the manner shown in Table 2.2, it is possible to calculate an expected UPA score. In the case of factor 5, the expected numbers have been calculated on the sample numbers in each ward, rather than those who are economically active, and the assumption made that the ratio of economically active patients to non-

Table 2.3 Numbers of sample patients expected to score for each factor for the 15 electoral wards shown. (Expected factor percentages, v*100%, are given below the two total lines; 1981 census ward populations are shown in brackets)

Electoral ward	#in ward	%ward pop	Expected number with each factor							
			1	2	3	4	5	6	7	8
CAMDEN										
Adelaide (7894)	3	0.04%	0.26	0.12	0.08	0.08	0.28	0.26	0.45	0.27
Bloomsbury (6901)	1	0.01%	0.11	0.03	0.01	0.07	0.08	0.13	0.27	0.15
Chalk Farm (5162)	2	0.04%	0.19	0.09	0.07	0.07	0.33	0.18	0.42	0.15
Regent's Pk (8437)	4	0.05%	0.38	0.17	0.12	0.24	0.42	0.50	0.46	0.47
WESTMINSTER										
* Baker St (4420)	265	6.00%	28.09	6.25	3.90	8.53	16.38	31.99	56.84	20.14
* Bryanston (4634)	87	1.88%	9.37	2.56	1.31	3.78	5.90	7.53	16.62	7.90
* Cavendish (6797)	250	3.68%	24.05	6.35	3.43	5.48	15.80	29.15	54.15	30.93
* Church St (9647)	36	0.37%	3.15	1.93	1.44	4.30	4.79	7.08	3.23	6.13
Hamilton Terr (5328)	13	0.24%	1.88	0.38	0.16	0.15	0.88	0.85	2.12	0.79
Harrow Rd (10 667)	1	0.01%	0.07	0.06	0.05	0.09	0.15	0.24	0.14	0.29
Hyde Park (7173)	1	0.01%	0.08	0.04	0.02	0.01	0.09	0.11	0.26	0.13
Little Venice (8268)	2	0.02%	0.17	0.07	0.06	0.11	0.21	0.28	0.33	0.18
Lords (5727)	6	0.10%	0.87	0.20	0.09	0.18	0.41	0.30	0.80	0.33
* Regent's Pk (8971)	99	1.10%	10.56	2.57	1.36	2.77	5.98	7.18	16.29	6.59
West End (5050)	3	0.06%	0.37	0.09	0.04	0.14	0.22	0.36	0.64	0.32
Total	773	0.74%	79.60	20.94	12.12	26.00	51.91	86.14	153.01	74.76
v*100%			10.30%	2.71%	1.57%	3.36%	6.72%	11.14%	19.79%	9.67%
Total of (*) Wards	737	2.14%	75.23	19.67	11.43	24.87	48.85	82.93	147.13	71.69
v*100%			10.21%	2.67%	1.55%	3.37%	6.63%	11.25%	19.96%	9.73%

economically active patients was uniform across the sample.

If all 15 wards are considered, an expected score of 17.22 is obtained. Taking only those wards in which the sample population exceeds 0.1%, a score of 16.89 results. As might be anticipated, given the way in which they were derived, both these scores are comparable with local ward scores (Table 2.4) but considerably lower than the score of 60.37 derived from the practice data. What differences in the UPA factors can account for the scores being so widely dissimilar?

Practice versus census score

Table 2.4 shows the percentage values for each factor for the five main local wards, as derived from census information, compared to those for the practice (MHC). The value of 3.62 for factor 1 of

the practice makes a negative contribution to the score (see Table 2.2), there being few 'elderly living alone' in comparison to national and local values. In contrast, factors 2, 3, 6 and 7 for the practice ('children under 5', 'single parent', 'overcrowding' and 'moved house'), are not only all very much higher than the surrounding wards but result in large positive contributions being made to the score. Likewise, the ethnicity factor contributes nearly 10% to the final score (see Table 2.2) and is second only in size to that of the Church Street ward.

DISCUSSION

This study shows that it is feasible to calculate a practice UPA score using a patient questionnaire. For the practice studied, the resultant score of 60.37 puts the needs of the practice on a par with those of areas

Table 2.4 The percentage values of the eight UPA factors, derived from 1981 census data, and UPA scores for the five main local wards, compared to practice derived values (MHC)

Electoral ward	% Factors (v*100)								
	1	2	3	4	5	6	7	8	UPA
Baker St	10.60	2.36	1.47	3.22	6.18	12.07	21.45	7.60	16.06
Bryanston	10.77	2.94	1.51	4.35	6.78	8.66	19.10	9.08	18.18
Cavendish	9.62	2.54	1.37	2.19	6.32	11.66	21.66	12.37	14.61
Church St	8.76	5.37	4.00	11.95	13.31	19.67	8.98	17.02	40.51
Regent's Pk (West)	10.67	2.60	1.37	2.80	6.04	7.25	16.45	6.66	10.01
MHC	3.62	12.55	5.05	6.21	9.34	26.91	43.21	14.75	60.37

such as Moss Side in Manchester (60.83) and St Mary's in Tower Hamlets (61.01) (Jarman 1988). In contrast, the local census derived ward scores are, with one exception, all under 20. The difference between these scores, it is proposed, results primarily from the characteristics of the practice population being studied and, only to a lesser extent, from the methodology which was used.

First, only new patients were included and this group would be expected to have different socio-demographic factors to those of established patients, most notably a greater likelihood to have moved recently. Indeed, as shown in Table 2.2, the mobility factor makes the largest contribution of any of the factors to the overall score. Recalculating the score using a mobility factor derived from census data (v=0.20), the practice score is reduced to 48.27 from 60.37 but nonetheless remains high. However, the fact that the sample group by the end of the study represented nearly 40% of the practice population would suggest that, apart from the mobility factor, the remaining factors were representative of the practice as a whole.

Established practices wishing to use the same method to calculate their own scores could randomly sample one in 10 of already registered patients and so would be able to minimise the effect from this variable.

Secondly, the practice had an 'open door' policy towards all local residents which is likely to have attracted a disproportionate number of disadvantaged people, compared to other established practices which may be more selective about

whom they register. Indeed 9% of all people joining the practice in the year following the study were registered as homeless and 25% were from ethnic minorities. The effect of this policy is reflected in the values of individual UPA factors (factors 2, 3, 6 and 8) being very much higher than those of the local ward scores (Table 2.4).

Although the nature of the practice is sufficient to explain the difference, it could be argued that the practice score is exaggerated for other reasons, such as the redefinition of the factors, or the method of its calculation from those factors. However, the latter is identical to that for calculating the local ward scores, and the redefinitions have resulted in an underestimate rather than overestimate of the practice score, as explained earlier. Also the fact that there was little change in the socio-demographic characteristics of London between the 1971 and 1981 censuses, suggests that changes in local population since 1981 are unlikely to have had much effect (Jarman 1983, 1988).

There are thus a number of good reasons to support the contention that a practice score calculated in this way does reflect practice workload. Its usefulness for a practice is that it provides data which can be used:

- to argue for more appropriate resources
- for consideration as to why such differences exist
- as a basis for planning.

For instance, the realisation that a disproportionate number of the practice population are from ethnic minorities might suggest the need for specialised services such as an interpreter and would provide an argument for extra funding.

An alternative method for calculating a practice score was put forward in 1987 by Hutchinson (Hutchinson et al 1987) who linked a practice population through its postcodes to the UPA scores of the local enumeration districts (EDs). However, as he pointed out, the correlation between postcodes and EDs is poor, with up to 50% inaccuracy. The Government has since decided not to calculate the UPA score on an ED basis (Information Management Group 1990).

This is the first study to use current information elicited direct from the patients, and highlights the sense of many general practitioners that the workload varies from practice to practice within the same area. As such, it provides general practitioners with a method to quantify such workload as well as the means by which to make realistic comparisons.

Further studies, employing the same methodology on other practices, would determine whether the discrepancy between the practice and census-derived UPA scores, as found in this study, is typical. If found to be the case, then where the discrepancies are large, such results could well be used by practices as a basis on which to renegotiate their deprivation payments.

ACKNOWLEDGEMENTS

The authors acknowledge Crown copyright in the use of 1981 census data provided through the Department of General Practice, St Mary's Hospital Medical School. They also gratefully acknowledge the helpful advice of and discussions with Professor Brian Jarman, Madhavi Bajekal and Pat White.

REFERENCES

Charlton J R H, Lakhani A 1985 Is the Jarman underprivileged area score valid? British Medical Journal 290 pp 1714–1716

Curtis S E 1990 Use of survey data and small area statistics to assess individual morbidity and neighbourhood deprivation. Journal of Epidemiological Community Health 44 pp 62–68

Department of Health and the Welsh Office 1989 General practice in the National Health Service. A new contract. 28

Foy C, Hutchinson A, Smyth J 1987 Providing census data for general practice. 2. Usefulness. Journal of the Royal College of General Practitioners 37 pp 451–454

Hutchinson A, Foy C, Smyth J 1987 Providing census data for general practice. 1. Feasibility. Journal of the Royal College of General Practitioners 37 pp 448–450

Information Management Group 1990 NHS review. Working for patients, framework for information systems. London Department of Health annex 12

Irving D, Rice P 1984 Information for health services planning from 1981 census 84/11. London, King's Fund

Jarman B 1983 Identification of underprivileged areas. British Medical Journal 286 pp 1705–1709

Jarman B 1984 Underprivileged areas: validation and distribution of scores. British Medical Journal 290 pp 1714–1716

Jarman B 1988 Primary care. London, Heinemann pp 101–106

Office of Population Censuses and Surveys 1981 Census 1981 definitions. London, HMSO

Office of Population Censuses and Surveys 1983 Small area statistics, 1981 census. London OPCS

THE IMPACT OF A VOLUNTEER COMMUNITY CARE PROJECT IN A PRIMARY HEALTH CARE SETTING

Vivien Webber
Veronica Barry
Peter Davies
Patrick Pietroni

This is a descriptive account of the setting up of a community care programme, based on patient participation, in an inner city health centre in central London. Using a questionnaire to establish patients' needs and interests, an outreach programme, a befriending scheme and a variety of patient group activities have been developed. These are now integral to the work of the Health Centre.

INTRODUCTION

The Marylebone Health Centre, a National Health Service primary health care practice opened in 1987, emphasises a multidisciplinary approach to patient care and to doctor–patient relationships. In addition to a core team of three general practitioners (GPs) and district nursing and health visiting staff, it provides educational activities, counselling, complementary therapies (acupuncture, massage, homoeopathy, and osteopathy) and a community care programme. These extra services have been supported by funding from the Wates Foundation, which has also funded research projects exploring new ways of delivering primary health care to an inner city population (Pietroni 1991).

This paper describes the development of the community care programme, including some of the problems which were encountered and the lesssons learnt. It reflects the various contributions made by staff and patients arising out of on-going discussions and the comments on earlier drafts. A principal aim of the project was to explore the possible impact that patient participation activities might have in reducing social isolation and enhancing patient's physical and psychological well-being.

BACKGROUND

The Marylebone Health Centre is based in the recently converted crypt of Marylebone Church alongside a Pastoral Centre and Music Therapy unit. The crypt has restaurant facilities and an activities hall. It is located in central London in the north east corner of Westminster, an area characterised by extremes of wealth and poverty.

The total patient population of 3800 is highly mobile. This is partly a result of the relatively large number of single people registered with the practice, but the many bed and breakfast hotels within the catchment area are also used by London boroughs as temporary housing for homeless people. Nearly 25% of people registered with the practice are from ethnic minority groups, many of whom live in this hotel accommodation. They are a cosmopolitan group comprising Asian, African, Bangladeshi, Chinese, Turkish and others.

Social support/health care research

It has long been held that social bonds and supportive interaction are important to a person's physical and psychological health. Researchers define and measure social support in different ways. Some use the concepts of social network, psychosocial assets, and perceived social support interchangeably, while others attempt a more precise definition. Mitchell (1969) describes a social network as the set of relationships of a particular individual. Schaefer (Schaefer et al 1981, Bloom 1990) distinguishes between social network and perceived social support, the latter focusing on the person's own evaluation of the nature of the interactions within a social relationship. These interactions include feeling loved, cared for, esteemed, valued and that one belongs to a network of mutual obligation.

Reprinted with permission from the Journal of Social Work Practice: 5(1) pp. 83–90 1991, published by Carfax Publishing Company, PO Box 25, Abingdon, Oxfordshire OX14 3UE.

Schaefer also distinguishes between informational (advice/problem-solving), tangible (direct aid or service), and emotional support, and that all are important in determining health and well-being. Turner (1981) suggests that social support may act as a buffer against life stress rather than directly contributing to physical and psychological outcomes. House et al argue that social support is important in its own right, that it is most important in stressful circumstances, and that it varies across class groupings (House et al 1988). Clearly, there is scope for further research to clarify the causal processes through which support influences health outcomes (Bloom 1990).

In the planning stages of the project, the experiences of other patient participation groups (De Maeseneer & Debunne 1986) and neighbourhood care schemes were reviewed.

Patient participation programmes

The idea of a community care programme corresponds with the view that an integrated approach to primary health care should include participation of local residents and should not just be restricted to one-to-one doctor–patient interactions. Indeed, the National Association for Patient Participation (NAPP) was established upon this premise (RCGP 1981, Pritchard 1983, Hutton & Robins 1985, Richardson & Bray 1987). The history of the patient participation movement is one of success and frustration, but despite the struggles the nationwide expansion of such groups is an acknowledgement of their potential worth (Richardson & Bray 1987). The basic model of such groups is:

1. To act as a planning tool by providing the practice staff with feedback about policy-related matters.
2. To provide education and discussion on health-related topics of interest.
3. To extend patient involvement and to act as a support for the practice by organising voluntary care in the community (RCGP 1981).

Neighbourhood care schemes

Many neighbourhood care schemes have been established in recent years. Such schemes set up a variety of volunteer programmes and networks based on local needs and resources in different settings. These schemes have wrestled with the terms 'community' and 'volunteer' (Sheard 1986, Hatch & Hinton 1986). Opinions differ, but the literature concedes that the term 'community' has a 'broad usage that deprives it of exact meaning but conveys togetherness with people and indicates a widespread unease at the disjunction between the formal organised world of service providers and the informal world of service recipients' (Hatch & Hinton 1986). Such a view presupposes a latent community of interest. Similarly, the term 'volunteer' implies a degree of formal organisation and the presence of a formal channel through which potential volunteers are linked to someone in need of care. Schemes must provide for reciprocity: those who help must get something out of the scheme and those who receive must have something to give in return.

The literature also identifies financial resources, staff structures and geographical catchment areas as organisational issues for consideration. A permanent coordinator must be employed (Abrams et al 1986). This is important because creating and sustaining mutual support structures consumes energy and needs to adapt to changing circumstances.

THE MARYLEBONE COMMUNITY OUTREACH PROGRAMME

The approach that the Marylebone Health Centre took to the community outreach programme—and indeed to the project overall—was based partly on that of other neighbourhood and patient participation groups and was partly influenced by local needs as highlighted by the results of a patient questionnaire.

It was acknowledged that there would always be vulnerable users. For example, the elderly aged over 75 would probably need direct provision of care without the possibility of reciprocating in any way; likewise for some young parents. The homeless/hotel residents were regarded as a similar group in that their needs were often greater than their ability to give and, furthermore, they were dispersed and isolated, living on the margins of the community around them.

The more concentrated attention that such groups require, and the knowledge that they often make little use of traditional models of health care, resulted in the development of the community outreach component of the project. A community service volunteer and social work students on placement in the Health Centre participated in home visits with a view to introducing vulnerable people to crypt-based activities, to befriending volunteers, or to other organisations, as appropriate. It was also hoped that by developing a community outreach component, the traditional volunteer/client divide characterised by office-based schemes would be alleviated to some extent (Hedley 1984).

The practice has close links with other health agencies, voluntary bodies and local social services. The emphasis has been to work in partnership with such agencies and to complement rather than overlap with their different functions.

Patient questionnaire

The project began by assessing patients' health and social needs and resources using a questionnaire devised at the Health Centre. The responses to the questionnaire formed the framework for the different activities of the project. The questionnaire was initially piloted amongst a sample of users attending the surgery, then revised to include a prompt list of tasks. These ranged from befriending to practical activities such as reading, letter writing and decorating. Users were asked to indicate which activities they were interested in helping with, and which they wished to benefit from. An additional prompt list was included with the aim of gauging volunteer interest in such activities as education, an ideas/policy group, a practice newsletter, self-help groups and social events. Patients were requested to indicate the time they could commit to such a scheme, as well as the regularity with

which they might need support. This questionnaire was initially mailed to the 600 users who had joined the practice when the project started. It was subsequently offered to patients to complete as they registered. Details of each completed questionnaire were entered and collated on a computer in the Health Centre and patients who expressed an interest in offering or receiving regular help were sent volunteer application forms and referral forms respectively. On the form they were encouraged to give as much or as little time as they wished. It was thought that the volunteers' commitment to the project would be better guaranteed if they completed an application form which also requested two references.

Running simultaneously with the distribution and collation of the questionnaires, the community service volunteer and social work students began home visits to vulnerable users, with a view to linking them with volunteers or other appropriate resources.

The initial questionnaire, mailed to 600 patients, only produced a return of 25%. Subsequently, patients were encouraged to complete the questionnaire on registration. Findings from both sets of responses (n=479) showed most interest in the Health Centre's educational activities (47%) with less interest for the volun-

Table 2.5 Percentage of patients completing the questionnaire (n=479), who offered help or needed help for the tasks listed

	% offering help	% requesting help
Listening/befriending	31.52	8.98
Shopping/errands	14.61	3.76
Legal advice	0.84	7.93
Transporting in car	5.64	2.51
Housing advice	1.04	6.05
Babysitting	7.72	4.95
Job/career advice	5.43	5.85
Childminding	6.26	4.38
Social security advice	0.46	3.97
Sitting with frail adults	8.56	1.04
Language interpreting	8.98	2.71
Decorating	5.43	3.13
Literacy	10.86	0.63
Letter writing	20.46	3.34

tary mutual support scheme (23%). Of the activities based at the Health Centre, people responded most positively to the opportunity to assist with self-help groups and social events.

Those offering help did so mainly in the areas of befriending, letter writing, shopping and literacy (see Table 2.5). A notable feature of the initial responses to the questionnaire was that the take-up of offers of help did not match initial expressed needs despite the use of concerted efforts and various means to advertise the project.

The most common requests for help came for specific tasks such as befriending, legal advice, job advice, social security advice, childminding and babysitting.

There was an inevitable shortfall between those who expressed an initial interest and those who completed application forms, but within a year of starting the project, 32 volunteers had committed themselves to an activity suggested on the questionnaire. A profile of the volunteer group reflected a primarily female interest and involvement and most were in the middle-aged or retirement groups. The majority were British with a sprinkling of white Europeans and other ethnic groupings.

On average, the volunteers were prepared to offer one or two hours each week and most volunteers expressed an interest in undertaking more than one activity. A roughly equal number expressed an interest in befriending as in some of the practically-oriented aspects of the scheme, particularly reading to people and teaching writing and literacy skills. A committee comprising staff and patients was formed to provide ideas for educational activities, fundraising, improvement of service delivery and social support activities.

One unexpected and encouraging result of the project was that people who had been referred by the GPs because they needed help had, on occasions, met that need through becoming a volunteer. In one or two cases, they subsequently became volunteers following a period of counselling or practical support from the social worker or social work student.

The befriending scheme

A sustained interest in the befriending aspect of the scheme, both on the part of 'givers' and 'receivers', gradually emerged. As a result of the interest expressed through the community outreach programme and GPs' surgery consultations and counselling assessments, befrienders are now matched with isolated patients in need of company and emotional support. Sometimes, practical problems arise to which the befriender also responds. The matching process takes into account the amount of free time that a befriender has, as well as personality and experience.

Group supervision for the befrienders is provided on a monthly basis. This has provided containment and support, supervision on individual patients and an opportunity for befrienders to learn some counselling skills. As they have gained more confidence in their role and more trust in each other, so they have begun to assert their needs more openly, in particular their need to discuss their patient contact directly with the GPs. They have also shown increasing honesty about the difficulties of working with individual patients, recognising that feelings stirred up in the group often reflect the feelings between themselves and their patients.

Health Centre-based activities

One of the first activities undertaken by volunteers, with some input from the coordinator, was the production of a newsletter. This is distributed to each household on a quarterly basis. Volunteers have also established groups in the crypt centre. A parents' self-help creche consisting of nine core members started as a result of a social work student's visits to young parents. Practical difficulties associated with running the group on a self-help basis have meant that it is now coordinated by an older volunteer. An over-50s 'movement to music' group was also started by another volunteer with dance teaching experience. More recently, a reminiscence group has been started by another social work student on placement. Volunteers have also supported a music-making and listening group organised jointly by the Pastoral Centre and Music Therapy Units, and with crypt social functions. Latterly, they have also been involved in fundraising activities as well as providing some of the necessary clerical and administrative support to manage and expand the community care programme. As a result of these activities, spontaneous friendships have arisen between volunteers who now meet outside the Health Centre.

DISCUSSION

Although the relationship between social support and physical and psychological health has not been adequately researched (Bloom 1990), after 3 years of development work, the Health Centre now has a community care framework that encourages participation and a sense of feeling supported, and fosters social ties and interaction amongst its patient population.

From its start it was considered important that the framework could be reproduced in a similar form in other NHS primary health care settings. Unlike many other schemes, this project has the advantage of a clearly defined catchment area and a clearly defined group of users. The practice was also new and had a comparatively low number of registrations at the time of opening. However, other practices could focus on a core group of registered users and start a similar project by offering a questionnaire to draw in new people as interests arise.

As the project has evolved, a variety of organisational and clinical issues and dilemmas emerged for discussion amongst the staff multidisciplinary team. These issues emphasised the need for adaptability on the part of both staff and volunteers if the scheme was to survive and grow. The areas of concern are as follows:

- funding
- confidentiality
- professional/personal boundaries
- trust and mistrust
- homelessness.

Each of these concerns is now dealt with in turn.

Funding

The model cost comparatively little, having relied on one paid worker with some administrative support. The costs of the community service volunteer were offset by income from the social work student-placing agency, and the practice newsletter costs were partially met by local advertising. Clearly, to run a scheme on this level of funding creates pressure. As the project has developed, so has the practice's dependence on volunteers' fundraising activities.

The problem of being bound by limited finances conflicted at times with the need for continuity. For instance, community service volunteers, whose costs were low, did not necessarily want to commit themselves for long periods of time. Social work placements inevitably came to an end. This meant that community outreach visits lost momentum as volunteers were replaced and new workers spent time familiarising themselves with local resources and with organisational aspects of the project.

Confidentiality

The staff sometimes expressed unease that the befrienders' support group shared personal information about other patients with each other. This is a problem with no easy solution. An attempt was made as far as possible to respect boundaries of confidentiality by eliminating mention of names. Befrienders were also required to inform and gain permission from the person befriended before discussing him or her in a group context. Such procedures acknowledged that the befrienders worked in good faith and helped to meet some of the understandable concerns of GPs and other staff. In addition, neither befrienders nor volunteers acting in a clerical capacity in the Health Centre had access to clinical notes. The use of a community service volunteer to cover outreach overcame this problem.

Professional/personal boundaries

Boundaries were a particular issue for the staff, who were exploring staff/patient relationships in other areas of work. How should they, for instance, respond to volunteers who wanted to discuss their treatment outside surgery hours? While the staff valued the notion of reciprocity and wanted to convey a sense of real appreciation for volunteer help, this was a problem that sometimes arose. However, for the most part, volunteers did not have such expectations and felt their needs were met by a sense of belonging and involvement in purposeful activity. Indeed, here was an example of reciprocity since some volunteered as a means of conveying personal gratitude for the service they received. The Health Centre came to recognise the need for reciprocity by offering priority access to educational courses. This avoided tension in the more sensitive clinical area.

Trust and mistrust

An unexpected problem was the low number of people who, having completed the questionnaires, actually came forward to ask for help, even after a further follow-up letter had been sent out. This is also the experience of some other neighbourhood care schemes. Studies indicate that most requests for help come via a third person referral and that help is limited to once-only requests (Abrams et al 1981). These studies indicate a reluctance on the part of individuals to ask for help out of a sense of pride and independence. In addition, in a geographically mobile area people may need, first of all, to lay down their roots. Perhaps, too, a community care scheme has itself to become rooted before people can trust it sufficiently to come forward, as either givers or receivers. Indeed, experience of the project suggested that personal contact was a key feature to its growth. Volunteers often needed encouragement to take responsibility. Personal contact with the coordinator and other members of staff helped them to gain trust and confidence in increasing their commitment to the scheme.

Trust in the project was also an issue for some members of staff. In the early stages, staff had differing and incomplete understandings of the nature and purpose of patient empowerment. This possibly resulted in limited involvement

and the lack of much needed impetus. Patients also commented on the lack of publicity for the scheme. Fortunately, some early successes with the project and further discussion saw these problems resolved.

Homelessness

The outreach visits highlighted the fact that the terms 'reciprocity' and 'community' are inappropriate when looking at the needs of people living in bed and breakfast accommodation. The community service volunteer found a group for whom housing and finance were top priorities over and above health. The stresses of a bed and breakfast lifestyle often lead to isolation, to an unwillingness to view the situation as more than temporary and to depression. Within the homeless group, ethnic minorities and women seemed particularly isolated. The homeless were therefore an essentially needy group unable to commit themselves to anything. In addition, largely as a result of the temporary nature of their residence, any attempts at building relationships or finding any sense of continuity were often frustrated. Once again, trust was an issue when considering the success or otherwise of the outreach visits. Clearly, the face-to-face contact helped to break down some mistrust, but nonetheless this marginal group understandably tended to keep themselves to themselves.

These conditions inevitably raise the question of whether a Health Centre can do more than provide people, on arrival, with a list of useful contacts in the new area and direct them on to groups more equipped to deal with their needs. Or would that once again lead to 'disintegration' and further exclusion of an already marginal group? Without doubt, a flexible approach is essential when working with this group.

Consideration must also be given to the possibility that the Health Centre was over-ambitious in attempting to set up an outreach programme and a core volunteer group at the same time. This inevitably meant that an expressed need could not always be matched with appropriate volunteer help.

CONCLUSION

The community care project at Marylebone coincides with the current political and professional climate which places increased emphasis on the neighbourhood as a key unit for service management and delivery (Kivell et al 1990). A primary health care practice is not only strategically located but is also a gateway for a local population in a way that social services and most voluntary organisations are not.

The model described is one which combines elements of service with elements of network, one which is concerned to respond to the needs of its patient community and one which adopts the ideas of participation, reciprocity, empowerment, relationship and a sense of belonging as important components of social and psychological health.

Clearly, a number of problems were encountered in setting up the project. However, the firm roots of its structures, for instance, the befriending and other group activities, in combination with the influences just described has resulted in a decision to give it a more central role. In order to integrate the community care programme and to focus more concentrated attention on the most vulnerable groups, money has been diverted from some of the clinical and educational activities to the employment of a permanent outreach worker, as well as a coordinator. Using the lessons learnt so far, it is hoped that efforts will continue to be made to link patients in mutual interest and support.

ACKNOWLEDGEMENTS

The authors acknowledge the help of Rodney Hedley of the London School of Economics for his helpful comments on the patient questionnaire and on the overall development of the project. The authors also acknowledge the valuable contribution made by the patients.

REFERENCES

Abrams P, Abrams S, Humphrey R, Snaith R 1981 Action for care. Volunteer Centre, Berkhamstead

Abrams P, Abrams S, Humphrey R, Snaith R 1986 Creating care in the neighbourhood. Advance, London

Bloom J R 1990 The relationship of social support and health. Social Science and Medicine 30: 5 pp 635–637

De Maeseneer J, Debunne M 1986 Community participation, patient participation groups. Paper given to the World Organization of National Colleges

Hatch S, Hinton T 1986 Self-help in practice community care. Joint Unit for Social Services Research, University of Sheffield

Hedley R 1984 Neighbourhood care in practice. London Voluntary Service Council, London

House J S, Lands K R, Umberson D 1988 Social relationships and health. Science 241 pp 540–545

Hutton A, Robins S 1985 What the patient wants from patient participation. Journal of the Royal College of General Practitioners 35 pp 133–135

Kivell P T, Turton B J, Dawson B R P 1990 Neighbourhoods for health service administration. Social Science and Medicine 30 pp 701–711

Mitchell J C 1969 Social networks in urban situations. Manchester University Press, Manchester

Pietroni P C 1991 Wates Foundation primary health care research project—final report. Marylebone Centre Trust

Pritchard P 1983 Patient participation in general practice. In: Perira G D (ed) Medical Annual. Bristol, Wright pp 227–238

Richardson A, Bray C 1987 Promoting health through participation. London, Policy Studies Institute

Royal College of General Practitioners 1981 Occasional Paper no 17. London, Royal College of General Practitioners

Schaefer C, Coyne J C, Lazarus R S 1981 The health related functions of social support. Journal of Behavioural Medicine 4 pp 381–401

Sheard J 1986 The politics of volunteering. London, Advance

Turner R J 1981 Social support as a contingency in psychological wellbeing. Journal of Health and Social Behaviour 22 pp 357–367

THE RELATIONSHIP BETWEEN PASTORAL CARE AND PRIMARY HEALTH CARE

Patrick Pietroni

INTRODUCTION

Primary health care has grown out of General Practice which itself grew out of hospital medicine. The foundation stone to these disciplines that operate in the community or, as Vickers (1967) put it, 'the world of the well', has been the medical model with its emphasis on identifying pathological cause with symptoms presented by individuals who seek help from doctors. It is increasingly fashionable to be critical of what is now perceived to be an unacceptable model for responding to the needs in the community. Increasingly, the term 'primary health care' is being supplanted by the term 'primary health and social care' (PHSC), and we may soon accept conceptually if not organisationally that even PHSC is itself a sub-section of community care. Most general practitioners will accept that whether or not their training was based on the hospital concept of disease, the reality of their practice is that they are presented daily with problems that do not have 'pathological causes' and that cannot be fitted with neat diagnostic labels. Crombie, in his study, found that in over 300 consecutive consultations, a specific medical diagnosis was arrived at in only 150 and that treatment was commenced even though the problem(s) presented would not fit any of the classical medical diagnoses (Crombie 1963). TATT (tired all the time) or ACOPIA (failure to cope) are not topics to be found in any undergraduate medical curriculum, and are difficult to find in vocational training schemes, but they are the

Reprinted with permission from the Primary Care Management: 4(4) pp. 3–5 April 1994, published by Churchill Livingstone.

stuff of General Practice. The trainee, who on entering General Practice said 'Take my prescription pad and referral letter away from me and what else have I been taught?' may well be tempted, like another trainee, to ask for his money back from the medical school and vocational training scheme that had so let him down.

PASTORAL CARE

Is the missing ingredient pastoral care? If it is, what is it? John Berger's *A Fortunate Man* (Berger & Mohr 1967) or David Widgery's *Some lives: the GPs East End* (Widgery 1991) demonstrate that pastoral care has always been part of General Practice both in rural settings and in the deprived inner cities, but can it survive? Is one of the penalties of the purchaser–provider split the loss of altruism on which it would appear this aspect of care is based? What is the unit cost of compassion? How can we evaluate its effectiveness? More importantly, can it be incorporated in the curriculum and does it rely on doctors or can it be more effectively delivered by other members of the primary health care team? Some would say pastoral care is alive and well and being delivered by the 'secret heroines and heroes' of the Health Service, as Virginia Bottomley put it. These are the 6 000 000 or so carers who provide daily, nightly, weekly and monthly care for their elderly infirm, handicapped husbands/wives/mothers/fathers, who do so with rarely a break or holiday, who do so unpaid, and who do so largely unrecognised even by their general practitioners. If pastoral care is part of primary health care, it may be that all that is required is the recognition of this large 'voluntary' workforce and its recruitment as part of our expanded primary health care team. Before doing so, let us explore in some greater detail what we mean by pastoral care. Is it the same as spiritual care? Is it less or is it more? Some years ago, I compared the work of pastors (priests, rabbis, imams) with that of a general practitioner and identified what I then thought were examples of pastoral care that occurred in General Practice (Table 2.6).

The term 'pastoral care' appears preferable to that of 'spiritual practice' but it carries an

Table 2.6 The role of priest and the role of general practitioner

Spiritual practice	General practice counterpart
1. Providing a sanctuary	Consulting room as a 'safe space'
2. Confessional	Active listening
3. Interpret tribulation	Give meaning to stressful life events
4. Source of ritual and ceremony	Repeat prescription
5. Provide support and comfort	Teamwork
6. Increase spiritual awareness	Give permission for spiritual discussion
7. Laying on of hands Prayer and meditation	Use of touch Relaxation and quiet time
8. Communion	Self-help groups/patient participation

element of paternalism that has become almost politically incorrect. Balint (1957), one of the great influences on British General Practice, termed this the 'apostolic function'—the idea that somehow the doctor knows what's best for the patient and sets about telling him so. This interpretation of pastoral care, with all its moral overtones, has become unacceptable as a method of interchange, although I am sure it still forms part of many consultations. The recent introduction of the computer has enabled us to classify our patients by age, sex and occupation—the traditional social parameters. These are no doubt useful for much of the clinical work that is undertaken in primary health care, but it leaves out probably the most important factor that determines health-seeking behaviour, to use the sociological term, and that is health-belief, or more importantly, health-need. Needs assessment certainly forms part of the new Community Care Act and is the basis for many health surveys that are undertaken to help plan the allocation of resources. In the consulting room, these methods may be of little help in addressing the needs of the individual patient and I have found a modification of Maslow's (1987) hierarchy of need of more immediate value. It has helped me to think of the patients I see in one of the following three groups, all having different expectations and needs.

Survivors

These are patients who are barely 'surviving', hanging on to daily and nightly life by their finger-tips, not only in a physical way but in a psychological/social and spiritual way. They are overburdened with housing, family, financial problems. They may be from an ethnic minority and suffering prejudice and discrimination. They are our elderly, single patients living on the third floor of a tenement building, isolated and living a social death whilst waiting for their physical death.

Conspicuous consumers

This is probably the largest group of patients who see and use the health centre as a modified supermarket store. They want easy access, long opening hours, courteous attention and a wide range of products on sale. They would like information so as to get the 'best buy', and often, like supermarkets, fashion plays a large part in their needs/demands—annual cholesterol check, osteopathy for back problems, repeat prescriptions within 24 hours, annual 'flu jabs, and so on.

Self-actualisers

This is a small 10–15% of the practice population and may depend on the geographical area, but seems not to be related to social class structure. This group's need is for 'meaning' and relationship. Individuals wish to be more involved in their health/spiritual care and search for explanations that will allow them to be empowered and fulfilled. They are willing to talk about dying and accept a level of uncertainty and ignorance from their doctors.

Interchangeability

It is also true that patients are not necessarily 'stuck' in one of these groupings and often it is important to recognise that someone in group 3 may want to be treated as someone in group 1. Although pastoral care in its widest sense can be a model for working with all three groups, it is probably with the first group that the primary health care team, in a truly non-denominational and secular way, can begin to have an impact and has traditionally had a part to play as evidenced by the descriptions in the two books quoted earlier (Berger & Mohr 1967, Widgery 1991). Paradoxically, the computer—that most impersonal and high-tech instrument that has invaded all of General Practice—has now made it possible to plan and monitor pastoral care much more effectively.

ANTICIPATORY/PROACTIVE CARE

The emphasis on preventive care and health promotion, although clearly important, seemed to focus on identifiable disease and secondary prevention through the closer monitoring of chronic disease (hypertension/asthma). The focus on facts and figures required to demonstrate the effectiveness of this approach inhibited the awareness that General Practice was facing a major conceptual challenge. Traditionally and almost universally, General Practice has been a reactive-based model of medical care, i.e. patients initiate transactions and doctors respond. One of the features most prized by patients is the open access policy that allows them to determine when and where they seek a medical opinion. Tudor-Hart's research, amongst others, has demonstrated how much medical pathology is missed and his emphasis on the 'measurement of omission' and the 'rule of halves' (half the people with high blood pressure are not detected, half those detected are not treated and half those treated are not controlled) has highlighted the need to balance our reactive mode of care with a proactive one (Tudor-Hart 1988). This is a major sea-change for many GPs, for they are having to acknowledge and accept that not only should they provide individual care to their individual patients but they need to operate as mini community physicians (? pastoral care) to their population of 1700, or 10 000 if in bigger practices. This major attitudinal change is as yet not apparent and very few vocational training schemes have addressed the curricular changes required to ensure GPs are prepared for this task. The tools may be in place—age/sex registers, disease registers, percentage uptake of immunisations or cervical smears, audit cycles and audit protocols—but the realisation of what the shift from reactive to proactive care implies is as yet unclear. The two major implications are the need for Primary Health Care Centres to form closer liaison with community teams (HV, DN, CPN, care managers) and the need for anticipatory proactive care to embrace the notion of pastoral care. Thus it should be possible to ensure that each practice develops its own practice-based Jarman score (underprivileged area) (Chase & Davies 1991) Certainly this could be made a requirement for those practices in receipt of the extra allowance. Identifying the elderly, isolated patients, the homeless, the single parents, the vulnerable chronic sick and the unemployed, will allow the practice to address the social, psychological and pastoral needs of these vulnerable groups who probably fall into group 1 (survivors). Such pilot studies have been undertaken and all their reports are encouraging and helpful (Webber et al 1991). The factors that encourage success in such 'pastoral' or 'community care' schemes include:

1. the willingness of the practice to broaden its definitions of health care—not in name only
2. the expansion of the primary health care team to include colleagues from social care and the development of a teamwork ethos which does not privilege one form of care over another (i.e. body [physical/mind/psychological], soul [spiritual], environmental [social])
3. the designation of proactive care through outreach as being integral to the task of community care
4 the recruitment and active involvement of volunteers from the practice population
5. the encouragement and empowerment of all those active individuals to participate in the practice itself
6. the recognition of the unsung heroines and heroes present in each practice that have undertaken this form of care without support.

CONCLUSION

Of all the experiments undertaken at the Marylebone Health Centre, the one described above has been the most difficult, has taken the longest to demonstrate results but will probably turn out to be the most important for General Practice and Community Care—far more important than the introduction of alternative medicine for which our Centre has become known. We now have in place a series of programmes mostly run by patients but coordinated by an outreach worker (see Box 2.1).

The practice has also benefited in that we have a group of 12 or so active volunteers who help with clerical work (stuff envelopes, make up blank charts, transport specimens to the laboratory) and an active specialised group which helps with our informal complaints procedure.

None of these activities need interfere with the individual pastoral care that occurs 'when in the intimacy of the consulting room one human being in distress confides in another human being whom he trusts'. This 'individual package' of health care practice will always remain at the core of British General Practice—but times change and so must we.

REFERENCES

Balint M 1957 The doctor, his patient and the illness. Churchill Livingstone, London
Berger J, Mohr J 1967 A fortunate man: the story of a country doctor. Allen Lane, London
Chase D C, Davies P 1991 Calculation of a practice underprivileged area (UPA) score. British Journal of General Practice 41 pp 63–66
Crombie D L 1963 Diagnostic process. Journal of the Royal College of General Practitioners 6 pp 579–589
Maslow A H 1987 Motivation and personality, 3rd edn. Harper & Row, New York
Pietroni P C 1986 Spiritual interventions in a general practice setting. Holistic Medicine 1 pp 253–262
Tudor-Hart J 1988 A new kind of doctor. Merlin
Vickers G 1967 Community medicine. Lancet 29 April pp 944–949
Webber V, Barry V, Davies P, Pietroni P C 1991 The impact of a volunteer community care project in a primary health care setting. Journal of Social Work Practice 5 pp 83–90
Widgery D 1991 Some lives: the GPs East End. Sinclair–Stevenson, London

---

Box 2.1 Community care programmes at the Marylebone Health Centre

1. Transport service for patients and their relatives
2. Decorating and minor repair services
3. Befriending (sitting with elderly patients)
4. Telephone contact—once a month for all the over 75s.
5. Single parents club
6. Newsletter three times per year
7. Language interpreter service
8. Homeless accommodation service (we have a large population of refugee patients)
9. Crisis listening service (drop-in)
10. Swimming club
11. Movement to music
12. Choir singing
13. Elderly–toddler afternoons
14. Yoga classes
15. Reminiscence group

DISABILITIES ISSUES IN THE PROVISION OF HEALTH CARE: AN INITIAL INVESTIGATION

Christopher Pietroni
Patrick Pietroni

Access to the built environment is an issue close to the heart of anybody with mobility problems. It circumscribes the ways in which lives are lived and the degree to which people may be independent individuals. This is true of the health care environment no less than any other. Recent changes in the structure of health provision have allowed the issue of access to be placed high on the agenda as never before and yet there is still a lack of understanding and knowledge about disabilities issues within the health care professions. This is a situation that needs addressing urgently.

This document is an attempt to begin that process. It is not an authoritative piece of research into all or even many of the issues raised when considering access and the National Health Service. Rather it is a starting point. The aim has been to identify and explain some of the issues of relevance to the discussion of this field and to demonstrate, with empirical data where possible, what the genuine problems are. A few tentative suggestions are given as to the possible ways forward, but few conclusions are drawn. Research in this area is still very scanty—especially if compared with the USA—and much more study is needed before any firm decisions can be made.

DOES ACCESS MATTER?

It is far from self-evident that access to health care facilities for disabled people should be a matter of much concern to the planners of health services. Hospitals, after all, tend to have good access by their very nature and the domiciliary visit is a convenient way of reaching those who are not able to get themselves to primary health care facilities. It might seem, therefore, that disabled access is an expensive luxury that cannot be afforded. In reality, for medical, social and monetary reasons, it is in the best interests of both the individual patient/client and the providers of health care services to improve access to the NHS.

That access to primary health care facilities is poor can scarcely be denied. One study, carried out in Liverpool, suggests that one-quarter of all GP practices are entirely inaccessible to those using wheelchairs and a further quarter have only partial access (Ratoff et al 1992). Perhaps more worryingly, the study also indicated that even in a number of practices where adaptations had been made to improve access, provision remained poor. In conclusion the authors wrote that 'access to the disabled client group is disgracefully low'. There is no reason to suggest that the situation elsewhere in the country is significantly better although there has not been sufficient research to be sure of the exact level of provision nationwide.

This situation becomes a medical concern when it is taken in conjunction with other findings. In a survey conducted during 1990/91, North West Thames Regional Health Authority reported that the general health of people with a disability was consistently poorer than the rest of the population, a finding that came as little surprise to those in disabilities organisations. Other studies suggest that one contributing factor may be the inadequacy of the domiciliary visit as the sole means of contact between the GP and the patient. A study carried out in the Somerset Health District showed that 29. 3% of severely physically disabled adults had unmet needs and the prevalence was higher (40. 3%) among subjects whose sole contact with health services professionals was in the home (Williams & Bowie 1993). There is a clear suggestion that the general health of physically disabled people is enhanced if they are themselves in a position to initiate contact with a health care professional, on a regular basis and in a health care facility. This can only happen if health care facilities are fully accessible. If improved access to health care facilities benefits the physically disabled client group then so too does it benefit health care professionals. The domiciliary visit is a time consuming and expensive way to carry out health care and so, in the long term, improved access is a means of improving the efficiency as well as the quality of care provided (Davies & Langton-Lockton 1988).

There is one further context in which access to the

NHS for physically disabled people must be seen. In a very real way the NHS and Community Care Act 1990 (HMSO 1990) has revolutionised the form in which health care is provided. The whole thrust of the legislation, which is by now axiomatic, is that wherever possible health care provision should be in the community and should be needs based. The legislation was designed to 'enable people to live as normal a life as possible in their own homes or in a homely environment in the local community' (HMSO 1989). It is clear, therefore, that in order to fulfil this objective, as far as physically disabled people are concerned, access to primary health care facilities must be widespread. Similarly, if it is true that 'promoting choice and independence underlies all the Government's proposals' (ibid) then improving access can again be seen as absolutely in line with the current thrust of thinking on health care matters. Independence and choice are perhaps the two privileges that physically disabled people lack most frequently. Improving access to the built environment will not immediately make these privileges a reality but it will bring them a little closer.

DISABILITIES ACCESS AND INFORMATION PROVISION

An access directory for disabled people

One of the greatest access barriers for many people with physical disabilities is not so much the existence of inaccessible buildings but the lack of information about accessibility in general. An individual with certain access needs can make provision to avoid access barriers, or arrange ways of getting round them, only if they know that the barrier is there. It is with this in mind that Regional Health Authorities, Family Health Service Authorities (FHSAs) and other bodies have begun to produce literature aimed at providing just this sort of information for primary health care facilities. This move is to be welcomed since it not only allows people with physical disabilities to be more independent and to make informed decisions for themselves, but it also provides a body

of data about accessibility which can be used to campaign for improvements in the level and range of accessible primary health care facilities.

One such guide has been produced for Brent, North Kensington and North Westminster. The Access Directory for Disabled People (Parkside Health 1993) contains information about dentists, GPs, opticians and pharmacies in these areas. The type of information given includes distances to the nearest forms of public transport, how many steps there are at the entrance to a given building, whether there are handrails at the entrance and inside the building and what special facilities and services (if any) can be provided. The guide is the result of a collaboration by the Brent Association of Disabled People, Brent & Harrow FHSA, the Independent Living Team and Kensington, Chelsea and Westminster FHSA and was produced on behalf of Parkside Health. In theory this is exactly the kind of collaboration, involving both providers and consumers of services, that could act as a model for future projects. In the Foreword to the Access Directory, Nancy Robertson (Former Director of The Prince of Wales' Advisory Group on Disability) congratulates Parkside Health on its initiative and comments that 'accurate information, clearly presented is a vital element in the provision of many services'. It is clear that this is a sentiment with which few would disagree yet a close inspection of the document suggests that there may be a number of very serious flaws, inaccuracies and omissions which make it of little practical use. Indeed it might be argued that the document is worse than useless—it is positively harmful—since it misinforms while giving the impression of being authoritative.

In order to assess the accuracy of the Directory a study was undertaken into the 14 general practices listed which fall into the North Westminster area. Each of these was visited by an experienced access surveyor and a re-survey was attempted. Four of the practices could not be adequately surveyed (due to either an unwillingness on the part of the practice or an inability to gain access to the premises at all). Of the 10 practices that were surveyed all had at least one piece of inaccurate information about them in the Access

Directory (most had more) and seven had inaccurate information which was specifically related to access (number of steps, hand rails, door widths, etc). Some of the errors were trivial, for example the address of one of the practices was incorrect, while others were more serious. The number of steps at the entrance to the practices, as recorded in the Access Directory, was wrong in four cases (in one case there was flat access when there had been a step recorded) and handrails were commonly misreported. Perhaps the greatest flaw in the Access Directory is the fact that it gives no real indication of the level of access once inside the premises. Split levels are not recorded and even the fact that consulting rooms were up a flight of stairs was omitted. Added to this is the omission of dimensions for lifts or doors. In the case of a lift simply its presence or absence is noted and while it is true that doors are classed as 'wide enough for wheelchair access' or not, no definition of 'wide enough' is supplied. These are basic and fundamental errors in the way the Access Directory was conceived and written. Rather than providing hard facts about access, on the basis of which people should be able to make their own judgements as to whether or not the building will be accessible to them, the Access Directory is vague and full of half-truths. The errors that were found in it are summarised in Table 2.7.

There were also some specific and generic inaccuracies and omissions which are worth noting individually.

Travel

Approximate distances were provided for the nearest bus, underground and British Rail stops. However, it would have been more useful to record the name of these stations since all stations are not, by any means, equally accessible. One entry measured the distances in approximate walking time, information which is of little practical use to a disabled walker or someone who uses a wheelchair.

Parking

The area around North Westminster has little free off-road parking and indeed virtually the only parking available for practical purposes is through the use of parking meters. When parking was indicated as a facility this is what was meant and yet only two entries made this explicit. The reality of the situation is that finding a parking space would be, more often than not, impossible.

Entry bells

Six of the practices surveyed had entry bell systems which were used to gain entrance. All of these were out of reach of, for example, a wheelchair user and yet there was no mention of this in the guide.

Misrepresentation

There were three practices which had notably good access (flat or ramped entrances with flat access to reception and consulting rooms) and yet this was not presented clearly by the information contained in the guide.

Survey methods

Obviously it is not good enough to throw criticism at a document of this kind, which was written in good faith and with the best of intentions, without trying to understand why it should come to be so inaccurate. It seems that the root of the problem was the method of surveying used. Rather than being based on evidence provided by a survey carried out during a visit of the practices, the Access Directory was 'compiled only through information

Table 2.7 Inaccuracies, errors or omissions found in the Access Directory for Disabled People (Parkside Health 1993)

Practice	1	2	3	4	5	6	7	8	9	10
Parking	x	-	-	-	-	-	-	x	x	x
Transport	-	x	-	-	-	-	-	-	-	-
Steps at entrance	-	x	-	-	x	-	x	-	x	-
Steps inside	-	x	x	x	x	-	x	-	-	-
Hand rails at entrance	-	x	x	x	-	x	x	-	-	x
Hand rails inside	-	-	-	-	-	-	x	-	-	-
Door width	-	-	x	x	-	-	x	-	-	-
Lift	-	x	-	-	-	-	-	-	-	-

x denotes an inaccuracy, error or omission.

provided by the practitioners' (Parkside Health 1993). The guide relied on those working at the practices to fill in a form about the accessibility of their premises and did not verify its accuracy at a later date. While it seems hard to believe that any practice would have knowingly supplied false information, it seems clear that a number did supply information that was inaccurate. In some ways this is not surprising. It is never enough to rely on information produced by questionnaire surveys. With the best will in the world, people who do not have experience of surveying will make mistakes since they will not properly understand what is being asked of them. It seems that this is what happened in the case of the Access Directory.

It should be stressed that only a small fraction of the total number of entries in the Access Directory were surveyed in this study and it is therefore not possible to imply that the whole is as inaccurate as the sample. That said it is striking that every one of the premises that was surveyed was inaccurately recorded in the Access Directory. It seems from this evidence that access guides produced solely on the basis of a questionnaire, while being undoubtedly simpler and cheaper to produce, are scarcely worth the effort.

DISABILITIES ACCESS AND THE LAW

The development of building regulations

For many years the extent to which a given building was made accessible to those with physical disabilities was governed entirely by goodwill. This seems to have applied to health care facilities no less than other buildings to which the public have general access. More recently, however, the laws governing building regulations have been made more rigorous with regard to physical access. In Britain the main participants in the planning process are the Secretary of State for the Environment, the county councils, the district councils (including the 32 London Boroughs and the City of London) and the developers who must seek the permission of the rest. All these bodies are guided by various statutes (Chronically Sick and Disabled Persons

Act 1970 (HMSO 1970); Town and Country Planning Act 1971 (HMSO 1971); Building Regulations 1985 Approved Document Part M (HMSO 1985)). Each of these acts, with greater or lesser forms of coercion, has aimed to improve the accessibility of the built environment. The culmination of this process was the development of the building regulations known as Part M. This requires that 'reasonable provision be made to enable disabled people to gain access to all storeys of a building used as an office, shop premises, factory or school. Where sanitary conveniences are provided in such buildings reasonable provision must be made'. These regulations have been made successively more rigorous in new editions published in 1991 and 1992. Changes include:

- extending the definition of 'disabled people' to include those who have impaired hearing or sight
- extending the regulations to cover not only non-domestic buildings which have been newly erected but also those which have been substantially reconstructed and extensions to a building which includes a ground storey
- the latest regulations also give detailed guidance on the provision of handrails, wheelchair stair lifts and WCs.

Restrictive as Part M may initially seem it is still significantly flawed. First, it does not include listed buildings, housing, transport, leisure and tourist facilities and some public buildings are only required to be accessible at the main entrance. Secondly, and arguably more importantly, Part M is implemented by Building Control Officers (BCO) whose perspective is principally one of health and safety and whose background is tied up with the construction companies that they are trying to regulate. There is no appeal against the decision of a BCO which means that Part M is only really implemented on the basis of goodwill.

BUILDING REGULATIONS AND THE NATIONAL HEALTH SERVICE

Health care facilities, as buildings to which the public have access, are governed by Part M of the Building Regulations. There are clear guidelines, published by the Department of Health (1989a) in a document entitled Health Building Note 40, which relate to the level of adequate provision of access and facilities for those with physical disabilities in hospitals. However, there are no similar guidelines for primary health care facilities. Indeed, despite the recent shifts in emphasis towards consumer-led provision of health care, there has been little change in the level of access required by law from health care facilities. In effect primary health care providers are in exactly the same position as any other small businessman and cannot be required by law to adapt their premises unless they undertake substantial rebuilding or renovation. There is a statutory requirement for FHSAs to consider the 'need for access by handicapped persons using wheel-chairs' when approving the premises of general practices for reimbursement of rent and rates and the approval of cost-rent schemes (Department of Health 1989b). The reality of this requirement is that it is only put into force when a GP is building new premises or extensively refurbishing existing premises and thus the real problem—the number of existing premises which are inaccessible—is untouched.

The Patient's Charter begins to address this issue with National Charter Standard 2 which calls for 'arrangements to ensure everyone, including people with special needs, can use services . . . for example, by ensuring that buildings can be used by people in wheelchairs' (HMSO 1991). This, of course, has no legal authority as the National Charter Standards 'are not legal rights but major and specific standards which the Government looks to the NHS to achieve, as circumstances and resources allow' (ibid). It would be wrong to imply that these standards are of no use simply because they have no legal requirement and it appears that some movement in the direction of improved access to primary health care facilities has begun. For example, a number of Regional Health Authorities have collaborated with FHSAs and disabilities interest groups in producing access guides to the facilities in their areas. The accuracy and usefulness of these may, however, be doubted. This advance notwithstanding, it does seem that there may be a very high proportion of GPs surgeries which are not accessible to people with even a slight degree of mobility impairment and it seems to be Government policy to rely on persuasion rather than coercion to deliver accessible health care environments. It is the view of at least one council planning officer that:

the only solution is anti-discrimination legislation that would make access the first consideration for all buildings and not just something that is tacked on by accident. It is only with a completely new statute, covering all loopholes, that an accessible built environment will be possible rather than desirable (Bool 1994).

TRANSPORT: FROM AN ACCESS PERSPECTIVE

It is an obvious but easily overlooked fact that the key to good access is good and accessible transport. Many people with limited mobility may be able to negotiate the slight access barriers presented at buildings but not the greater ones presented by many systems of public transport. This is as true for users of health care facilities as it is for anyone else. Travel in London is perhaps particularly difficult since the problems presented by size, distance and congestion are almost insurmountable. At present there is very little statutory provision for non-emergency transport to health care facilities. Ambulances which will take people to out-patients' appointments, for example, are almost non-existent in some areas. The NHS will help with the cost of travel to hospital appointments for those who fall below a certain income bracket but this is about as far as the state provision goes. In most situations individuals need to arrange for their own transport by some other means. There is no provision on a national basis for transport to primary health care facilities regardless of mobility. Transport is, therefore, a key issue when considering access to the NHS for disabled people.

Public transport

The London Underground

Provisions for disabled people on public transport systems in London are not nearly as good as they are, for example, in Paris, New York or Washington DC (Couch 1989, 1993). Yet a survey conducted by GLAD in 1985 suggested that over 400 000 Londoners (roughly 7% of the population) had some degree of 'transport handicap' (GLAD 1985). Given this, the level of accessible public transport in London is disgracefully inadequate. According to London Regional Transport there are 40 stations on the Underground network which have 'some degree of step-free access' although nearly all of these are in suburban areas. In fact, according to LRT's Disability Unit, the only fully accessible stations in Central London are South Kensington, Olympia, Hammersmith and Liverpool Street. Until recently this paucity of accessible stations was aggravated by LRT policy which restricted the travel of wheelchair users to off-peak hours and by prior arrangement. Even then only the surface or near-surface sections of the network were officially open to those using wheelchairs. However this policy has now been reversed and from 1 October 1993 it has been up to individuals to decide which sections of the Underground they can use.

LRT does have a long-term policy to improve the accessibility of its Central London stations and there is a stated objective to adapt 20 'core' (i.e. central) stations so that they will be fully accessible. They also insist that as existing stations are refurbished and updated improved access will be considered a high priority. In addition, any new stations or sections of the Underground system must, by law, be made accessible.

However, despite these good intentions, it seems that the overall accessibility of the Underground network is unlikely to improve significantly since resources are being constantly squeezed. In recent years Government funding of LRT has been cut by one-third and this clearly has a direct effect on the amount of money available to invest in access improvements. Indeed, an unfavourable interpretation of the recent relaxation in travel restrictions for wheelchair users on the Underground might be that this change has finally been approved, after decades of campaigning, because it is inexpensive to implement at a time when resources are short. There are fears that LRT will now feel under less pressure to move quickly on fully adapting stations in Central London.

The London bus system

LRT also has responsibility for London's network of accessible buses—the so-called Mobility Buses. At present there are around 90 routes served by Mobility Buses, but again most of these are in the suburbs. They run only once or twice a week and only two or three times on those days. Thus the total provision is much less than it may at first appear. One system which does serve Central London is the Stationlink (previously Carelink). This is a fully accessible minibus, run by LRT which links 10 of London's British Rail stations and Victoria Coach Station. While this is a useful system—it runs 7 days a week—and is being increasingly widely used, it does have limitations. It is clearly a limited service in terms of the area that it covers and it does not run as frequently as regular London buses. Most importantly, however, buses only run in one direction along the route thereby severely limiting its potential usefulness.

While LRT is making efforts to improve its provision of accessible transport the network is still highly flawed and is likely to remain so. It is also unlikely that the system, as it stands at the moment, is of much practical use to people when trying to get to and from health care facilities. The difficulties involved in getting to and from Underground stations and bus stops may well rule it out for those with even a minor disability.

Other means of accessible transport

Dial-a-Ride

This service provides an invaluable and very useful door-to-door transport facility and is organised by individual London Boroughs. The cost of a trip is based on LRT bus prices and as such is a much more inexpensive means of transport than using taxis. However, it is of no practical use for transport to or from either health care or social services facilities since the system will not act as a transport service specifically for these. This is understandable, though regrettable, and means that one of the most useful and most accessible means of transport is taken out of consideration.

Taxicard

Taking all factors into consideration, this system seems the most likely to be used by people with mobility problems wishing to attend health care facilities. It is funded by 29 London Boroughs and enables card-holders to book and use adapted taxis at a reduced rate. For a flat rate of £1.40 a holder can make a journey which would normally cost up to £10.60. Once that ceiling has been reached any excess must be paid by the individual concerned. There are also some extra charges for extra passengers, bank holiday travel, etc. The criteria for acceptance to the scheme are:

- an inability to walk more than 100 metres without help
- an inability to stand at a bus stop for more than 15 minutes
- an inability to get on and off conventional buses and trains (including negotiating the steps at the station).

This system, as might be expected, is also flawed. For example, the taxi driver will start his meter as soon as the call is booked and may technically charge waiting time while an individual makes his way into the cab (a manoeuvre which for many disabled people may take some time). It is also essential to pre-book a taxi to be sure of getting one at a specific time. This is a

particular difficulty, for example, when returning from an appointment at a health care facility since precise times that consultations will end can rarely be given. These problems are quite apart from the concerns that may arise when a taxi driver is expected to physically aid someone with perhaps severe disability. The system effectively relies on the goodwill of the individual driver to function properly and it cannot be regarded as a suitable alternative to fully adapted systems of transport.

Voluntary agencies

The role of the voluntary sector in providing transport to and from health care facilities is considerable but little more than that can be said with certainty. There has been no systematic research into this field and indeed it is an area that could well do with more study. At present, national organisations such as the Red Cross and the St. John's Ambulance Service make a considerable contribution to helping increase the mobility of individuals who cannot use other forms of available transport. However, both organisations are under considerable financial pressure and cannot be expected to take on the role single-handedly. Indeed, with the demographic trend towards an ageing population the situation is set to get considerably worse in the years ahead and it would seem that these organisations are not equipped to cope.

Increasingly, volunteer transport schemes, organised on a local or community basis, are being used to assist. Again, there is no clear indication of the extent of these schemes across the country nor indeed of their effectiveness. It has been suggested, however, that this sort of community-based scheme is well suited to coordination from a primary health care setting. 'A primary health care practice is not only strategically located but it is also a gateway for a local population in a way that social services and most voluntary organisations are not' (Webber et al 1991). However, this study also suggested that volunteer schemes do run into certain problems. Primarily there may be significant difficulties in recruiting both volunteers to help and those in need of assistance. Coordinating needs with volunteered services can also be a complex and time consuming undertaking. Indeed, it was found that the appointment of full-time outreach workers and coordinators was necessary to facilitate the volunteer scheme. This at once reduces the simplicity and economy of the scheme—two of its most attractive qualities.

Even if the administrative problems of such a scheme could be surmounted it is still arguable that such a system of transport would not be desirable. It runs into many of the same objections as the first scheme especially since it would rely on untrained volunteers acting, at least partially, in the role of carers. There are also practical objections since the use of unadapted cars as a means of transport would exclude people with more severe physical impairment. However, when it is considered that only an estimated 5–8% of the disabled population use wheelchairs this may seem to be a less serious criticism. These objections notwithstanding, volunteer schemes organised through primary health care facilities do seem to be a viable, if limited, alternative to public transport.

Box 2.2 Conclusions and recommendations

1. It is clear that more information about the accessibility of primary health care facilities is urgently needed. At present it is hard to comment authoritatively let alone make recommendations for policy on the issue of accessibility since little is known save that the situation is bad.
2. The production of access guides for disabled people must involve them at every stage and must be based on information derived by visit. If either of these factors is absent the guide is likely to be inaccurate at best and wrong at worst.
3. Most commentators suggest that the only way to ensure the universal provision of accessible environments is via anti-discrimination legislation. This would affect the NHS no less than any other body or company. Even if this were to be enforced, however, it would be of little practical use if funds were not made available to adapt existing primary health care facilities. In the short term, clearer and more informed advice needs to be available for primary health care professionals who wish to improve their facilities.
4. Solving the problem of transport to and from health care facilities for disabled people is perhaps the most difficult issue of all. In the present economic and social climate the answer seems to lie in a combination of voluntary schemes run from the primary health care setting and, where possible, in-house services provided specifically for this purpose.

Primary health care 'in-house' systems

The possibility that health care facilities might purchase transport services on behalf of their patients/clients is becoming increasingly likely. With the new arrangements in primary health care it would be possible for a fund-holding GP, for example, to purchase a transport service for a patient who might otherwise be unable to visit the practice. However, the possibility and the likelihood of this happening are very different issues. Whether or not to provide this service would be essentially an economic decision since the service would probably be funded from the practice's administrative budget. There is every reason to believe that in this hypothetical situation the GP in question might prefer to carry out a domiciliary visit since this would be less expensive. In many ways, in-house services would seem to be in the best interests of disabled patients yet the reality of funding arrangements means that they are still some way away.

CONCLUSION AND RECOMMENDATIONS

This study was not undertaken with the intent of providing firm data on the basis of which clear recommendations for specific change could be made. However, the investigation into various issues relating to disability and the NHS have naturally suggested a number of areas which require further research and a number of places where there is room for improvemt. These are indicated in Box 2.2

ACKNOWLEDGEMENTS

The authors are indebted to Mr A Bool for his advice on issues relating to the legal requirements governing building regulations and for letting them quote liberally from his unpublished dissertation 'Geographical perspectives on disabled access and social justice' (1994) submitted to the School of Geography, University of Oxford. The authors acknowledge the useful comments and encouragement from Vivien Webber and Dr Peter Davies in the writing of this article.

REFERENCES

Bool A 1994 Geographical perspectives on disabled access and social justice. School of Geography, University of Oxford

Couch G 1989 Access in London. Nicholson, London

Couch G 1993 Access in Paris. Quiller, London

Davies A, Langton-Lockton S 1988 Access to surgeries for the disabled. Royal College of General Practitioners Members' Reference Book

Department of Health 1989a Health building note 40. In: Common activities spaces vol 4: design for disabled people

Department of Health 1989b Statement of fees and allowances payable to general medical practitioners in England and Wales from 1 April 1990

GLAD 1985 All change: a consumer study of public transport handicap in Greater London. GLAD, London

HMSO 1970 Chronically Sick and Disabled Persons Act. HMSO, London

HMSO 1971 Town and Country Planning Act. HMSO, London

HMSO 1985 Building Regulations Approved Document Part M. HMSO, London

HMSO 1989 Caring for people. p4 NHS and Community Care Act. HMSO, London

HMSO 1990 National Health Service and Community Care Act 1990. HMSO, London

HMSO 1991 The Patient's Charter. HMSO, London

Parkside Health 1993 Access directory for disabled people

Ratoff L et al 1992 Are you keeping the disabled out? Royal College of General Practitioners Connection 48(7)

Webber V, Barry V, Davies P, Pietroni P 1991 The impact of a volunteer community care project in a primary health care setting. Journal of Social Work Practice 5(1)

Williams M H, Bowie C 1993 Evidence of unmet need in the care of severely physically disabled adults. British Medical Journal 306(6870) pp 95–98

3

Patient participation and self-care

INTRODUCTION

The notion of patient participation is one that is becoming increasingly accepted in health care circles. The scope of the term is very broad and incorporates:

- self-care measures which patients may undertake, thus participating in their own health care
- opportunities and schemes which allow patients to participate in the process of the delivery of their health care services.

These two aspects of patient participation are reflected in the research interests of the Marylebone Centre Trust and the general approach to health care of the Marylebone Health Centre.

The opening up of this field is reflected in the growing debate over what is the correct term for what was at one time unquestioningly termed the 'patient'. This term has come under attack from all sides. There are those who reject it as part of a construct of health and disease which is imposed by a medical profession unable and unwilling to recognise its limitations. 'Client' may be preferred as a more accurate term and one which reduces the suggested power relationship inherent in the 'doctor/patient' construct. In an increasingly market oriented society—comprising consumers and not citizens—'clients' themselves are being replaced by 'users' and 'consumers'. Which of these terms is used is crucial to the way in which health and social care is thought about and therefore provided. The changing and developing relationships between those who seek and those who provide care need to be investigated if care is to be provided in the most successful way. It is clear that with the growing emphasis on the idea of patients as consumers of health care, it is they who will be increasingly leading the development of the delivery of health services.

While the notion of patient participation may be agreed to be desirable in theory, however, it may be far from trouble-free to implement. Pietroni & Chase (Partners or partisans? Patient satisfaction at Marylebone Health Centre, p. 76) describe the development of a scheme designed to involve the users of the Marylebone Health Centre in its foundation and subsequently in its operational and decision-making processes. While initial interest in and commitment to such a users' group was high, this began to fall off when the pressing issues arising from the founding of a new health centre had been largely resolved. It also became evident that expectations of the role of such a group were different for staff and for patients. This in turn contributed to a situation in which the users' group could feel undervalued and excluded from the 'real' decision-making process which they associated with the doctors. The doctors believed however that they had been open and receptive to input from the users' group whenever it had been forthcoming. Clearly this example illustrates that the field of patient participation is littered with issues that need addressing if such an arrangement is to work. For example:

- How involved can non-clinicians be in the management of primary health care facilities?
- What are the best ways of facilitating such involvement?
- How is tokenism in patient participation to be avoided and genuine involvement to be fostered?

Pietroni & Chase point the way to some possible answers based on their experience.

The ways in which users of primary health care facilities may participate in the running of those facilities are clearly broader than simply through direct involvement in management and decision making. Indeed for most people this is unlikely to be the way in which they participate. Rather, most people may contribute by evaluating and commenting on the nature and standard of the service they receive. Again, this is a field that is ever growing and is clearly a natural development from the idea of the patient as a consumer. This is nowhere more clearly shown than in the increasingly important area of complaints about service delivery. That such complaints are rising is perhaps unsurprising given a prevailing atmosphere that encourages the users of health services to be ever more critical of them. Addressing this issue Pietroni & Uray-Ura (Informal complaints procedures in general practice—a one year audit, p. 82) demonstrate that it is quite possible for general practices to establish informal complaints procedures which:

- are cheap and easy to run
- are quicker in producing a resolution than the existing formal complaints procedures associated with FHSAs
- help to maintain a high level of staff and patient morale.

The model they describe recognises that complaints may be made by staff about patients just as easily as by patients about staff and that both these types of complaint need to be validated and brought to a satisfactory resolution. The type of system which they describe has the added benefit of reducing the tendency and need for complainants to resort to litigation and as they point out, complaints procedures are really nothing more than an exercise in good customer relations. Far from leading to hostility this kind of patient participation can actually help to develop better relations between staff and users in primary health care settings.

The involvement of patients in the delivery and evaluation of their health care is something that is now widely accepted and to a certain extent implemented. This is not the case, however, for the issue of self-care. While many clinicians may be willing to act in partnership with their patients on what they consider to be essentially management issues, many still doubt that there can be a clinical partnership as well. The approach of the Marylebone Health Centre considers this to be a false distinction since empowering the patient means first and foremost empowering the patient to take responsibility for his own health.

McLean & Pietroni (Self-care–who does best?, p. 88) undertook a study to evaluate the efficacy of self-care as a clinical intervention and in particular to investigate whether patients' health beliefs had an effect on their long-term clinical progress within the context of self-care. Following Levin they define self-care as 'activities individuals undertake to restore and promote health, prevent disease and limit illness'. While, for methodological reasons, the research was inconclusive it was demonstrated that there was a predictive relationship between health locus of control beliefs and health improvement. Those who had an independent health locus of control tended to do better than those who had a chance health locus of control or a powerful others health locus of control. As the authors indicate, further study in this area is needed since the differences may also have been affected by social, racial and economic factors. Nevertheless, it seems clear that self-care programmes can be of genuine clinical benefit to a significant proportion of people seeking health care.

This finding is born out by the research of Harrison et al (A controlled trial of self-care classes in general practice, taught by staff members with a short training, to long-term users on anxiolytic, hypnotic and anti-depressant drugs,

p. 96). Their study was designed to investigate the effect of classes, which incorporate a number of different health care techniques, on the health, consultation and prescribing rates of patients in general practice who are long-term users of anxiolytic, hypnotic and anti-depressant (AHA) drugs. This research suggested that such an approach could lead to a reduction in patients' insomnia and, to a lesser degree, their somatic symptoms as well. It was also shown that during the study period the prescribing rates of AHA drugs for the patients' GPs also fell, although consultation rates remained constant. Significantly, the original benefits which had resulted from the self-care classes were not maintained until the 12-month follow-up and it is suggested that this was the result of a failure to continue with the self-care techniques which had been taught. It is also pointed out that the action of attending a class was itself therapeutic for a number of the subjects.

Given these findings, and while recognising the need for further investigation, it is no longer possible to consider self-care as an optional extra in a package of health care services. Rather, self-care should be seen as central to all clinical interactions and interventions and clinicians should be looking for new ways to involve people in their own care. Research should be undertaken to establish which people could most benefit from self-care and which methods are most beneficial. Philosophically, morally, economically and clinically self-care, as an element of patient participation, makes sense.

PARTNERS OR PARTISANS? PATIENT PARTICIPATION AND GENERAL PRACTICE: THE MARYLEBONE EXPERIENCE

Patrick Pietroni
Derek Chase

This paper outlines some of the issues for patients and professionals involved in patient participation projects at the Marylebone Health Centre in London. It describes the projects undertaken and focuses on the practical implications of working *with* rather than *for* patients. A number of dilemmas within patient participation are discussed, including the ways in which volunteers are rewarded, how doctors and patients can share knowledge, how participation is affected by professional boundaries, and why a regular group may not be the best way to involve patients in decision-making. The successes of patient participation are also highlighted.

INTRODUCTION

Participation is one of the developing tenets of primary health care, and yet it raises difficult issues for professionals and patients alike. During a recent discussion at the Marylebone Health Centre, a patient summarised the dilemma: 'What needs to be made clearer is the patient's role as a patient and his/her role as a participator in the running of the centre'. We talk of patient empowerment and patient participation, but what does this really mean in the context of a general practice in the centre of London? What issues do the concepts raise for staff and patients? How can some of the dilemmas be resolved?

Doctors' traditional position of authority has been challenged over recent years. The new focus on consumerism emphasises the role of patients as purchasers of a service and doctors as sellers, reversing the old pattern where doctors generally gave directions and the patient followed instructions (Haug & Lavin 1981). The patient is now more informed about health issues, and the competence gap between the patient and physician has narrowed (Haug & Lavin 1981). The nature of general practice is therefore changing, and there is increasing emphasis on working *with* patients rather than working *for* patients. Patients are being encouraged to participate in the clinical decisions made and the services provided. As the power relationship between doctor and patient changes, health care has been seen increasingly as a contract between doctor and patient in which both sides are equally powerful (Haug & Lavin 1981).

The National Association for Patient Participation was established in 1978 to foster the development of patient participation and to provide a link between patient participation groups. In general, the role of such groups has included planning, dealing with patients' complaints, providing health education, organising voluntary care in the community, and feeding back information on patients' needs to health care providers (Richardson & Bray 1987).

General practitioners have varying reasons for encouraging participation. Some see it as a way of providing help to their patients and emphasise the health education and voluntary activities which a patient participation group would develop. They see patients as 'an enormous resource'. Some are concerned to encourage self-care, and point to doctors' limitations in curing or preventing illness. Some are concerned to create a mechanism for consumer feedback about their practice. Other perspectives range from a concern about their relationship with patients to a commitment to much wider political ideals (Richardson & Bray 1987).

THE MARYLEBONE HEALTH CENTRE

The Marylebone Health Centre is based on a holistic, primary health care model which emphasises the need to empower patients and enable them to take more control of their health and well-being. Complementary therapies are provided alongside general practice and in-

Reprinted with permission from the British Journal of General Practice: 43 pp. 341–344 1993, published by the Royal College of General Practitioners.

house counselling is available. Patients can also be referred to a Christian counselling service provided by the Church in the crypt of which the centre is housed. Patients are encouraged to participate in education and community activities and to provide ideas and feedback on health centre services and management. The general practice is supported by the FHSA in the usual way. The 'extra' services were funded initially by a 5-year grant from the Wates Foundation, and are now supported by a charity, the Marylebone Centre Trust, donations from patients and various fund-raising activities.

Patients can take advantage of various classes covering self-care, stress management, massage, meditation and yoga. Alongside the team of doctors, complementary therapists, a social worker and administrative staff, a health educator is employed part-time to run the education and community programmes and to promote patient participation.

PATTERNS OF PATIENT PARTICIPATION

Users' groups

When the health centre was established in 1987, patients were invited to join a 'Users' Group'. The aims of the group were as follows:

1. To promote dialogue about current provision of primary health care and to encourage suggestions for improvement.
2. To plan and run jointly a health education and self-care programme with the aim of improving patients' health and increasing their responsibility for maintaining their own health.
3. To develop a voluntary, mutual self-help scheme.

The invitation to patients to attend the introductory meeting of the Users' Group stressed that 'the name Users' Group has been chosen, rather than Patient Participation Group, to emphasise health and partnership'.

The Users' Group consisted of eight patients, the social worker, the education officer, one GP and a representative from the Church. The group made recommendations about how the new health centre should be run, including how long appointments should be and when surgeries should be held. The education programme was largely driven by the education officer, but the group was asked for its ideas and opinions.

Volunteers

During the following two years, a successful volunteer scheme was established. Patients were encouraged to provide practical help to other patients, to support the health centre administratively, and to run some of the self-help groups, courses and social events.

Volunteers offered a range of services including letter writing, escorting, transporting, shopping, childminding, sitting with frail adults and reading. Potential volunteers were asked to complete an application form and to provide two referees. These references were taken up and the volunteer was interviewed before being accepted for the scheme (Webber et al 1991). This scheme continues to be a useful resource, and a database of volunteers is now held on the practice computer system for access during consultations.

A separate group of volunteers became 'befrienders', offering emotional support to isolated, usually elderly, patients referred by the practitioners. The befrienders themselves were supported with monthly meetings facilitated by the centre's social worker and another professional who was registered with the practice.

Other patients volunteered to help with the practice newsletter and to undertake administrative tasks such as typing, correspondence and filing. One patient initiated and taught a movement to music class (subsequently funded by the Adult Education Institute); others started a crèche one afternoon a week.

Ideas group

After 2 years, key issues about the day-to-day running of the centre had been resolved and there seemed to be little left for the Users' Group to discuss. Staff and patients' energy and enthusiasm in the group dwindled.

At the same time, evaluation of the education programme showed that most participants came from outside the practice—only 1% were actually registered at MHC. More energy was needed to develop an education and activity programme specifically for patients at the practice. Thus, the Users' Group was disbanded and an 'Ideas Group' formed. This would continue the work of the Users' Group, but its main function would be to plan and promote a patient education programme.

The Ideas Group was introduced at an evening meeting to which all patients were invited. Most of the Users' Group chose to continue their involvement, but new faces also appeared. About 25 patients attended the introductory meeting, and eight of them opted to meet regularly as the Ideas Group.

The Ideas Group was chaired by the health educator. The group decided that no doctor should attend meetings unless specifically invited, since it was felt that patients could speak more freely if the doctors were not present.

Feedback from the Ideas Group was channelled into the Management Group, which consisted of two patients from the Ideas Group, the practice director (a general practitioner), the practice manager, and the health educator. A separate fund-raising group, with the same members of staff but two different patients (members of the Ideas Group), also met regularly.

Following an initial burst of energy, the Ideas Group had a similar experience to the Users' Group and other patient participation groups around the country. Once a patient education programme had been established and means for more effective patient feedback (a suggestions box) provided, there were not enough issues to maintain group discussions every 6 weeks. As one member of the group put it, 'there's nothing to get our teeth into anymore'.

As services increased, the practice was under pressure to raise funds, and discussion of fund-raising activities began to take over the meetings. This was frustrating for patients who had joined the group out of an interest in health, and who wanted to be involved in policy-making.

However, staff felt that it was difficult to involve the group in decisions on policy issues which might require 'medical knowledge'.

The decisions the group did make were small but useful. For example, they decided where the patient suggestions box should be sited, and ways in which information about classes and activities could be more widely disseminated. There was, however, a feeling—not unique to Marylebone—that the doctors did not hear what was discussed and were not interested in the group and its views. Minutes of meetings were distributed to staff, but one patient commented, 'I don't think they know we exist'. Others in the group excused the doctors: 'they were so busy, no more could be expected from them'.

The group's comments about not being heard were greeted with genuine bewilderment by the doctors, who felt that the group had not made many suggestions but when it had its ideas had been acted upon. This bewilderment was exemplified by the practice director's comment, 'When have I ever said 'no'?' In a national survey on patient participation, few staff said they had ever refused to do something they had been asked to do (Richardson & Bray 1987).

The health educator who was running the programme became something of a 'buffer' between the patients and staff. The patients could say things to the health educator that they felt unable to say direct to the doctors. While this enabled them to say more, it also meant that they felt less 'heard' and did not receive information direct from the source. There was a tendency on both sides to doubt the feelings being relayed by the 'go-between'. (The member of staff co-ordinating the Befrienders Group had a similar experience).

The Ideas Group has now been dissolved, by mutual consent. It has been replaced by evening meetings twice a year to which all staff and patients are invited. The meetings provide an opportunity for staff and patients to get to know each other socially, and provide a forum for direct discussion between professionals and patients. A fund-raising group continues to meet and a steering group to implement the Patient's Charter has been established. Patient representation at staff meetings is also under discussion.

WORKING TOWARDS SOLUTIONS

Formal and informal meetings with patients and staff have highlighted some of the issues involved in patient participation at Marylebone. In many instances, staff and patients had different expectations of participation:

- staff were concerned about confidentiality and the patient/professional boundary
- volunteers were sometimes unclear about their role
- patients were disappointed that they had not been involved in 'real' decision-making.

Also, in the end, only a handful of patients had participated. Was it really worth all the effort? How could these issues be resolved and more patients be encouraged to participate?

Is volunteering a gift or a contract?

It appears that the schemes which have succeeded most at Marylebone are those which provide patients with clearly defined tasks and regular support. For example, the Befrienders Group, which meets once a month, has increased in size and continues to provide an important service for isolated patients.

However, professionals and patients frequently have different criteria for success. For patients, these criteria usually depend upon why they became involved in the first place. Professionals comment that patients who volunteer have particular needs which are met through volunteering. However, many patients maintain that they volunteered because they wanted to give something back to the health centre, having benefited from its services themselves. Others want to be 'part of the team' and are interested in being involved in the 'different' model of health care Marylebone offers.

Some volunteers are also 'professionals' in their own right, and offer their professional services free to the health centre. If the service offered does not fit in with health centre staff's plans and is turned down, the volunteer can feel rejected and unvalued—particularly if he/she feels that it is a service which the health centre should be offering anyway.

Feedback and professional involvement

Volunteers must feel that the doctors value their opinions and judgement. Feedback mechanisms are important. For example, doctors referred patients for befriending, but sometimes appeared uninterested in any feedback. On occasion, the befrienders felt nervous about going in to the doctor to report back information about the befriendee. The befrienders had to fit in with the professional's agendas. To redress the power balance, one of the general practitioners now attends the monthly Befrienders Meeting at regular intervals.

Professionals' involvement is important. To patients, doctors are still the 'king-pins' in general practice, and patients need direct contact with them to feel that they are really participating. It does not seem to be enough to have an intermediary member of staff playing 'go-between'. Despite the fact that the Ideas Group had decided not to include a doctor at the meetings, in retrospect the group would have felt more powerful if a doctor had attended the meetings. Equally, if patients are to organise fund-raising events, it is important that professionals from the practice attend, join in, and thank and congratulate the volunteers involved.

In an attempt to clarify the role of volunteers at the health centre, anyone—patient or non-patient—who volunteers at Marylebone is now given a brief job description. This is negotiated with the volunteer and describes the tasks they are expected to complete and what they can expect from the health centre in return. One member of staff is allocated as a support/supervisor for each volunteer. A full-time patient liaison officer—who is not registered with the practice—has also been employed to coordinate and support the volunteers.

Professional boundaries

Working alongside patients as volunteers raises issues of professional boundaries for the staff involved—particularly the clinicians. It was confusing for doctors if volunteers asked them about medication or treatment when they met in reception. Doctors felt that such discussions should be dealt with in the consulting room. Volunteers were sometimes hurt by this attitude on the doctors' part. Such situations are also difficult for the doctors, who are not used to wearing different 'hats' at different times.

Issues of confidentiality—particularly with befrienders—have also caused concern. Befriendees are not referred to by name at the monthly meetings. Nor are patients registered with the practice allowed to deal with the patient filing system or patient correspondence.

Professionalisation: who has the final say?

Perhaps the biggest issue for professionals is how to involve patients in decisions which require 'medical knowledge'. For example, can you involve patients in decisions about budgeting or allocation of resources? Who should decide which complementary therapies are made available?

As Adams points out, professionalisation is a problem:

not because professional judgements and skills should be undervalued, but knowledge must be shared and made available, not used to have undue influence over others. Professionals have one kind of knowledge and ability and citizens have another—both are valid and should be utilised (Adams 1989).

The literature suggests that there is an inherent reluctance on the doctors' part to take patient participation groups seriously. 'It was not so much that doctors actively hindered the progress of the group, but they did not do so very much to help it along' (Richardson & Bray 1987). It is important that the group should be proactive as well as reactive. As well as commenting on suggestions made by professionals, the group must be encouraged to make suggestions of its own, and these suggestions should be considered seriously by staff.

Professionals must be wary of creating expectations which are unrealistic and cannot be fulfilled. They may feel that creating an environment in which issues can be raised and discussed is an achievement in itself and that the process is as important as the end result. But this is not necessarily the perception of the patients involved.

One of the biggest challenges to patient participation is how to bring doctors and patients together in a 'neutral' setting where both groups feel equally powerful and can discuss their needs and visions without becoming defensive or feeling 'one-down'.

A group is not necessarily the answer

A patient participation group may work well in the early stages of establishing a health centre. But as the number of issues to discuss decreases, it is difficult to sustain interest in a group which meets regularly. It is particularly difficult to sustain interest if the group feels peripheral and uninvolved in 'major' decision-making.

An established group also taps into the same few people time and again; those outside the group may feel excluded, and it is difficult to introduce new 'voices'.

The newly introduced twice-yearly meetings at Marylebone should enable more patients to participate. Patients are invited to come and share a glass of wine and to meet staff informally, out of office hours. The meetings provide an opportunity to build relationships, to discuss both staff and patients' expectations, to encourage each other and consider suggestions for change, and to make key decisions. They also provide a regular opportunity for review.

New models for evaluation

If patients are to participate in planning and implementing services, they should also be involved in evaluating them. A Patients' Satisfaction Study, undertaken by the Marylebone Centre Trust, has attempted to allow patients to participate in evaluating the health centre. Unstructured interviews with patients set the agenda for a questionnaire which was circulated throughout the patient population. This study is reported in a separate paper currently in preparation.

CONCLUSION

As Brownlea points out:

participation may be seen as a way of broadening the range of inputs to a decision, but in fact may represent a kind of tokenism. The input is received, but very quickly discarded as of little or no consequence. The motions have been gone through. The democratic ideal has been observed, but there is little power behind the participants' input' (Brownlea 1987).

The expected difference that participation is supposed to achieve might well vary between those drawn into the system to participate and those already in the system who have the ultimate decision-making power. Rather than influencing a decision, participation may provide a platform for the acceptance of a decision made elsewhere in the system. As such, participation may validate or legitimate the status quo rather than promote change (Brownlea 1987).

There are clearly many lessons to be learnt from the Marylebone experience. Patients are most able to participate when there are clearly defined roles for them to undertake and when they have a specific member of staff to whom they are responsible and with whom they can work.

Beyond this specific voluntary activity, patients and staff must meet regularly to negotiate the role that patients are to have. The hopes and expectations of both parties must be discussed and taken into account. Opportunities to take stock and assess progress together must also be created.

Participation is ultimately about moving away from a 'them' and 'us' mentality towards a partnership which, as reported in a National Association of Patient Participation newsletter, can be of mutual benefit to all parties.

REFERENCES

Adams I 1989 Healthy cities, healthy participation. Health Education Journal 48 pp 179–182

Brownlea A 1987 Participation, myths, realities and prognoses. Social Science and Medicine 25 pp 605–61

Haug M, Lavin B 1981 Practitioner or patient—who's in charge? Journal of Health and Social Behaviour 22 pp 212–230

Richardson A, Bray C 1987 Promoting health through participation. Research report 659. Policy Studies Institute, London

Webber V, Barry V, Davies P, Pietroni P 1991 The impact of a community care project in a primary health care setting. Journal of Social Work Practice 5 pp 83–90

INFORMAL COMPLAINTS PROCEDURES IN GENERAL PRACTICE—A ONE-YEAR AUDIT

Patrick Pietroni
Sybilla de Uray-Ura

Objective:
This discussion paper identifies and evaluates the findings of an informal patient complaints system using a strong patient participative programme.

Design:
Audit of an informal complaints procedure (ICP).

Setting:
The Marylebone Health Centre, London.

Subjects:
39 complaints received over the audit period.

Main outcome methods:
1. Types of complaints
   1. 1 Administrative
   1. 2 Doctors/medical care
   1. 3 Health centre staff about patients
   1. 4 Mixed
   1. 5 Other
2. Resolution of complaints: how patient complaints were dealt with and their resolution.

Results
An informal complaints procedure is more cost-effective than the cumbersome FHSA complaints system. Out of 39 patient complaints, 37 complaints were resolved within a 2-week period. Two complaints that were sent directly to the FHSA, with patients' agreement, were resolved by using the Informal Complaints Procedure. The procedures for administering a two-way patient complaints system are relatively straightforward and do not require major organisational restructuring.

Conclusion
The use of an informal complaints procedure within general practice is an effective way of dealing with patient complaints, giving patients a faster turn-around time for dealing with complaints and an explanation of where things have seemed to have gone wrong. The Informal Complaints Procedure improves morale of health centre staff as the complaints sytem is a two-way process rather than the usual one-way complaints system.

Reprinted with permission from the British Medical Journal: 308 pp. 1546–1549 11 June 1994.

INTRODUCTION

The increase in the number of complaints has been the subject of numerous recent publications both within medicine and in the national press (Owen 1991, Department of Health 1991–1992, JRCGP 1993, Mori Poll 1993, Panting 1993, Stütte 1993). The Secretary of State's recent decision to set up a working party (BMA 1993) highlighted the need for a rethink as to how both the public and the professions can arrive at a mutually agreed system which protects both sides from the resource implication, both financial and personal, of this development. Surveys within the defence organisation reveal that 'between 1980 and 1992, there has been a ten-fold increase in the number of complaints received and that over 30% of such claims are successful' (MDU 1993). 'Female GPs under the age of 50 have 50% fewer claims made against them than their male colleagues but over the age of 50, female GPs are at slightly greater risk' (MDU 1993). Several factors have been identified as the cause of this increase, not least the Secretary of State's much quoted statement that 'complaints are to be encouraged'. The GP press has itself undertaken several surveys that underpin the stress doctors feel with regard to complaints and the recent suicide of a well-liked doctor illustrates the cost in more tragic personal terms.

Other factors arise out of the new contractual obligation, the Patient's Charter and the more active involvement of Community Health Councils. The purchaser/provider split, with the emphasis on the patient as customer, no doubt has effected a change in public perception although there is no evidence that the increase in complaints reflects a decrease in standards. FHSAs have, perforce, found themselves at times overwhelmed with complaints and several have set up joint working groups with LMC representatives in an attempt to establish new guidelines for handling what can only be described as a crisis. Both formal and informal reports that have been published agree that more locally based procedures need to be developed and that the rather cumbersome and time-consuming formal FHSA hearing needs to be supplemented with additional procedures. In discussing this matter, it is important to remember that comparative surveys reveal that within the UK the medical profession as a whole still carries a very low professional negligency indemnity insurance in comparison to other professional bodies. In the USA, for example, doctors have to carry negligence indemnity five times greater than is carried by the average UK doctor (Stütte 1993). It is to prevent the trend to a more legalistic and costly system that experiments in informal procedures are so necessary.

BACKGROUND

The Marylebone Health Centre was established as an experimental primary health care centre to explore new ways of delivering care to an inner city population. The practice has a patient list size of approximately 5000 with a 30% turnover. The socio-demography of the patients is very mixed—34% of the patients do not have English as their first language and over 200 patients are classified as homeless. A practice-based UPA (Jarman score) was undertaken and revealed a figure of 61.4 (ward average 17.2) (Chase & Davies 1991).

Part of the brief was to encourage patient participation and patient empowerment. During the course of this, a 'Users' Group' was established in 1987 which proved very popular with patients and staff alike. The aims of the group were as follows:

1. To promote dialogue about current provision of primary health care and to encourage suggestions for improvement.
2. To plan and run jointly a health education and self-care programme with the aim of improving patients' health and increasing their responsibility for maintaining their own health.
3. To develop a voluntary, mutual self-help scheme.

A fuller description of this programme is given by Pietroni & Chase (p. 76). The patient Users' Group met every 2 months to discuss patient complaints and was made up of 12 patients (users).

METHOD

In 1991, a Patient Liaison Worker (PLW) was appointed to supervise all aspects of the practice's non-clinical relationship with patients. She reported directly to the Practice Manager under the guidance of the Practice Management Group. Her training was in quality assurance, medical audit and hospital accreditation: this was a full-time post funded by the FHSA.

The Informal Complaints Procedure (ICP) was designed to provide complainants with an explanation of the circumstances surrounding an adverse event. It was decided from the beginning of the experiment that the ICP should be a two-way process available to both staff and patients, i.e. staff could report an adverse event concerning a patient to the ICP. The ICP did not replace or prevent access to the Formal Complaints Procedure (FCP). Explanatory leaflets and posters were distributed at the reception and waiting room area of the practice and patients were also informed through the practice newsletter.

A committee was established comprising volunteers from the larger Users' Group and a complaints form was designed to be completed for each incident. Two of the patients on the committee had lodged complaints previously with the health centre and therefore had a full understanding of the ICP. A flow chart (Fig. 3.1) illustrates the procedures which were followed once a complaint was received.

FINDINGS

The in-house complaints procedure was designed to provide complainants with an explanation of the circumstances surrounding an adverse event. All patient complaints were treated as separate cases and an audit was undertaken. A total of 39 complaints were processed during the experimental period and were divided into the following five categories:

1. Administrative: a complaint involving administrative procedures including repeat prescriptions, telephone system, receptionist, administrative staff action/inaction, appointment procedures.

Figure 3.1 Flow chart of the informal complaints procedure.

How complaints are dealt with

Health Centre is notified of complaint which is directed at once to Patient Liaison Worker

↓

Patient Liaison Worker responds within 3 days with acknowledgement of complaint (verbally/letter)

↓

If complainant is amenable to immediate resolution via meeting with practice staff, Patient Liaison Worker arranges such a meeting, supplies complainant with an information leaflet and arranges for complainant to complete an in-house complaint form

↓

Patient Liaison Worker helps complainant to identify clearly nature and extent of complaint. Patient can call in own representative or representative of Patient Complaints Committee to assist

↓

Patient Liaison Worker investigates complaint. Nominated GP for clinical matters.
Member of Complaints Committee for patient related matters
(Policy: an investigation should take no longer than 2 weeks, only in some cases more time may be required)

↓

Patient Liaison Worker discusses complaint (provided no problems of confidentiality arise) to ensure complainant's case is fully understood

↓

Patient Liaison Worker makes a factual report, incorporating any investigative work from health centre staff advice and comments from Patient Complaints Committee, and offers a written explanation to complainant

Resolution of complaint

Patient Complaints Flow Chart © Marylebone Health Centre 1993

2. Doctors/medical care: complaints directed at individual doctors and/or medical care at the health centre.
3. Complaints from health care staff about patients: this included health centre staff complaints directed at individual patients, e.g. rudeness, repeated failed appointments.
4. Mixed: an individual complaint involving two or more of the five categories.
5. Other: a patient complaint which did not fit into any of the above four areas including patient complaints directed at other NHS services, and waiting lists for treatment.

Table 3.1 Number of complaints in each category during audit year

Outcome	Number
Administration	5
Doctor's medical care	14
Complaints from health centre staff about patients	10
Mixed	5
Other	5
Total	39

Table 3.2 Outcome and resolution (if any) of 39 complaints

Category	Number
Received letter of apology from health centre	17
Received letter of explanation and clarification of health centre procedures	17
Resolved via a meeting with GP, patient, patient representative	3
Received explanation from hospital to which the complaint was addressed	1
No resolution (no response from hospital out-patient department)	1
Total	39

DISCUSSION

Like all new syndromes when first identified, there is a tendency to find many new examples. In the preceding 5 years the practice had received two formal complaints, one involving the medical defence organisation. In the one year of the experimental scheme, 39 complaints were recorded, 10 of which were generated from staff (Table 3.1).

More complaints were therefore received once the ICP was instituted (Fig. 3.2).

The vast majority of these complaints were resolved within 3 days of receipt and only two required an investigation period of 3 weeks before the complaints were finally resolved (Table 3.2).

The total time spent and correspondence involved was, even so, less than the time spent on the two complaints received in the preceding 5 years, reducing the personal stress experienced considerably. Two complaints sent directly to the FHSA during this experimental period were directed, with the patients' agreement, to the ICP, thus reducing FHSA time and involvement. The two complaints were satisfactorily resolved by the ICP.

The procedures for administering such a scheme are relatively straightforward, and do not require a major organisational restructuring. The recruitment of a Patient Liaison Worker to pilot and manage such a scheme was no doubt a major factor in its success, but it is possible for existing Practice Managers to undertake this task within existing job descriptions. The recruitment of patient representatives as members of the complaints panel ensured there was equity and protected the complainant from feeling that he/she was unrepresented and that the procedures were there to 'protect' the practice staff.

For the staff and GPs, the reciprocity of the scheme ensured that their own grievances and complaints about patients could be acknowledged and were validated as appropriate by other 'independent' persons. There was also an improvement in morale through the reciprocity of the scheme.

Many of the complaints resulted in an investigation of existing practice procedures, the development of practice protocols and the setting of standards. For example, staffing arrangements were altered following a complaint regarding a delay in answering the telephone at those times when the greatest number of incoming calls were received.

When establishing an informal complaints procedure issues of confidentiality need to be properly addressed, especially when the complainant is not the patient. Consent forms need to be issued and confidentiality statements signed by patients, patient representatives and all staff involved in investigation of the complaints.

The cost implications of a practice-based informal complaints procedure are minimal when one compares the cumbersome and lengthy procedures currently in place. FHSAs may well wish to finance the initial start-up costs of similar schemes through developmental budgets and Patient's Charter initiatives: they will no doubt benefit from the reduced workload.

Finally, the term 'complaints procedure' may be an inappropriate wording for what could be viewed as 'good customer relations'. Patient complaints have allowed the organisation to reflect on its performance and have encouraged the development of policy and procedural changes.

Figure 3.2 Investigation form used for informal complaints.

COMPLAINT INVESTIGATION FORM

To: ....

   ....

Re: ....

   ....

Date: ....

From: ....

   ....

Please find attached a complaint received from:

   ....

   ....

❏ Please could I have any information about the attached complaint.

❏ Please could you give me a statement below so that we can amalgamate this information and address the issues raised in this letter of complaint. Please return to me within 14 days.

Statement:

   ....

   ....

   ....

   ....

   ....

   ....

   ....

   ....

   ....

   ....

Signature: ....

ACKNOWLEDGEMENTS

We would like to thank Dr Sally Hargreaves of the Kensington and Chelsea and Westminster FFHSA for her support of this project.

REFERENCES

BMA 1993 Evidence to the NHS Complaints Review Committee

Chase D, Davies P 1991 Calculation of a practice under-privileged area score. British Journal of General Practice 41 pp 63–66

Department of Health 1991–1992 Health service indicator. Department of Health, London

Journal of the Royal College of General Practitioners 1993 Handling complaints in NHS general practice

Medical Defence Union 1993 Coping with patient complaints in general practice. p. 2

Mori Poll 1993 East London GP services. East London FHSA

Owen C A 1991 Formal complaints against general practitioners. British Journal of General Practice 41 pp 113–115

Panting G 1993 How to establish an in-house general practice complaints procedure. Medical Protection Society Casebook 2 pp 6–9

Pietroni P C, Chase D Partners or partisans? Patient participation at Marylebone Health Centre (Discussion Paper). British Journal of General Practice 43 pp 341–344

Stütte P 1993 What the complaints survey means for GPs. Medical Defence Union

SELF-CARE—WHO DOES BEST?

Julienne McLean
Patrick Pietroni

A clinically evaluated study to assess the benefits of a
self-care programme in general practice is described.
There was significant improvement in psychiatric morbidity at the 6-month follow-up, which was maintained at
one year. The capacity of Multidimensional Health Locus
of Control scales to predict long-term clinical improvement was demonstrated, suggesting that a predominantly internal control of reinforcement appears to be crucial
to the successful adoption of self-care practices. The
clinical and educational benefits of such programmes in
dealing with a wide range of psychophysical problems in
primary care is discussed.
   Key words: health locus of control, self-care, general
practice.

INTRODUCTION

There is now widespread interest among health
professionals in encouraging self-care practices.
Levin [1] defines self-care as activities that individuals undertake to restore and promote health, prevent disease and limit illness, and range from self
medication to taking care with diet and exercise.
There have been few reports of organised approaches to self-care, particularly relating to
stress management, in general practice, and often
these have been limited by small sample sizes
and short-term evaluation. In a pilot study
involving 35 patients, Teare Skinner [2] described the
clinical benefits of introducing a self-help course
in anxiety management skills to primary care
patients. Kiely & McPherson [3] followed up 27
patients for 3 months, and demonstrated significant advantages for patients receiving stress self-
help leaflets during GP consultations over
control patients. In a comprehensive study, Long
& Bourne [4] reported the successful fusion of
professional and self-help initiatives for anxious
and agoraphobic patients. Psychologists have

Reprinted from Social Science and Medicine 30 (5) pp.
591–596 with kind permission from Elsevier Science Ltd, The
Boulevard, Langford Lane, Kidlingron OX5 1GB, UK.

also effectively developed adult education classes
teaching psychological self-help techniques [5].

Psychological studies of personality and attitudes to self-care are becoming more frequent
particularly those which examine the concept of
locus of control and its usefulness in predicting
specific features of health behaviour. The health
locus of control questionnaires, developed from
Rotter's social learning theory, are designed to
tap people's beliefs about the source of reinforcements
for their health behaviour across three separate
factors. The internal health locus of control orientation (IHLC) measures the degree to which
people perceive health outcomes to be contingent on their own decisions and actions, whilst
an external orientation relates to generalised
expectancies that the factors which determine
health are more related to chance (CHLC) or
under the control of powerful others (PHLC) [6].

Levenson [7] has demonstrated the construct
validity of the scales in identifying diagnostic
differences in psychiatric patients. Strickland [8]
reported that the majority of research studies on
locus of control and precautionary health practices had showed a positive correlation, reinforcing
theoretical assumptions that individuals having
predominantly internal as opposed to external
expectancies were more likely to assume responsibility for their health. However, a number of
later studies failed to find correlations between
health locus of control beliefs and a wide range
of health behaviours [9].

Our study had the following two major aims:

1. To measure the clinical outcome of a group of
   patients 12 months after their participation in
   a self-care programme in an inner London
   health centre.
2. To investigate whether patients' beliefs about
   the control of their health could be related to
   their long-term clinical progress.

METHOD
Procedure

We initially conducted a feasibility study investigating
the professional and clinical issues involved in
introducing a self-care programme into the existing

medical services in an inner London health centre [10]. After its successful implementation, the programme was incorporated into the routine services at the health centre, and the clinical research study was set up.

The self-care programme consisted of six 90-minute weekly classes incorporating a multidimensional approach, combining group behavioural methods with active health promotion. The components included the following:

1. An educational section, based on Selye's model of General Adaptation Syndrome, emphasising the relationship between stress and disease/ill health, mind/body integration and the importance of self awareness and responsibility in maintaining positive health [11].
2. Training in diaphragmatic breathing and progressive muscular relaxation techniques [12].
3. Meditation and visualisation exercises [13].
4. Nutritional counselling and physical exercise [14].

A comprehensive booklet was prepared which included information about stress and its causes, descriptions of the exercises, a programme of home-work and references for further reading. Weekly follow-up relaxation sessions were available after completion of the 6-week course.

A referral system was established, and the GPs (both at the health centre and locally) were asked to refer patients to the study by completing the appropriate referral card. Self referrals were also accepted. The two main categories of referral were:

1. Patients whose medical condition was felt to have a stress-related basis, e.g. headaches, hypertension.
2. Patients who identified themselves, or whom their GP identified, as having difficulties coping with anxiety and tension.

Assessment

On referral, each patient was invited to attend for a preliminary interview and assessment. All participants were asked to complete two questionnaires at the initial interview, and at follow-up assessments at 6 weeks, 6 months and 1 year.

The Multidimensional Health Locus of Control scale (MHLC) [6] is a self report measure, and assesses health beliefs according to 'internal', 'chance' and 'powerful others' factors, each of which comprises eight items arranged in a six-point Likert format ranging from strongly agree to strongly disagree, e.g. 'If I become sick I have the power to make myself well again' (internal), 'When I become ill, it's a matter of fate' (chance), 'I can only maintain my health by consulting health professionals' (powerful others) (see Box 3.1). Statistical analysis used t-tests for independent samples.

Box 3.1   MHLC scales

IHLC

1. If I become sick, I have the power to make myself well again.
6. I am directly responsible for my health.
8. Whatever goes wrong with my health is my own fault.
12. My physical well-being depends on how well I take care of myself.
13. When I feel ill, I know it is because I have not been taking care of myself properly.
17. I can pretty much stay healthy by taking good care of myself.

PHLC

3. If I see an excellent doctor regularly, I am less likely to have health problems.
5. I can only maintain my health by consulting health professionals.
7. Other people play a big part in whether I stay healthy or become sick.
10. Health professionals keep me healthy.
14. The type of care I receive from other people is what is responsible for how well I recover from an illness.
18. Following doctor's orders to the letter is the best way for me stay healthy.

CHLC

2. Often I feel that no matter what I do, if I am going to get sick, I will get sick.
4. It seems that my health is greatly influenced by accidental happenings.
9. When I am sick, I just have to let nature run its course.
11. When I stay healthy, I am just plain lucky.
15. Even when I take care of myself, it's easy to get sick.
16. When I become ill, it's a matter of fate.

Box 3.2 DSSI/sAD

(The anxiety items are indicated by an asterisk.)

*1. Recently I have worried about every little thing.

2. Recently I have been so miserable that I have had difficulty with my sleep.

*3. Recently I have been breathless or had a pounding of my heart.

*4. Recently I have been so 'worked up' that I couldn't sit still.

5. Recently I have been depressed without knowing why.

6. Recently I have gone to bed not caring if I never woke up.

*7. Recently, for no good reason, I have had feelings of panic.

8. Recently I have been so low in spirits that I have sat for ages doing absolutely nothing.

*9. Recently I have had a pain or tense feeling in my neck or head.

10. Recently the future has seemed hopeless.

*11. Recently worrying has kept me awake at night.

12. Recently I have lost interest in just about everything.

*13. Recently I have been so anxious that I couldn't make up my mind about the simplest thing.

14. Recently I have been so depressed that I have thought of doing away with myself.

The Bedford Foulds Personal Disturbance scale (DSSI/sAD) consists of seven state of anxiety items, and seven state of depression items (see Box 3.2). Every item is scored 0, 1, 2 or 3 according to the degree of distress experienced by the respondent, i.e. a little, a lot or unbearable. On totalling the scores from all questions answered, there are three categories of differentiation. Totalled scores between 0 and 2 are considered to be within the normal range (designated as non-personally disturbed or PD), totalled scores between 3 and 6 are considered to be within the borderline range (personally disturbed or PD), and totalled scores of 7 or above are considered within the psychiatric, or chronic, range (personally

ill PI). Research has demonstrated that the DSSI/sAD scale can reliably discriminate between normal and psychiatric patient groups [15].

In order to test our hypothesis regarding patients' beliefs about their health, we conducted a post hoc analysis of their MHLC scores across the three health factors—internal, powerful others and chance—according to whether their anxiety/depression scores indicated significant clinical improvement over the course of a 1-year period, i.e. from the psychiatric to normal range, or whether their scores had remained at the psychiatric level of morbidity over the same length of time. Therefore, at the 6-month and 1-year follow-ups, the differences in their MHLC scores were compared according to whether they could be categorised at the 1-year follow-up as either improved or chronic. For further comparison, the MHLC scores for patients who had remained in the normal range, as well as in the borderline range, are also included.

RESULTS

150 patients initially entered the study. Of this original sample, there were two main groups of patients who subsequently dropped out. The first group of patients dropped out after the preliminary interview and assessment, having either declined further involvement in the study, or just did not turn up to any of the classes in the programme (N=39). The other group of patients dropped out during the course of the follow-up assessments—patients who had either left the area or who were otherwise uncontactable (17 patients at the 6-month and 20 patients at the 12-month follow-up) (N=37). Therefore, at the

Table 3.3 Psychiatric morbidity at 1-year follow-up (Bedford Foulds scale)

	Baseline (N=111)	6 weeks follow-up (N=111)	6 months follow-up (N=94)	Year follow-up (N=74)
Normal (PD)	13	37	40	39
Personally disturbed (PD)	20	32	19	16
Personally ill (PI)	78	42	35	19

Chi square=54.02 (df=6). P<0.001.

Table 3.4 Comparison of anxiety and depression mean scores (Bedford Foulds scale)

	Baseline (N=111)	6 weeks follow-up (N=111)	6 months follow-up (N=94)	Year follow-up (N=74)
Anxiety scores (mean)	6.67	3.96*	3.45*	2.81*
Depression scores (mean)	4.08	1.78*	1.61*	1.52

*P <0.01 (Wilcoxon non-parametric statistical test).

1-year assessment, we only had 50% of our original sample as assessed at baseline—and in view of this rather high rate of dropouts, the analysis of results must be considered to be based on a somewhat biased sample of patients.

Table 3.3 demonstrates a significant difference between the psychiatric morbidity levels (PI) at baseline testing, and the 1-year follow-up (P <0. 001, chi-square), with 70% in the PI category initially (N=78), compared to 26% (N=19) of the remaining sample 1 year later. Table 3.4 shows the anxiety and depression scores, as measured

on the Bedford Foulds questionnaire, separately, where the mean scores assessed after the 6-week intervention were significantly lower than the baseline scores (P <0.01, Wilcoxon non-parametric), this trend continuing at the subsequent follow-up assessments.

Table 3.5 analyses the scores according to patients' clinical change a year later. 30 patients demonstrated clinical improvement at the 12-month assessment, where their questionnaire responses indicated a shift from the psychiatric level of morbidity (PI) at baseline to normal

Table 3.5 Means of locus of control scores by clinical improvement at the 12-month follow-up

	N	Internal	Powerful others	Chance
Patients who *initially* dropped out of study	39	21.73*	17.97*	17.90
Baseline testing				
Total number of patients	111	25.02	17.41	17.75
Patients whose scores remained *normal* at 1 year	9	28.56	16.67	16.56
Patients whose scores *improved* at 1 year	30	25.56*	16.92	18.23
Patients whose scores remained *borderline* (PD) at 1 year	16	25.31	16.37	14.69
Patients whose scores were at the *chronic* level (PI) at 1 year	19	23.95	18.95	20.63
Patients who *dropped out during* the study (at 6 and 12 months)	37	24.86	17.59	17.32
6-week follow-up				
Total number of patients	111	25.79	17.68	16.98
Normal at year	9	29.00	15.78	16.00
Improved at year	30	27.03**	17.59	16.56
Borderline at year	16	25.87	16.43	14.81
Chronic at year	19	24.00**	19.68	19.21
Dropped out	37	25.37	17.27	17.22
12-month follow-up				
Total number of patients	74	25.57	16.55	16.38
Normal at year	9	29.67	13.11	14.67
Improved at year	30	26.23	16.21	16.47
Borderline at year	16	26.43	15.06	14.06
Chronic at year	19	23.57	18.53	18.21

*P <0.005; **P <0.05 (independent t-tests).

levels (PD) at 1 year—termed 'improved patients'. The scores of 9 patients remained in the normal range (PD) from baseline throughout the year. Therefore, of the patients who entered the study (N=111), 12 months later, approximately one-third had improved (N=30), approximately one-third had stayed the same or deteriorated (N=35, borderline and chronic), and one-third had dropped out (N=37).

Differences between patients who improved and patients who dropped out initially

A significant difference (P <0.005) between both the baseline, and the 6-week follow-up scores (mean = 25.56, 27.03) on the internal scale of the MHLC, and the baseline internal MHLC scores of those patients who had initially dropped out (mean = 21.73) was demonstrated. This trend continued at the 6-month and 12-month follow-ups for those patients who had improved (in terms of their higher internal scores), but not at statistically significant levels. It could be argued

that the two groups of patients who dropped out (those initially, and those throughout the follow-up) are demonstrably different in their locus of control scores, and, by implication, in their attitudes to self-care—where there is a substantial difference between the mean total internal score (25.02), the mean score of the initial dropout group (21.73), and the mean score of the latter dropout group (24.86) at baseline testing.

Differences between patients who improved and patients who remained at the chronic level

In a similar fashion, the internal scores for the improved patients were also consistently higher than for those who had remained chronic (PI category), this difference only reaching statistical significance at the 6-week testing (P <0.05). On the other hand, the external scores of the chronic patients, both the chance and powerful others scores, were consistently higher than the scores for the improved patients throughout each of the follow-up assessments, although not at statistically significant levels.

Table 3.6 Analysis of demographic variables across morbidity groups

		N	Improved (%)	Chronic (%)	Dropped out (%)	Total (%)
Sex	Male	27	23	16	31	24
	Female	84	77	84	69	76
				(P <0.05)		
Age (yrs)	20–29	13	17	5	28	12
	30–39	36	43	21	18	32
	40–49	25	17	32	21	22
	50–59	20	17	21	15	18
	60+	17	7	21	18	15
				(P <0.001)		
Marital status	Single	47	47	37	36	42
	Married	40	37	37	49	36
	Div/sep/wid	24	17	26	15	22
				(P <0.01)		
Socio-economic class	Prof.	11	0	5	5	10
	Inter.	54	43	64	49	48
	N/Mskil.	31	37	26	26	28
	Manskil.	12	20	0	15	11
	Part-time	3	0	5	5	3
				(P <0.001)		
Referral	GP health centre	46	37	42	38	41
	Local GP	37	33	37	20	33
	Self	28	30	21	43	25
				(P <0.02)		

Chi-squared analysis.

Further analysis of the demographic variables between the three groups revealed significant differences (Table 3.6). A higher proportion of men and patients in the 20–29 age group dropped out, compared to those who completed the programme, and who were followed up at 12 months. The majority of the chronic patients were aged over 60 years (21%), with a higher proportion separated, divorced or widowed (26%), compared to the improved patients (17%), and the patients who dropped out (15%). The majority of the improved patients were aged between 30 and 39, with only 7% aged over 60, and nearly 50% being single. There were significant social class differences as well (P <0.001, chi-square)— nearly 70% of the chronic patients were in the upper two social classes (professional and intermediate) compared to 43% of improved patients. The highest proportion of patients who dropped out at the initial test were self referred.

DISCUSSION

Self-care is concerned with facilitating and promoting changes in patients' perceptions about themselves, and their enhanced role and responsibility in health care decision-making, as well as a more conscious involvement in the process of restoring and maintaining positive levels of well-being. Self-care relies more heavily on a systemic, or holistic, conception of health—as a multidimensional phenomenon involving interdependent physical, psychological and social aspects. The programme that we conducted at the health centre encouraged the innate capacity of individuals to help themselves through learning and applying the relaxation, breathing and meditation skills, alongside accepting greater responsibility and active involvement in their own patterns of diet, exercise, relationships, communication and the environment within which they lived and worked. The integration of self-care approaches is particularly important in general practice. Most authorities agree that anxiety-based problems are the most common psychological conditions to be found in primary care, notwithstanding difficulties of definition and classification. Various sources estimate that

approximately 10% of the population consult a doctor about tension at some time. Skegg [16] found that amongst registered patients, more than 20% of women and about 10% of men had received at least one prescription for a psychotropic drug during any one year, the figure rising to 30% amongst 45-year-old women. Our results show significant improvement in psychiatric morbidity, which was maintained at 1 year, in a representative group of patients participating in a programme that was both clinically effective and easily incorporated into the routine medical services of the health centre.

When these scores were further analysed, according to clinical progress, the results show clear differences in the health beliefs between the three groups. The low internal HLC scores of the patients who dropped out at the initial testing stage of the programme suggests that they believed that self-care practices would have minimal effect in helping them to manage their symptomatology. The consistently higher internal HLC scores of the improved patients concurs with the theoretical assumption that this group would exhibit more positive attitudes towards self-care, and take greater personal responsibility for their own health care, believing that improvement is related more to their own action than primarily to external factors. As expected, the patients who remained at the chronic level at the 1-year follow-up believed significantly more than the improved patients that external factors controlled their health, and that improved health is primarily dependent on luck and chance. There is a possibility that the influence of the demographic differences identified between the groups has exercised a confounding effect. Further work is required to understand the relationship between locus of control and age, sex and social class differences.

The goal of self-care programmes is often seen, implicitly, as primarily encouraging internal beliefs in individuals' abilities to influence and change themselves and their environment, and is supported by the bulk of research on locus of control, which has concentrated on individual differences to the exclusion of important demographic factors, e.g. economic or political differences, and can sometimes be interpreted as a subtle form of 'victim blaming'. It is vital that the advocates of self-care approaches in health do not allow such approaches to mask social, racial and economic inequalities, and to encourage a forum which justifies political and ideological differences.

However, self-care approaches are attracting increasing attention, among both professionals and the public. There are numerous cultural and historical changes which have contributed to the present emergence of self-care—the rise in chronic disease morbidity in the past two decades with the resulting shift from cure to care, an increasing awareness of the effect of lifestyle on many chronic diseases, the increasing difficulty of 'high technology' medicine to deal with long-term chronic illness alongside the increasing exploration of 'alternatives' to the philosophical assumptions of traditional Western medicine.

The introduction of the self-care programme offered a far wider range of resources to both the health care professionals and the patients at the health centre than were previously available. Self-help booklets have been used successfully in general practice for other problems, and their use in commonly occurring conditions has been advocated [17]. The extensive educational materials were integral to the programme, as were the numerous self-help strategies which were taught and encouraged, the emphasis being on practical skills, and were not physician/therapist dependent. In addition, the social support network generated by the group activity was not inconsiderable. Rather than specialist referrals, such programmes can offer a greater continuity of community care for patients by providing a combination of educational, preventative and clinical modes of health care. With the increasing interest in holistic approaches, the provision of adult classes, study groups and reliable self-care information and materials is even more necessary as an integral part of normal primary care services.

One major criticism of this approach has been its unsuitability in general practice due to the shortage of time available to the GP to run such programmes. The role of psychologists as teachers of self-management skills alongside a greater preventative focus of intervention is being increasingly recognised [18].

Our study demonstrated a predictive relationship between health values and beliefs and clinical improvement. It appears that an inner directed or internal orientation is vital for the successful utilisation of self-care and self-help approaches in health. Further research is needed to investigate the relationship between changes in the health values and beliefs, the causation and prognosis of disease and the maintenance of positive health.

SUMMARY

In conclusion, the major findings of the study are as follows:

1. A self-care programme has been demonstrated to be effective in helping patients in general practice cope with symptoms of psychosocial stress.
2. Patients with higher scores on measures relating to internal locus of control more often remained in and benefited from the programme.
3. Significant socio-demographic differences were demonstrated which characterised the patients who benefited from the programme.
4. There was a highly consistent, but non-significant, trend for patients with external beliefs to benefit less often from the programme.

REFERENCES

1. Levin L. S. Self-care in health. A. Rev. Publ. Hlth 4, 181–201, 1983.
2. Teare Skinner P. Skills not pills: learning to cope with anxiety symptoms. J. R. Coll. Gen. Pract. 34, 258–260, 1984.
3. Kiely B. G., McPherson I. G. Stress self-help in primary care: a controlled trial evaluation. J. R. Coll. Gen. Pract. 36, 307–309, 1986.
4. Long C. G., Bourne V. Linking professional and self help resources for anxiety management: a community project. J. R. Coll. Gen. Pract. 37, 199–201, 1987.
5. Butcher P., de Clive Lowe S. Strategies for living: teaching psychological self help as adult education. Br. J. Med. Psychiat. 58, 275–283, 1985.
6. Wallston K. A., Wallston B. S. Development of multidimensional health locus of control scales. Hlth Educ. Monogr. 6, 160–170, 1978.
7. Levenson H. Multidimensional locus of control in psychi-

atric patients. J. consult. clin. Psychiat. 41, 397–404, 1973

8. Strickland B. R. Internal external experience and health related behaviours. J. Consult. Clin. Psychol. 46, 1192–1211, 1978.

9. Wallston K. S. A., Wallston B. S. Who is responsible for your health? The construct of health locus of control. In: Social psychology of health and illness (edited by Sanders A. and Suls A.). Lawrence Erlbaum, Hillsdale, N. H. , 1982.

10. Pietroni P., McLean J., Walton N. A self care programme in general practice—a feasibility study. The Practitioner 231, 1226–1230, 1987.

11. Everly G. S., Rosenfeld R. The nature and treatment of the stress response. Plenum, New York, 1981.

12. McLean J. The use of relaxation techniques in general practice. The Practitioner 230, 1079–1084, 1986.

13. Sheikh A. (ed.) Imagery—current theory, research and application. Wiley, London, 1983.

14. Ballentyne R. Diet and nutrition—a holistic approach. Himalayan Institute, Pa, 1978.

15. Bedford A., Foulds G. A. A new personal disturbance scale (DSSI/sAD). Br. J. Soc. Clin. Psychiat. 15, 387–394, 1976.

16. Skegg D. , Doll R., Perry J. The use of medicines in general practice. Br. Med. J. 1, 1561–1563, 1977.

17. Anderson J. E. , Morrell D. C. , Avery A. J., Watkins C. J. Evaluation of a patient education manual. Br. Med. J. 281, 924–926, 1980.

18. Espie C. A., White J. The effectiveness of psychological intervention in primary care: a comparative analysis of outcome ratings. J. R. Coll. Gen. Pract. 36, 310–312, 1986.

A CONTROLLED TRIAL OF SELF-CARE CLASSES IN GENERAL PRACTICE, TAUGHT BY STAFF MEMBERS WITH A SHORT TRAINING, TO LONG-TERM USERS OF ANXIOLYTIC, HYPNOTIC AND ANTI-DEPRESSANT DRUGS

Clare Harrison
Peter Davies
Patrick Pietroni

A longitudinal randomised controlled trial assessing the effect of self-care classes on the general health, consultation and prescription rates of long-term users of anxiolytic, hypnotic and anti-depressant (AHA) drugs in general practice is described. The classes were educational in their approach and were taught by practice staff who had received a short training. The classes significantly decreased patients' insomnia and, to a lesser degree, their somatic symptoms, with the benefits diminishing over the following year. Whilst there was no change in consultation rates, prescription rates of all participants decreased significantly over the 12 months of the study. Possible implications of the findings are offered. It is proposed that self-care classes taught by practice staff could provide general practitioners with a valuable means of supporting and helping long-term AHA drug users.

INTRODUCTION

Over the last few decades, the use of all psychotropic drugs in the long-term management of patients presenting in general practice with psychological symptoms has become a prominent issue (Catalan & Gath 1985). Although the use of psychotropic drugs has decreased since the 1970s, every year 14% of adults take a benzodiazepine and 40 million prescriptions for psychotropic drugs are issued (Medawar 1984). In 1975, these drugs cost the Department of Health £22 057 000 (Department of Health 1977), approximately 15.3% of the annual drug budget (Trethowan 1975).

The cost of these drugs is not merely financial. Side-effects include drowsiness, sedation and impairment of memory, sensory functions, perception, and cognitive and motor skills (Clayton 1976, Greenblatt et al 1983, Angus & Romney 1984, Smiley & Moskowitz 1986). Risks of dependency and problems of withdrawal have been widely documented (Petursson & Lader 1981, Ashton 1984) and seem to be greatest among long-term users (more than 12 months) (American Psychiatric Association 1990). Evidence collected towards the end of the 1970s suggested that sedative hypnotics maintained their therapeutic effect for only between 3 and 14 days (White House Office of Drug Policy and National Institute on Drug Abuse 1979) and that tranquillisers and benzodiazepines used in the treatment of anxiety rarely had an active effect for more than 4 months (Committee on the review of medicines 1980).

Concern over the use of psychotropic drugs has led to a search for viable alternatives, many of which have, to some degree, embraced a philosophy of self-care, described by Levin (1983) as 'those activities individuals undertake in promoting their own health, preventing their own disease, limiting their own illness and restoring their own health'. As such, non-drug interventions have often adopted an educational as well as, or rather than, a therapeutic approach. Studies in general practice introducing anxiety management (Cormack & Sinnott 1984, Skinner 1984, Butler et al 1987, Lindsay et al 1987), cognitive therapy (Blackburn et al 1981, Teasdale et al 1984, Salkovskis et al 1986, Lindsay et al 1987) behaviour therapy (Koch 1979, Robson et al 1984, Blakey, 1986) and/or counselling (Anderson & Hasler 1979, Gath & Catalan 1986) have generally concluded that such interventions can be beneficial to some long-term psychotropic drug users, but are less effective for patients being prescribed major tranquillisers and anti-psychotics (Woodward & Jones 1980, Gath & Catalan 1986, Butler et al 1987, Long & Bourne 1987). These studies have focused almost exclusively on patients presenting with one particular psychological symptom, such as anxiety or depression, and on one form of intervention with any given patient, such as cognitive or behaviour therapy. They have depended on professional experts to provide these interventions.

AIM

The aim of the present study was to assess the effect of classes, incorporating a number of different self-care approaches, on the health, consultation and prescription rates of patients in general practice who were long-term users of anxiolytic, hypnotic and anti-depressant drugs, when classes were taught by practice staff who had received a short training.

METHOD

The study was a longitudinal, randomised, controlled trial involving six general practices in the Greater London area. In the light of the research referenced above, it was decided to limit the criteria for participation to patients who had received a prescription for an anxiolytic, hypnotic and/or anti-depressant drug from their general practitioner on at least three different occasions over the previous 12 months, and to exclude those who were taking major tranquillisers or anti-psychotics. All of the patients were aged 18 years or over.

Study intervention

The classes had been developed over a number of years as part of a larger research project exploring different ways of delivering primary health care (Pietroni 1992). Each class offered both a presentation and then discussion concerning experiences of stress, followed by teaching of a relaxation technique. They are described in an earlier study (Pietroni et al 1987) on which the present study is based. In that study, they were found to lead to a 30% decrease in the medication and to improve, greatly or to some extent, the symptoms of patients suffering from a wide range of stress-related symptoms and illnesses.

Key workers

The classes were taught by people involved in the practices (two community psychiatric nurses, one practice nurse and health adviser, and one doctor's wife) and, where this was not possible, by people who had some experience in self-care classes. It was hoped that by providing someone already involved with the practice with the skills to teach such classes, practices would have the option of continuing to offer such classes to any patient group at minimum cost and inconvenience. The 'key workers' all received 2 days' intensive training in the classes, followed by a series of six supervision sessions held during the period in which they were teaching. The emphasis of the classes was educational rather than therapeutic. On completion, each key worker filled in a feedback form concerning his/her training in and teaching of the classes.

Participants

282 patients were identified as being aged 18 years or over and having received a prescription for an anti-depressant, hypnotic and/or anxiolytic drug from their general practitioner on at least three different occasions over the previous 12 months. 166 (59%) agreed to participate, of whom 32% were men and 68% women; their ages ranged from 24 to 85 years, with a mean of 61 years (SD=13. 25). 52% were married, 20% single, 16% widowed and 12% divorced or separated. 86% were British, 8% Irish and 6% were of other nationalities. According to the Registrar General's Classification, 2% were from social class I, 24% from II, 24% from IIIN, 20% from IIIM, 3% from IV and none from V. In addition, 7% were unemployed, 16% said they were a housewife and 4% gave no response. 19% of the patients said they had first been prescribed an anxiolytic, hypnotic or anti-depressant (AHA) drug up to 2 years ago, 16% between 2 and 5 years ago, 16% between 5 and 10 years ago and 49% more than 10 years ago.

Questionnaires and outcome measures

All patients were asked to fill in two questionnaires:

- the 28-item General Health Questionnaire (GHQ) (Goldberg & Hillier 1979)

- the Hospital Anxiety and Depression Scale (HADS) (Zigmond & Snaith 1983).

These questionnaires were completed on four different occasions over a 12-month period. The first occasion (T_1) was at the beginning of the study. Patients were then randomly allocated into one of two groups. Members of the control group (n=84) were sent the questionnaires on three further occasions. Members of the experimental group (n=82), in addition to being sent the questionnaires, were invited and recommended by a letter from their GP to attend a series of self-care classes at the practice. This letter made no reference to the questionnaires and the study in which they were participating. All patients filled in the questionnaires for the second time (T_2) immediately after the self-care classes had finished, approximately 3 months after the commencement of the study. Questionnaires were then completed at 6 months (T_3) and 12 months (T_4) from time T_1. In addition to the GHQ and HADS, all patients filled in a questionnaire at time T_1 which provided demographic information and details of how long ago any doctor had first prescribed an AHA drug.

Information was also collected on the consultation and prescription rates of the sample, for both the 12 months prior to the study and the 12 months of the study period. Prescription rates were collected for both the number of drug items prescribed overall and, separately, the number of AHA drug items.

Analysis

Of the 82 patients invited to attend the classes, 47 attended no classes and 35 attended at least one class. For the purposes of analysis, therefore, patients were divided into one of three groups:

1. Group I—those who were not invited to the classes (the control group (n=84).
2. Group IIa—those who were invited but did not attend any of the classes (n=47).
3. Group IIb—those who were invited and attended between one and six of the classes (n=35).

Table 3.7 Attendance of the self-care classes by patients in group IIb

Class no.	No. attended	% attended
1	30	85.7
2	27	77.1
3	25	71.4
4	20	57.1
5	24	68.6
6	21	60.0

Table 3.7 illustrates the number of patients from group IIb who attended each of the six self-care classes and the variation in attendance rates.

Analysis was carried out on a mainframe computer using the statistical package SPSSx. A one-way analysis of variance (repeated measures) was the main statistical test used. Use of a two-way analysis of variance was limited to group by doctor, as there were no patients in some of the categories when applying this test to other variables. A significance level of 0. 05 was adopted throughout.

RESULTS

Questionnaires

Response rates to the three sets of follow-up questionnaires were as follows

1. Time T_2 82.5% (137/166)
2. Time T_3 90.1% (145/161)
3. Time T_4 91.0% (142/156).

No significant difference was found between those allocated to the control group (group I) and the experimental group (group II) in the severity of symptoms as measured on the GHQ and HADS, at the commencement of the study, time T_1. There were also no significant differences at time T_1 between those who subsequently chose to attend none of the classes (group IIa) and those who attended up to six of the self-care classes (group IIb).

122 of the initial sample of 166 (74%) completed the questionnaires on all four occasions. Analysis showed there to be no significant differences between the scores of this group, for whom the questionnaire data was complete, and

the whole sample (n=166) at time T_1. So that data can be compared for the same group of people over the four time periods, results of the questionnaires given below are for this smaller group. In terms of the distribution of patients between the three groups, this changed as follows:

	Group I	Group IIa	Group IIb
n=166	84	47	35
n=122	69 (82.1%)	25 (53.2%)	28 (80.0%)

Analyses indicated a significant difference in the GHQ anxiety and insomnia scores of participants from the three different groups across the four different time periods (p=0.028). As illustrated in Table 3.8, the scores of those in group IIb decreased significantly at T_2 and gradually increased up to T_4. A similar pattern was found in the somatic symptom scores which approached significance (p=0.053). These contributed to a significant difference in the total GHQ scores of people from the three different groups across time (p=0.034).

No significant differences were found by group in the social dysfunction and severe depression scores as measured by the GHQ, nor in either the anxiety or depression measures of the HAD Scale.

Neither were any significant differences found over the four time periods by patient age, sex, social class, practice attended and time since first prescription of an AHA drug.

Further analysis of the questionnaire scores was carried out to try and determine whether or not there was a significant difference in the degree to which the scores of those in group IIb decreased according to the number of classes they had attended. It was not worthwhile carrying out analyses on each of the six sub-groups of group

Table 3.8 Questionnaire results by group from a two-way analysis of variance

Group	Variable	Mean (SD) at time T_1	T_2	T_3	T_4	FOR ENTIRE POPULATION Between-subjects p= By group	Within-subjects p=	interaction p=
I	GHQ							
	Somatic Symptoms	1.75 (1.97)	2.16 (2.27)	2.06 (2.16)	1.62 (2.24)	.843	.931	.053
	Anxiety & Insomnia	1.90 (2.27)	1.96 (2.46)	1.84 (2.45)	1.65 (2.33)	.754	.853	.028
	Social Dysfunction	2.13 (2.32)	1.91 (2.35)	1.96 (2.48)	1.74 (2.36)	.985	.712	.303
	Severe Depression	1.15 (2.16)	1.15 (2.10)	1.19 (2.19)	0.99 (2.00)	.561	.590	.393
	Total	6.93 (7.24)	7.17 (7.76)	7.04 (7.99)	6.00 (7.83)	.993	.902	.034
	HADS							
	Anxiety	8.97 (5.75)	8.26 (5.38)	8.81 (5.76)	8.20 (5.82)	.569	.847	.767
	Depression	6.57 (4.93)	6.79 (4.88)	7.12 (5.21)	6.68 (5.35)	.772	.486	.861
IIa	GHQ							
	Somatic Symptoms	2.28 (2.41)	2.52 (2.38)	2.48 (2.24)	2.44 (2.66)			
	Anxiety & Insomnia	1.96 (2.11)	2.60 (2.68)	2.36 (2.75)	2.28 (2.54)			
	Social Dysfunction	2.16 (2.46)	2.44 (2.45)	2.20 (2.55)	2.16 (2.73)			
	Severe Depression	0.84 (1.43)	0.84 (1.72)	0.84 (1.68)	1.08 (2.10)			
	Total	7.24 (5.67)	8.40 (7.80)	7.88 (7.55)	7.96 (8.60)			
	HADS							
	Anxiety	9.80 (4.98)	10.16 (5.85)	9.48 (6.13)	9.64 (5.26)			
	Depression	6.57 (4.93)	6.79 (4.88)	7.12 (5.21)	6.68 (5.35)			
IIb	GHQ							
	Somatic Symptoms	2.21 (1.97)	1.39 (1.91)	1.82 (2.06)	2.11 (2.46)			
	Anxiety & Insomnia	2.75 (2.30)	2.00 (2.06)	2.18 (2.44)	2.43 (2.74)			
	Social Dysfunction	2.32 (2.13)	1.82 (2.18)	2.07 (2.19)	2.21 (2.41)			
	Severe Depression	1.04 (1.45)	0.89 (1.83)	0.75 (1.60)	1.11 (2.08)			
	Total	8.32 (5.68)	6.11 (6.30)	6.82 (6.70)	7.86 (8.11)			
	HADS							
	Anxiety	10.64 (4.67)	10.25 (4.21)	10.50 (4.72)	10.29 (5.25)			
	Depression	6.18 (4.24)	6.46 (4.09)	7.21 (4.63)	6.82 (4.72)			

Table 3.9 Consultation, overall prescription and anxiolytic, hypnotic and anti-depressant (AHA) drug rates by group and by doctor (one-way analysis of variance)

Group	Variable	12 months pre-study Mean (SD)	12 months post-study Mean (SD)	FOR ENTIRE POPULATION Between-subjects p= By group	Within-subjects p=	Interaction p=
I	Consultations	1.71 (2.05)	1.70 (2.31)	.647	.249	.681
	All prescriptions	8.07 (7.53)	7.31 (6.91)	.807	.001	.598
	AHA Pres.	2.81 (1.91)	2.42 (2.68)	.490	.000	.538
IIa	Consultations	1.49 (1.35)	1.34 (1.09)			
	All prescriptions	8.74 (7.62)	7.26 (6.04)			
	AHA Pres.	3.11 (2.72)	2.38 (2.47)			
IIb	Consultations	1.45 (1.66)	1.18 (1.27)			
	All prescriptions	7.59 (4.69)	6.53 (4.76)			
	AHA Pres.	2.56 (1.67)	1.85 (1.30)			
Practice No.				**By doctor**		
1	Consultations	0.58 (0.63)	0.71 (1.13)	.000	.662	.064
	All prescriptions	6.88 (5.60)	4.14 (4.22)	.001	.000	.087
	AHA Pres.	2.17 (2.22)	1.47 (1.98)	.484	.000	.156
2	Consultations	1.49 (0.97)	1.75 (0.93)			
	All prescriptions	10.16 (7.24)	7.95 (4.92)			
	AHA Pres.	3.26 (1.83)	2.03 (1.27)			
3	Consultations	2.23 (2.28)	2.21 (2.28)			
	All prescriptions	5.69 (3.84)	5.33 (5.28)			
	AHA Pres.	2.57 (2.21)	2.11 (3.18)			
4	All prescriptions	10.57 (9.31)	9.94 (7.40)			
	AHA Pres.	2.93 (2.04)	2.89 (2.34)			
5	Consultations	0.87 (0.68)	0.26 (0.36)			
	All prescriptions	11.38 (8.92)	9.21 (7.90)			
	AHA Pres.	3.57 (2.72)	2.43 (2.04)			
6	All prescriptions	5.47 (2.70)	5.36 (3.30)			
	AHA Pres.	2.49 (1.32)	2.18 (1.67)			

IIb, as numbers were too small. However, an analysis in which patients from group IIb were divided according to whether they attended between one and three (n=6), four and five (n=9) or all six of the classes (n=13) indicated that there were no significant differences in the degree to which their GHQ anxiety and insomnia scores decreased (p=0.343), nor their GHQ somatic symptoms scores (p=0.466), nor their GHQ total scores (p=0.685).

Consultation rates

Consultation data, compiled from patients' notes, was found to be incomplete for practice numbers four and six and therefore was excluded from analyses of consultation rates.

Consultation rates did not differ significantly by group, although there was a significant difference between the doctors in their individual consulting patterns (p=0.000) as illustrated in Table 3.9.

There were no significant differences in consultation rates according to age group, sex, social class or length of time since participants had first been prescribed an AHA drug.

Prescription rates

Both the overall prescription rate (p=0.001) and the AHA drug rate (p=0.000) of *all* participants decreased significantly during the 12 months of the study. This represented an average decrease of 12.5% in the overall prescription rate and 19.4% in the AHA drug rate. Although prescribing rates for each of the doctors varied significantly both for overall prescription rates (p=0.034) and AHA drug rates (p=0.002), all doctors decreased their prescribing rates by the same degree.

Table 3.10 Decrease in overall prescription and anxiolytic, hypnotic and anti-depressant (AHA) drug rates over the study period by time since first AHA prescription

Time since first AHA prescription	Mean rate 12-months pre-study	Mean rate 12-months post-study
Less than 5 years		
All prescriptions	8.69	6.92
AHA drugs	2.34	1.70
More than 5 years		
All prescriptions	8.22	7.71
AHA drugs	3.01	2.53

There were no significant differences in the extent to which overall prescription and AHA drug rates decreased according to group, age, sex, social class or time since first AHA prescription.

Although prescription rates of participants who had been taking AHA drugs for more than 5 years decreased to the same extent, the overall AHA drug rate of this group was 37.08% higher than for those who had been taking AHA drugs for less than 5 years. The corresponding figure for their overall prescription rate was 2.08%. Table 3.10 gives details of the reductions in overall prescription and AHA drug rates by time since first AHA prescription.

DISCUSSION

The study looked at the feasibility and possible benefits when key workers with a minimum of training provided self-care classes for a group of long-term AHA drug users in a general practice setting. The sample was predominantly made up of elderly female patients who had been on AHA drugs for over 5 years. From feedback obtained from the key workers, many of the patients also had considerable physical disabilities and illnesses. Comments from practice staff indicated that the sample included many of their 'most difficult' patients.

Response and attendance rates

The high response rate to the questionnaires indicated a keen motivation, but this was not extended to class attendance. Whilst care was taken in the scheduling of the classes, many were held during the evenings of winter months, which, given the characteristics of the patient group, may have contributed to the low attendance rate. A further explanation may be gained from comments to the key workers and research assistant which suggested that at least some patients' willingness to participate was driven by what they perceived to be their doctor's interests rather than by their own. Attendance might have been greater if the patients had been told that the classes were part of the study for which they were completing questionnaires. This was deliberately avoided, however, in order to avoid possible bias in their questionnaire responses.

Benefits of the classes

The feedback forms completed by the key workers indicated that what the patients gained from the classes above all was a greater awareness and insight into their lives and lifestyles and how these affected their sense of well-being. This awareness, it was felt, laid the foundations for potential development and changes. From the results of the General Health Questionnaires, the classes improved the patients' anxiety and insomnia and, to a lesser extent, their somatic symptoms. Since the anxiety scores from the Hospital Anxiety and Depression Scale did not decrease significantly, one may speculate that it was primarily, if not exclusively, the patients' insomnia which improved as a result of the classes, rather than their anxiety. The classes had no obvious effect on patients' symptoms of depression or social dysfunction.

The classes introduced a number of different approaches to self-care in the hope that they would be of benefit to patients experiencing a wide range of symptoms and that patients would be able to incorporate into their own lives those aspects of the classes which meant most to them personally. The experience of the present study suggests that when running the classes for long-term AHA drug users, it may be useful to decrease the amount of material introduced. One way of doing this would be to allocate more time to learning and practising relaxation techniques and less time to information-giving. Since the improvements in insomnia and somatic symptoms that the patients gained from the classes in the present study did not seem to be maintained at the 12-month follow-up, it may also be useful to increase the number of classes offered or to offer follow-up sessions to those who have attended the classes. Comments from the key workers support these two recommendations.

Further analysis of the patients in group IIb suggested that there was no significant difference in the degree to which their symptoms improved according to how many of the classes they attended. Although the numbers involved in this analysis are too small to enable one to draw any reliable conclusions, the results do suggest that attending classes had a therapeutic effect for all, regardless of the number of classes attended. From this, it is possible to speculate that the content of each class was comprehensive enough in itself for participants to gain something without having to attend previous or subsequent classes. The support they may have felt from meeting with other people, from having a key worker who showed a genuine and practical interest in their well-being, or from simply knowing that the classes were continuing to run and were available to them, may also have contributed to participants' increased sense of well-being.

In view of the potential benefits gained from the classes, it would be useful to find ways of encouraging greater attendance of the classes.

Consultation and prescription rates

The lack of change in the consultation rates may be accounted for both in terms of patients continuing to make appointments to see their general practitioner and general practitioners calling patients in for regular consultations. This may be more likely with this particular patient group who receive regular prescriptions.

Prescription rates for *all* the patients participating in the study reduced significantly over the 12 months of the study period, including those for AHA drugs. There were no significant changes in the number of times the patients consulted their general practitioner.

Participation in the study may have provided sufficient intervention in itself to effect patients' consumption of the drugs, which might imply that a visible review of the patients by the doctors on a regular basis may itself help reduce prescription rates. Similarly it may have affected the attitudes and behaviour of the general practitioners. This is supported in a study by Harris et al (1984) which showed that when doctors' attention is simply drawn to their prescribing rates and patterns, a significant reduction in their prescribing habits occurs.

However, other factors also need to be taken into account. On a national level, general practitioners have been under increasing pressure to decrease their prescriptions not only of psychotropic drugs, but of all drug groups. The Prescription Pricing Authority's quarterly production of Prescribing Analyses and Cost (PACT) figures illustrates this pressure.

Key workers as teachers

Of the three practices which provided their own key workers, all have gone on to run further classes at their respective health centres. They felt that the training they received in the self-care classes was sufficient and that they particularly benefited from the supervision sessions provided whilst they were running the classes at their practices. As was stressed in their training, the key workers confirmed that their ability to teach the classes was substantially enhanced if they themselves practised the relaxation techniques and were personally committed to the material they were teaching. It was also enhanced if they had done additional reading around the subjects. In their feedback, many key workers said they would have liked to know something of the patients' physical illnesses and disabilities prior to teaching the classes.

CONCLUSION

From the experiences of the present study, it would seem that self-care classes have a valuable contribution to make to the management of AHA drug users in a primary health care setting, and that they can be run effectively and efficiently by practice staff who have received minimal training. The present classes had particular benefit for patients experiencing insomnia and, to a lesser degree, somatic symptoms. It is proposed that with minimal revision of the classes, their effect could be both longer lasting and of benefit to patients experiencing a broader spectrum of symptoms. Reducing the number of approaches to self-care covered, allowing more time to practise relaxation techniques, ensuring that the teachers are themselves personally committed to the material they are sharing, and offering some form of follow-up support to those who attend the classes may all enrich future self-care classes offered to this patient group.

ACKNOWLEDGEMENTS

The authors gratefully acknowledge the cooperation of the doctors whose practices were involved, the key workers who ran the classes and Dr David Peters for training the key workers. They are also grateful to Dr Doreen Asso and Michael Davey at Goldsmith's College, London.

REFERENCES

American Psychiatric Association (task force report) 1990 Benzodiazepine dependence, toxicity and abuse. American Psychiatric Association, Washington D. C.

Anderson S, Hasler J C 1979 Counselling in general practice. Journal of the Royal College of General Practitioners 29 pp 352–356

Angus W R, Romney D M 1984 The effect of diazepam on patients' memory. Journal of Clinical Pharmacology 4 pp 203–206

Ashton H 1984 Benzodiazepine withdrawal—an unfinished story. British Medical Journal 288 pp 1135–1140

Blackburn I M et al 1981 The efficacy of cognitive therapy in depression: a treatment trial using cognitive therapy and pharmacotherapy, each alone and in combination. British Journal for Psychiatry 139 pp 181–189

Blakey R 1986 Psychological treatment in general practice: its effects on patients and their families. Journal of the Royal College of General Practitioners 36 pp 209–211

Butler G, Cullington A, Hibbert G, Klines I, Gelder M 1987 Anxiety management for persistent generalised anxiety. British Journal of Psychiatry 151 pp 535–542

Catalan J, Gath D H 1985 Benzodiazepines in general practices: time for a decision. British Medical Journal 290 pp 1374–1376

Clayton A B 1976 The effects of psychotropic drugs upon driving related skills. Human Factors 18 pp 241–252

Committee on the review of medicines 1980 Systematic review of the benzodiazepines. British Medical Journal 280 pp 910–912

Cormack M A, Sinnott A 1984 Psychological alternatives to long-term benzodiazepine use. Journal of the Royal College of General Practitioners 33 pp 279–281

Department of Health 1977 Health and personal social services. Statistics for England. HMSO, London

Gath D, Catalan J 1986 The treatment of emotional disorders in general practice: psychological methods versus medication. Journal of Psychosomatic Research 30 pp 381–386

Goldberg D P, Hillier V F 1979 A scaled version of the general health questionnaire. Psychology and Medicine 9 pp 139–145

Greenblatt D J, Shader R I, Abernethy D R 1983 Drug therapy: current status of benzodiazepines (second of two parts). New England Journal of Medicine 309 pp 410–416

Harris C M, Jarman B, Woodman E, White P, Fry J S 1984 Prescribing—a suitable case for treatment. Royal College of General Practitioners Occasional Paper 24

Koch H C H 1979 Evaluation of behaviour therapy intervention in general practice. Journal of the Royal College of General Practitioners 29 pp 337–340

Levin L S 1983 Self-care in health. Annual Review of Public Health 4 pp 181–201

Lindsay W R, Gamsu C V, McLaughlin E, Hood E M, Espie C A 1987 A controlled trial of treatments for generalised anxiety. British Journal of Clinical Psychology 26 pp 3–15

Long C G, Bourne V 1987 Linking professional and self-help resources for anxiety management: a community project. Journal of the Royal College of General Practitioners 37 pp 199–201

Medawar C 1984 Social audit: the wrong kind of medicine? Hodder & Stoughton, London

Petursson H, Lader M H 1981 Withdrawal from long-term benzodiazepine treatment. British Medical Journal 283 pp 643–645

Pietroni P 1992 Wates Foundation primary health care research project: final report. Marylebone Centre Trust, London

Pietroni P, McLean J, Walton N G 1987 A self-care programme in general practice: a feasibility study. The Practitioner 231 pp 1226–1230

Robson M H, France R, Bland M 1984 Clinical psychologist in primary care: controlled clinical and economic evaluation. British Medical Journal 288 pp 1805–1808

Salkovskis P M, Jones D R O, Clark D M 1986 Respiratory control in the treatment of panic attacks: replication and extension with concurrent measurement of behaviour and pCO_2. British Journal of Psychiatry 148 pp 526–532

Skinner P T 1984 Skills not pills: learning to cope with anxiety symptoms. Journal of Royal College of General Practitioners 34 pp 258–260

Smiley A, Moskowitz H 1986 Effects of long-term administration of buspirone and diazepam on driver steering control. American Journal of Medicine 80 pp 22–29

Teasdale J, Fennell M J V, Hibbert G A, Amies P L 1984 Cognitive therapy for major depressive disorder in primary care. British Journal of Psychiatry 144 pp 400–406

Trethowan W H 1975 Pills for personal problems. British Medical Journal 3 pp 749–751

White House Office of Drug Policy and National Institute on Drug Abuse 1979

Woodward R, Jones R B 1980 Cognitive restructuring treatment: a controlled trial with anxious patients. Behavioural Research Therapy 18 pp 401–407

Zigmond A S, Snaith R P 1983 The hospital anxiety and depression scale. Acta Psychiatry Scand 67 pp 361–370

4

Extending the range of clinical interventions

INTRODUCTION

The range and number of therapies now available to patients is greater than ever before. In part this is the result of the development of medical technology which is constantly producing new and better forms of diagnosis and treatment for conditions ranging from cancer to the common cold. Equally important, however, is the recognition of the role of psychosocial factors in determining health which has led to an understanding of the importance of and potential benefits arising from counselling, and other forms of one to one support. It is also the case that what were once termed 'alternative' or 'complementary' therapies are now firmly part of the range of interventions which people call upon to help resolve their perceived ill-health. All these approaches to the treatment of ill-health are adopted at the Marylebone Health Centre and are a natural, indeed necessary, part of the 'whole person' approach which the Health Centre practises.

Since nearly one million people a year seek out a complementary therapist of one kind or another, and since there are an estimated 30000 complementary therapists practising in Great Britain, the so-called complementary therapies clearly have a place in this extended range of interventions. Yet it is still the case that complementary therapies are not widely available on the NHS, and this despite the fact that there is evidence to suggest that significant numbers of GPs are actively interested in these approaches as clinical interventions. Pietroni (The interface between complementary medicine and general practice, p. 108) suggests that this is in part to do with the nature of the profession which acts as a tribe attempting to protect itself from a perceived threat. In part also this is the product of a good deal of ignorance and misunderstanding. For example, Dr Pietroni argues that the British Medical Association report on complementary therapies was poorly researched. No member of the committee of inquiry was a complementary therapist and, as a result, the committee was not fully competent to investigate the field. Even so, the report did recognise the weight of descriptive evidence to support the successful use of particular complementary interventions such as the use of acupuncture to relieve pain and osteopathy in the treatment of back complaints. Given this, it seems strange that such hostility still remains.

However, it must be recognised that extending the range of clinical interventions available to the patient is not of itself a positive act. Just as the mechanising of medicine may be seen to have had detrimental effects on the type of health service provided, so making ever more therapies available without any real understanding of what it is hoped they may achieve, will not necessarily be of benefit to either the patient or the Health Service as a whole. Rather, it is important to evaluate the usefulness of all therapies so that resources may be allocated effectively and the best possible service provided. Just as doctors need to look at their referral and prescribing rates, so other clinicians need to investigate the genuine improvements that their therapies may effect.

Four such studies were carried out at the Marylebone Health Centre which aimed to investigate the usefulness and applicability to a general practice setting of traditional Chinese medicine (TCM), massage, counselling and a musculoskeletal clinic run by a GP with training in osteopathy, medical acupuncture and intralesional injections. Each of these clinical interventions was available to patients on the NHS and referrals were usually carried out by the GP. In the case of counselling (Counselling in an inner city general practice: analysis of its use and uptake, Webber et al, p. 132), referrals were sometimes carried out by one of the other clinicians. The studies into TCM (Traditional Chinese medicine in general practice:

an audit of one year's referrals, Desser et al, p. 112) and the musculoskeletal clinic (Musculoskeletal clinic in general practice: a study of one year's referrals, Peters et al, p. 138) showed that it was possible to use these interventions cheaply and to the added benefit of the patient. In the case of the musculoskeletal clinic, referrals from the practice to hospital physiotherapy and rheumatology departments were lower than national figures would have predicted, although orthopaedic referrals in general were not significantly lower. The study into the use and uptake of counselling stressed the need for flexibility in the counselling interaction if the service was to be as useful as possible. The Marylebone Health Centre was able to provide this by the use of a social work student, a trainee counsellor and a befriending service in addition to the 'official' counsellor. For example, at times it was deemed useful for the patient to receive support in a more general and on-going sense and the befriending service was able to meet this need. It also became clear that many of the people referred to the counsellor were in need of information about local support and social services and this too could best be provided by members of the befriending group who were themselves local.

The report on the introduction and use of massage (Massage: a review of its introduction as a therapeutic intervention in general practice, McCormack & Pietroni, p. 119) was of a more subjective nature but nevertheless demonstrated that a very high proportion of those patients who had received massage at the Health Centre believed that they had received a high level of benefit from it. It also indicated that massage was an effective intervention for a very wide variety of complaints ranging from stress and depression to chronic pain.

One aspect to emerge from all the reports is the importance of good interprofessional communication if multidisciplinary approaches to health care are to be effective. For example, it was recognised that GPs often made referrals to the TCM practitioner as a last resort, when they felt that they had nothing to lose, rather than on the basis of a clear understanding of the diagnostic methods and healing potentialities of TCM. As a result it was possible for the TCM practitioner to resent these referrals, feeling that he had lost his clinical autonomy. Insufficient communication between practitioners was also deemed to be important in the continued rates of referral to hospital orthopaedic departments despite the presence of the in-house musculoskeletal clinic. In the case of massage it was recognised that this intervention was very widely applicable and that rather than having one massage therapist, other co-workers, especially practice nurses, were in a good position to integrate the use of massage into their own clinical practices.

An extended range of clinical interventions can be introduced successfully into a primary health care setting with benefits for both the patient and the practice as a whole since it has invariably been found that the integrated use of these therapies leads to a saving of resources which can then be effectively reallocated. A similar finding emerged from the work of Bridge et al (Relaxation and imagery in the treatment of breast cancer, p. 146). The research was undertaken to see if stress could be alleviated in women with early breast cancer by the use of relaxation and/or relaxation and imagery techniques. Using the profile of mood states questionnaires as a means of evaluating stress and anxiety, the authors found that relaxation techniques which concentrated on individual muscle groups did indeed reduce stress but that stress was reduced even further when this technique was used with an approach in which the women were also encouraged to imagine peaceful scenes. It was stressed to the women taking part in the study that these scenes were a resource which they could draw upon whenever they liked, and in this way the technique may be seen as one which empowers the individual and encourages her to believe that she can contribute to the management of her illness. Whether this belief, which suggests a high internal health locus of control, is common to many of the people who use 'complementary' therapies is unclear. Harrison et al (The expectations, health beliefs and behaviour of patients seeking homoeopathic and conventional medicine, p. 153) have shown that this is the case for patients attending a dermatological or rheumatological clinic seeking homoeopathic rather than conventional medi-cine. However they doubted that these findings could be applied to other groups seeking other forms of 'complementary' therapies. Either way it was clear from Bridge et al (p. 146) that relaxation techniques did indeed have a role to play in the management of stress in women being treated for early breast cancer.

That the mind and the body are inextricably linked is a notion that few would now question. Many of the 'complementary' and other therapies in the extended range of clinical interventions recognise this to be the case and work on the premise that by helping the mind so you will help the body. Yet a holistic approach to life recognises the importance and interrelatedness not only of these two aspects of human beings, but also of the spirit. As Dr Pietroni points out ('Spiritual' interventions in a general practice setting, p. 157) the definitions of the soul are many and varied and will depend on the beliefs of the individual. In whatever way the soul is conceived of, Dr Pietroni suggests, there are interventions common to all religions which also have a place in the consulting room of a GP. He demonstrates that 'religious' actions, such as confession, also occur in the secular setting of a consultation and that for a GP to properly treat a patient acting in such a way he must pay attention to the individual's spiritual dimension. This approach raises some very difficult questions for individual GPs about the nature of their own beliefs and how they relate to those of others, but these are questions which need to be addressed and answered if the medical profession is indeed to treat patients as a whole—mind, body and spirit.

The holistic approach of the Marylebone Health Centre and the Marylebone Centre Trust has been all too often equated with the use of alternative or complementary therapies. In many ways this is unsurprising and indeed an approach to care that insists on treating the whole person will necessarily be concerned to stretch the boundaries of traditional Western medical practice. However, it must be remembered that crucial as all the therapies and interventions included in this chapter are, they can no more provide definitive answers than can 'orthodox' medicine. If a truly innovative and responsive range of interventions is to be maintained there can be no ossification of old alternatives into new orthodoxies.

THE INTERFACE BETWEEN COMPLEMENTARY THERAPY AND GENERAL PRACTICE

Patrick Pietroni

Keywords: Complementary/alternative medicine, general practice.

INTRODUCTION

One of the problems facing all of us in debating this subject is that there is no clear definition of words such as *alternative, complementary, holistic, natural* or *fringe*, words which are often used to describe vastly dissimilar activities. Much confusion arises from the belief that holistic medicine and alternative medicine are the same thing. There are many more general practitioners who apply the principles of an holistic approach to their patients than there are acupuncturists who don't. The term 'alternative' or 'complementary medicine' is used as a 'catch all' definition for 'anything not taught at a Western medical school'. It is thus a definition by exclusion and as helpful a term as the word 'foreign'. An Englishman setting out to comment on 'foreigners' would be as accurate in his description of foreigners as most doctors are in their understanding of alternative therapies. The Englishman's commentaries on foreigners would tell us more about the prejudices of being English than the characteristics of non-English people. The most helpful classification that I use divides this vast area of complementary therapies into the following four distinct groups (Pietroni 1988):

1. Complete systems
2. Diagnostic methods
3. Therapeutic modalities
4. Self-care approaches.

Reprinted with permission from the Journal of the Royal Society of Medicine: 87 (2) pp. 28–30 1994.

Some of these categories require 4 years' full-time training akin to undergraduate medical school, whilst others can be learnt and applied after a few weekend seminars. It is inappropriate, and does reasoned debate an injustice, to lump all these categories together under one definition and respond with a prejudiced stance.

HISTORICAL BACKGROUND

The history of 'outsider' or alternative medicine is as long as history itself. It could be said that for a while general practice was viewed as alternative medicine or as an unacceptable alternative to medicine. Many of us were told that we were 'selling ourselves short' or that 'we had fallen off the ladder' if we embarked on a career in general practice. Lord Moran's comments on the establishment of the College of General Practitioners in the 1950s still rankles with our senior colleagues. 'O'er my dead body' he said. We, of all disciplines, should be sensitive to the views of colleagues in complementary medicine who experience the same arrogance and ignorance from doctors. This antipathy, however, has a much longer history and the language used is much richer:

But our Empirics and Imposters, as they are too ignorant either to teach or to practise Physic ... and too insolent, and too arrogant to learn of the Masters of that Faculty, or to be reduced into order: so are they most dangerous and pernicious unto the Weale public .... These Crocodiles, disguised with the vizard of feigned knowledge and masking under the specious titles of Physicians and Doctors, not attained in Schools, but imposed by the common people, do with their Absoloniçall Salutations steal away the affections of the inconstant multitude, from the Learned Professors of that Faculty, with their Loablike Imbracings, stab to the heart their poor and silly patients, ere they be aware or once suspect such uncouth Treachery (Beier 1987).

THE CURRENT POSITION

The medical profession, like all professions, acts as a tribe. First, it determines who can or cannot enter the profession and methods are developed for expelling a member who has transgressed the accepted code of conduct. Secondly, it attempts to maintain a clientele that is dependent on the services that only it is able to provide. Thirdly, it attempts to protect its special status and privilege by ensuring its autonomy and right to determine its own methods of accountability. We have seen how our hold on the health of the nation and our influence on government has been challenged and, in my view, overturned in this last decade, led not only by politicians, but, by consumers demanding a greater say in their health care, by nurses wanting to prescribe, by pharmacists setting up surgeries for minor complaints, by midwives achieving independent status and, increasingly, by alternative practitioners achieving recognition and legislative protection from the government. If I may express a personal view, our roots may be in medical schools, our identity may well be that of general practitioners, but our future lies as members and, at times, leaders of an expanded primary health and community care team, which must now include complementary therapies. Nevertheless there will always be a form of health care that is alternative to the orthodoxy—soon it may be the doctor who is willing to prescribe valium and sleeping tablets who will be considered alternative.

A number of questionnaire surveys revealed an interest amongst doctors which was unrecognised. Reilly (1983) found a positive attitude in 86 out of 100 general practitioner trainees towards alternative medicine. Wharton & Lewith (1986), in their survey of 200 general practitioners in the Avon District, found that 38% had received some additional training in some of the alternative therapies, and 76% had referred patients to colleagues practising some form of alternative or complementary medicine. The last major survey in the UK in 1982 identified a total of 30 000 practitioners of one sort or another (Fulder & Monro 1981). Subsequent developments have suggested a growth of 10% a year which would make the figure nearer 50 000. However, in what is considered the mainstream of alternative medicine, there are no more than 3000–4000 practitioners. If the figure of 20 000 spiritual healers is correct, it suggests that most of the public seeks help from alternative practi-

tioners because scientific, rational medicine does not address itself to problems of the spirit. Surveys as to why patients seek alternative medicine do not always provide a coherent set of answers. The consumer magazine *Which?*, in its survey of almost 2000 readers, found that one in seven had visited a complementary/alternative practitioner in the previous year, 82% claiming to have improved or been cured. 81% of patients identified dissatisfaction due to poor symptom relief as the main reason for seeking help, 71% sought help for joint or pain problems, 15% sought help for psychological problems (*Which?* 1981).

A more recent survey in the UK carried out by MORI in 1989 shows that 74% of the sample surveyed (1826 adults) would like to see some forms of alternative medicine introduced into the Health Service. However, 69% had not had any experience of alternative treatments and only 10% had tried either homoeopathy or osteopathy (Mori Poll 1989).

ALTERNATIVE THERAPY: THE BMA REPORT

As a direct result of the Prince of Wales's intervention, the BMA appointed a Scientific Committee to report on the efficacy of alternative medicine in England. Its precise remit was : 'To consider the feasibility and possible methods of assessing the value of alternative therapies, whether used alone or to complement other treatments' (BMA Board of Education and Science 1986).

The membership of the working party was drawn from within the BMA and surprisingly contained no person familiar with the subject and no general practitioner. The Committee sent out requests to a number of different bodies asking for information. Initially the time given for these bodies to respond was very short (8 weeks) and many of the established groups declined to take part. Over 600 submissions were received and the Committee also heard oral evidence. At the end of 1984, after a number of revisions, it produced its report and conclusions. It would be very easy to dismiss the validity of the report given that it was conducted in such a haphazard way.

Equally, the lack of any informed member on the Committee made it almost impossible for the group to assess the relative merit of the evidence submitted. Nevertheless the report identified certain factors which it believed were common to a number of alternative therapies and which were important to acknowledge. These factors were:

1. Time: alternative practitioners were able to offer patients more time to listen—the complaint that doctors were too busy was heard over and over again.

2. Compassion: as well as being given time, patients felt alternative practitioners were more caring and concerned. They treated the 'whole person' and not the disease.

3. Touch: in many of the alternative therapies, touch was used: e.g. massage, reflexology, acupressure, laying on of hands. This very fundamental method of communicating healing was thought by the BMA to contrast with the technology of modern medicine which got in the way of the doctor and the patient.

4. Authority and charisma: as medicine had become more familiar, it seemed important for patients to seek out practitioners who appeared 'magical'. Many of the alternative therapies with their strange words and unfamiliar practices conveyed the atmosphere of a magical cult which was a very powerful healing force.

As one can see from the above description, the BMA, whilst acknowledging that alternative medicine was growing in popularity, thought it was doing so because modern medicine was failing to give patients something they wanted. The Committee generally felt that the scientific validity of the therapies themselves was almost impossible to demonstrate. Partly this was because the sorts of problems seen by alternative practitioners were episodic (they relapsed and recurred naturally) and were non-life-threatening. The Committee was unable to find clear evidence of a *scientific* kind to prove, for instance, that acupuncture worked in asthma or that homoeopathy was of help in psoriasis. It also felt that to conduct such studies would be difficult and

costly. However, it did acknowledge that the weight of descriptive evidence for acupuncture in pain relief and osteopathy and chiropractic in back problems was so great that it accepted that these therapies did indeed have a place in the proper management of these disorders. Similarly, the Committee supported hypnotherapy, biofeedback and some forms of dietary therapy, in a limited set of circumstances.

CONCLUSIONS

What then should our attitude to our patients be if they seek some form of complementary medicine? It is difficult to advise from ignorance, and if you are ignorant, it is far better to say 'I don't know' than to say something prejudicial. The guide here is 'Keep an open mind but not so open that your brains fall out'.

The major ethical issues relate to life-threatening illness, especially cancer where the vulnerability and fearfulness of the patient may be exploited by unscrupulous practitioners, especially if the patient refuses potentially curative medical and surgical treatments. The whole area of cancer and complementary therapy is riven with strife, accusation and malpractice on both sides. A recognition of our own failures would help the debate. Nevertheless, if faced with such a patient, the facts and research studies do help to guide the advice we can now give. There is only one study of which I am aware that, as yet, has not been replicated, suggesting that survival time can be increased with the use of complementary therapies (Speigel et al 1989). Anecdotal accounts of remission are common and will always beckon as a torch to those who wish to follow. My advice to patients is simple. You may well get a lot of care and understanding about your cancer if you see a counsellor, relaxation therapist, and so on. The diets may make you feel better— sometimes they are awful and make you feel a lot worse. The herbs and home remedies will do little harm—Laetrile can be dangerous. The injections have not been shown to be helpful. Extra vitamins occasionally are required but none of these interventions will, I am afraid, cure or indeed reduce the progress of your cancer.

However, if I had cancer, I certainly might consider some of these interventions because, having used them, so many of my patients seem to manage their disease better, feel stronger in themselves, rediscover their own joy, lose some of their fear, develop a sense of the mystery and awe-fulness of life and, eventually, die as a more peaceful and contented person. How I wish I could say that modern oncology could offer such care.

I would like to finish on an equally difficult subject—that of research. The following argument is used: alternative therapies cannot be accepted as effective approaches because they have not been subjected to rigorous study, clinical trials, etc. If alternative practitioners were willing to undertake such trials and studies then we as doctors would have no difficulty in accepting them as valid, for we are an objective, rational, scientific-based group of professionals. Let them research their approaches like we do, *but*, when they do put forward protocols and grant applications, it is unethical to grant them money and support because their methods are unscientific and unproven!

Therapists who claim to treat the 'whole person' will require methodologies that allow for comparability of results whilst respecting the uniqueness of every human being. The nature of scientific inquiry and its limitations has been a point of debate and exploration amongst 'pure' scientists and 'social' scientists for several decades. The medical profession, which is so well-placed between both extremes has, for the most part, not entered the debate, and has attempted to resolve the conflict by identifying with the 'pure' form of analytic science, which strives to reject the indeterminate, relies on Aristotelian logic and considers the nature of scientific knowledge to be impersonal, value-free, precise and reliable. These therapies should be properly studied by doctors and scientists willing to enter into an honest debate where the high ground of 'rigour' is eschewed for the messy swamp of relevance.

REFERENCES

Beier 1987 Sufferers and healers—the experience of illness in seventeenth-century England. Routledge and Kegan Paul, London

British Medical Association Board of Education and Science 1986 Alternative therapy

Fulder S, Monro R 1981 The status of complementary medicine in the United Kingdom. Threshold Foundation

Mori Poll 13 November 1989. The Times

Pietroni P 1988 Alternative medicine. Journal of the Royal Society of Arts, October pp 791–801

Reilly D 1983 Young doctors' views on alternative medicine. British Medical Journal 287 pp 337–339

Speigel D, Bloom J R, Kraemer H C, Gottheil E 1989 Effects of psychological treatment on survival of patients with metastatic breast cancer. Lancet II pp 888–891

Wharton R W, Lewith G 1986 Complementary medicine and the general practitioner. British Medical Journal 292 pp 1498–1500

Which? August 1981 Magic or medicine?

TRADITIONAL CHINESE MEDICINE IN GENERAL PRACTICE: AN ANALYSIS OF ONE YEAR'S REFERRALS

Arnold Desser
Peter Davies
Derek Chase
Patrick Pietroni

A one-year retrospective analysis was undertaken of patients referred to a practitioner of traditional Chinese medicine (TCM), who was a member of a primary health care team in an inner-city NHS general practice. Of the 47 patients referred, 27 had respiratory, musculoskeletal or dermatological complaints and over half of all the patients referred had had their problem for 2 or more years. Patients with the same Western diagnosis (e.g. asthma) received different kinds of treatment, specific to their individual symptoms. Of the 37 patients who were treated, just under a quarter were assessed as having had their complaints resolved. The advantages and initial difficulties of incorporating TCM into general practice are described and guidelines suggested for making appropriate referrals.

INTRODUCTION

The Marylebone Health Centre, an NHS general practice in London's West End, has for the last 5 years undertaken a study of the methods and effects of incorporating the services of a practitioner of traditional Chinese medicine (TCM) into daily general practice. The TCM practitioner was part of a multidisciplinary team comprising one full-time general practitioner (GP), two part-time GPs, a GP trainee, practice nurse, counsellor, homoeopath, osteopath, and two massage therapists. In treating patients, the TCM practitioner used acupuncture, herbs, nutrition and instruction in physical and meditative exercises. He was contracted to provide nine sessions per month, mostly for clinical work, with some time for research, teaching and meetings.

There is an increasing national interest in the use of non-conventional therapies, by both patients and professionals whether in private health care, hospital medicine, or general practice (Wharton & Lewith 1986, Budd et al 1990,

Thomas et al 1991). This is also reflected in the increasing number of literature reviews (Aldridge & Pietroni 1987, Prance et al 1988) and research papers in peer review journals (Lewith 1984, Jobst et al 1986, correspondence in the Lancet 1990).

Several authors researching TCM have discussed the problems of designing outcome studies within the framework of conventional research methodology (Wharton & Lewith 1986, Aldridge & Pietroni 1987, O'Dowd 1988). The practitioners involved in this study undertook a one-year retrospective analysis in order to describe TCM's use in a general practice setting and as a first step towards evaluating its potential clinical role. The questions asked included:

- What criteria were GPs using for referrals?
- What was the age, sex and morbidity of the patients?
- How often and how frequently were patients seen?
- What was the range of treatments used?

The referral process

Patients did not have open access to the TCM practitioner and in all cases were referred by one of the GPs—occasionally at the patient's request. The general practitioners maintained their usual role as 'gate-keepers', partly to control demand on a limited resource but also to ensure medical responsibility for delegating patient care. When referring, the GP made a brief note in the patient's records, giving the symptoms and, wherever possible, a diagnosis. Patients then made an initial appointment with the TCM practitioner. At the first consultation, a treatment plan was mutually agreed and future appointments booked. In a few cases, it was explained that treatment would not be useful and the patient was referred back to the GP.

METHOD

The analysis covered patients referred to the TCM practitioner between 1 September 1989 and 31 August 1990. Patients' age, sex and dates of consultation were derived from computer records. Information about reasons for referral, conventional and traditional Chinese diagnosis, and treatment methods were obtained from patients' notes and then transferred onto a computer spreadsheet for analysis. 6 months after the completion of treatment the referring GP, the patient and the TCM practitioner recorded their subjective impression of clinical outcome, using a simple three point scale.

RESULTS

Patients

Of 47 patients referred, 18 (38%) were male and 29 (62%) were female, the same ratio as patients consulting GPs in the practice over the analysis period. Just under half the patients referred (49%) were aged 20–44 years, reflecting the large numbers of registered patients in this age group. With the exception of the 0–4 and 10–19 years age groups, percentages of patients referred for each group were consistent with percentages of patients consulting a GP. However, relatively more children aged 0–4 years were referred than for any other age group (see Table 4.1). The eldest patient was aged 77, the youngest aged 1.

Table 4.1 Age/sex details of patients referred to the TCM practitioner, with comparison between percentages of patients seen by TCM practitioner and patients seen by a GP during the analysis period

	Male %	Female %
Patients seen by TCM practitioner	38.30	61.70
Patients seen by GP	37.75	62.25

Years	Male	Female		TCM %	GP %
0–4	4	3	(7)	15	8
5–9	1	0	(1)	2	2
10–19	1	0	(1)	2	6
20–29	3	10	(13)	28	32
30–44	2	8	(10)	21	23
45–59	5	2	(7)	15	14
60–74	2	4	(6)	13	10
75+	0	2	(2)	4	5
Total	**18**	**29**	**(47)**	**100**	**100**

Problems referred

Of the problems referred, the largest group (see Table 4.2) was for respiratory complaints (11/47), almost half of whom (5/11) were children aged between 1 and 3. Although acupuncture is increasingly thought of for the treatment of pain, only seven patients were referred for joint pain and one for sciatica—probably because of the presence of an osteopath in the practice. A further seven patients were referred for skin problems, four patients for gynaecological problems, four for polysymptomatic complaints related to fatigue and stress, three for digestive problems, two for mental/emotional problems, two for genito-urinary problems and the remainder (five) for problems ranging from hypertension to headache and smoking. One patient was referred for HIV+ related symptoms. Secondary problems were noted in 30 patients of whom over a third (11/30) reported chronic depression and/or anxiety.

Treatment

Two of the patients referred were found to be unsuitable for treatment; one was referred in order to stop smoking but in the event did not want to stop, the other because of a reluctance to accept that a staple diet of Coca Cola and coffee might well be having an effect on her skin, menses and moods, the reasons for the referral.

Eight of the referrals were for assessment only, three of whom were uncertain about having treatment and decided not to proceed, the remainder being referred by the GP for a second opinion.

Thus, of the total 47 patients referred, only 37 were actually treated. Of these, 36 received acupuncture and nearly half were prescribed herbal medicine (see Table 4.3). With 15 patients, dietary advice was given in keeping with the traditional Chinese medical perspective on seasonal foods and their effect on basal metabolism. For instance, patients who had poor peripheral circulation or who complained of the cold were advised to eat 'warming' foods (not only cooked foods, as opposed to raw fruit and vegetables,

Table 4.2 Primary problems referred, broken down by major disease category

Middle section shows number of patients receiving treatments shown. (**A**=acupuncture, **H**=herbs, **HB**=herbal baths, **Mox**=moxibustion, **D**=diet, **M**=massage, **C**=counselling, **Cup**=cupping.)

Right hand section shows numbers of patients according to evaluation of outcome. (**R**=resolved, **Rr**=resolved but expect recurrence, **I**=improved, **NC**=no change, **OG**=on-going, **AO**=assessment only, including two patients who were unsuitable for treatment. N.B. (*) one patient treated in conjunction with practice's osteopath.)

Primary problem	Number	Treatment								Evaluation of outcome					
		A	H	HB	Mox	D	M	C	Cup	R	Rr	I	NC	OG	AO
RESPIRATORY	11														
asthma	4	4	4	2	-	3	2	1	-	-	1	-	1	2	-
wheezing	3	2	1	1	-	2	1	-	-	-	2	-	-	-	1
rhinitis	2	2	2	-	-	1	-	1	-	-	-	-	1	1	-
hayfever	1	-	-	-	-	-	-	-	-	-	-	-	-	-	1
catarrh	1	1	1	1	-	1	1	-	-	1	-	-	-	-	-
MUSCULOSKELETAL	9														
joint pain:															
knee	2	1	-	-	1	-	-	1	-	-	1	-	-	-	1
low back	2*	2	-	-	1	-	-	-	1	-	2	-	-	-	-
shoulder	1	-	-	-	-	-	-	-	-	-	-	-	-	-	1
wrist	1	1	-	-	1	-	-	-	-	1	-	-	-	-	-
polyarthritis	1	1	-	-	1	-	-	-	-	-	-	-	1	-	-
sciatica	1	1	-	-	1	-	-	-	-	1	-	-	-	-	-
heel spur	1	1	1	-	-	1	-	-	-	-	1	-	-	-	-
SKIN	7														
eczema	3	3	-	1	-	1	-	-	-	1	1	-	1	-	-
acne	2	2	1	-	1	2	-	1	-	-	-	1	1	-	-
impetigo	1	1	1	-	-	1	-	-	-	1	-	-	-	-	-
warts	1	-	-	-	-	-	-	-	-	-	-	-	-	-	1
GYNAECOLOGICAL	4														
endometriosis	1	1	1	-	-	-	-	-	-	1	-	-	-	-	-
leucorrhoea	1	-	-	-	-	-	-	-	-	-	-	-	-	-	1
polycystic ovaries	1	-	-	-	-	-	-	-	-	-	-	-	-	-	1
menopausal	1	1	1	-	-	1	-	1	-	-	-	-	-	1	-
POLYSYMPTOMATIC	4														
fatigue	3	2	-	-	-	-	-	1	-	-	1	-	-	1	1
stress	1	-	-	-	-	-	-	-	-	-	-	-	-	-	1
DIGESTIVE	3														
constipation	1	1	-	-	-	-	-	-	-	1	-	-	-	-	-
irritable bowel	1	1	1	-	-	1	-	-	-	-	-	1	-	-	-
obesity	1	1	1	-	-	-	-	1	-	-	-	1	-	-	-
MENTAL/EMOTIONAL	2														
bereavement	1	-	-	-	-	-	-	1	-	1	-	-	-	-	-
anxiety/depression	1	1	-	-	-	-	-	1	-	-	-	-	-	1	-
GENITO-URINARY	2														
polyuria	1	1	1	-	1	-	1	-	-	1	-	-	-	-	-
pruritus	1	1	-	-	-	-	-	1	-	-	-	-	1	-	-
CARDIOVASCULAR	1														
hypertension	1	1	1	-	-	-	-	-	-	-	-	-	1	-	-
OTHERS	4														
HIV+	1	1	1	-	-	1	-	-	-	-	-	-	-	1	-
head pain	1	1	-	-	-	-	-	1	-	-	1	-	-	-	-
headache	1	1	-	-	-	-	-	-	-	-	1	-	-	-	-
smoking	1	-	-	-	-	-	-	-	-	-	-	-	-	-	1
TOTAL	**47**									**9**	**11**	**3**	**7**	**7**	**10**

Table 4.3 Numbers and percentages of patients (n=37) receiving different kinds of treatment. (Note that nearly all patients received more than one kind of treatment)

Treatment	No. (n=37)	%
Acupuncture	36	97.3
Herbal medicine	18	48.7
Dietary advice	15	40.5
Counselling	11	29.7
Moxibustion	7	18.9
Herbal baths	5	13.5
Massage	5	13.5
Cupping	1	2.7

but also domestic herbs and spices like ginger and cinnamon).

Moxibustion, a technique involving the burning of *Artemisia vulgaris* to heat external areas of the body, was used for seven patients where there was pain or discomfort which could be alleviated by warmth. It was also used to strengthen those weak patients who were sensitive to the cold and was applied to some of the patients with musculoskeletal disorders.

Herbal baths were prescribed for five children with respiratory and skin complaints.

Of the five patients who received Chinese massage, four were children aged 3 years or less, all of whom had respiratory complaints. Their mothers received instruction to enable them to massage their children at home and thereby help sustain the effects of needling between appointments.

The one case in which cupping was used (a treatment in which suction is applied to specific areas of the body) was for the treatment of low back pain.

Treatment time

Of the 37 patients treated, seven had not finished their treatment by the end of the year. In the case of three of these, treatment spanned the entire year at 6-weekly intervals. Of the remaining 30, five patients were treated in one consultation, 24 patients received between two and nine treatments (average of five) and only one patient failed to complete the course of treatment. For the most part, treatments were given either weekly or fortnightly. In two cases, patients were re-referred for additional treatment because of relapse.

Outcome

Because of the variety of complaints referred it was not possible to obtain objective measures of outcome. However, through discussion with the referring GP, patient and TCM practitioner 6 months after completion of treatment, it was possible to arrive at a subjective evaluation of outcome. It was agreed that an outcome would be assessed as 'resolved' if the symptoms were no longer present (R); 'resolved' but a recurrence could be expected (Rr); or 'improved' where the symptoms had significantly lessened (I). Where there was no improvement, then outcome was assessed as 'no change' (NC). These mutually agreed, albeit subjective, evaluations are presented in Table 4.2.

Of the 37 patients treated, nine (24%) were judged to have had their complaints resolved; in the case of the patient with endometriosis, remission was confirmed by a hospital consultant. The symptoms of 11 patients (30%) were resolved, although a recurrence was expected, especially in cases where there had been an acute episode (e.g. acute low back pain) overlying a chronic problem, or where a child's eczema was part of an alternating pattern with asthma. Three patients (8%) were assessed as having improved, that is while their symptoms had not been resolved, the treatment was found to be beneficial, and seven patients (19%) experienced no change. Treatment was still on-going at the end of the year for seven other patients.

DISCUSSION

Not only is there increasing interest in complementary medicine, but with over three quarters of general practitioners, at least in Avon, being prepared to refer to such practitioners (Wharton & Lewith 1986) and with mechanisms now existing for their funding, e.g. health promotion clinics, staff reimbursements and budget holding, it is increasingly important to consider the role of such practitioners within general practice.

In this study, the GPs referred a wide range of problems, reflecting the overall morbidity of the practice population. However, each GP had a distinct referral pattern. While one GP referred mostly children, the second GP sent a disproportionate number of patients with polysymptomatic undifferentiated problems, and the third referred only women with chronic problems overlying considerable emotional distress. These patterns may have resulted from the GPs' lack of experience in making such referrals, combined with a lack of knowledge about TCM, which has quite different diagnostic and treatment criteria. In such a situation one might expect GPs to make 'safe' referrals where, from their perspective, there is nothing to lose and possibly something to gain. This is borne out by the observation that a surprisingly large proportion of the patients referred had long-standing problems. Over half the patients (53%) had had their problem for 2 years or more (Table 4.4) while only 11% had had their problem for between 1 week and 1 month.

However, it was recognised that there were additional reasons for referral, some of which were not always acknowledged. For instance, GPs were occasionally referring for their own personal support since the 'chronic group' is one of the most demanding (O'Dowd 1988, Gerrard & Riddell 1988). Also, some patients

requested referral in the belief that 'complementary treatment' would work where orthodox treatment had 'failed'. Clearly, more work is required to identify the exact reasons.

Although the efficacy of TCM in treating specific conditions or types of patient in a general practice was not formally assessed, it does appear that the chronic conditions of a small number of patients were resolved. In one case, this was subsequently confirmed by a hospital consultant. Others were able to reduce their intake of drugs and there was a small number of patients for whom periodic treatment aided the management of their discomfort and anxiety and gave their GP some support. Some patients experienced no change, but no-one appeared to deteriorate.

There were, however, occasional differences of opinion over what constituted an 'improvement'. An example of this was where a child appeared to have responded to treatment and the mother was much relieved. The father, who accompanied the family to the surgery for the last treatment, angrily insisted, however, that his son was no better.

While multidisciplinary work is rewarding both for the patients by providing a wider range of therapies and for the professionals by providing mutual support, it is not without its challenges. One such challenge comes from the process of the referral itself, in which the GP, by determining the type of problem or patient to be referred, is in a powerful position with respect to the TCM practitioner—particularly if he/she is also the employer (Reason 1991). This is particularly relevant for TCM practitioners whose tradition is one of diagnostic autonomy and of being able to treat a wide range of conditions. Another challenge is the patient who presents to the TCM practitioner symptoms different to those reported by the GP in the referral. In such a situation, it is vital that good communication is maintained between all the parties involved (Reason et al 1992).

At Marylebone, much time and energy was committed to meeting both formally and informally and discussing such issues, from which some guidelines for referral were drawn up (see Box 4.1).

Table 4.4 Duration of primary complaint for 44 of the 47 patients referred

Duration of primary symptom—less than one year (n=17)

Duration	No.	Male	Female
1w–1m	5	3	2
2m–4m	7	3	4
5m–12m	5	2	3
Total	**17**	**8**	**9**

Duration of primary symptom — more than one year (n=27)

Duration	No.	Male	Female
1y	4	2	2
2y–5y	16	4	12
6y–10y	6	3	3
21+	1	0	1
Total	**27**	**9**	**18**

Box 4.1 Referral guidelines

'Good' referrals would be those patients:

1. not responding to drugs or other conventional treatment
2. for whom drugs or surgery are contraindicated
3. not wishing to have drugs or surgery
4. whose complaint indicated a change in function rather than organic change
5. who experience their illness energetically, e.g. report feeling 'out of balance'
6. who are polysymptomatic
7. who wish a preventive and participative approach
8. who have previously responded to TCM.

Those for whom there is less likelihood of a successful outcome are:

1. older patients weakened by wasting diseases
2. patients on systemic corticosteroids (including oral contraception, hormone replacement therapy and long-term users of inhalers)
3. patients who do not report a characteristic aching, numb, distended or heavy feeling around the area being needled.

Treatment is contraindicated for:

1. diabetics who are unreliable in monitoring themselves
2. patients who are taking phenothiazines or lithium carbonate
3. patients who are inebriated, or 'high' on drugs.

Caution must be exercised with:

1. pregnant women in their first trimester
2. patients who require close monitoring while under a course of treatment.

One of the difficulties of such guidelines is that the diagnostic and treatment components of TCM are specific to individual patients rather than to their diseases; thus different patients with the same Western diagnosis may, to a TCM practitioner, require different treatments. In TCM, 'asthma' can be differentiated into six or more clinical entities, each one referring to a different pattern of dysfunction (e.g. 'respiratory', 'digestive', 'constitutional', 'hot' type, 'cold' type, 'excess' or 'deficient' types, or some combination of these). Each pattern requires a different kind of treatment. Thus, although in Table 4.2, all four patients referred for asthma were given acupuncture, the points used were tailored specifically to each patient's particular pattern of asthma. Similarly, the herbal prescriptions took into

consideration the specific pattern being treated.

Some patterns can be less amenable to treatment than others. Obviously, a TCM differential diagnosis is of no more use to the GP than the broad rubric of 'asthma' is to the TCM practitioner in making certain clinical decisions. What was found useful was a brief discussion between the referring GP and the TCM practitioner, concerning the duration and severity of the problem, the type and dosage of the drugs used and the constitution of the patient.

General practice is as much about the management of people with illnesses as it is about the cure of their diseases. Consequently, when considering the role of TCM in general practice, as much emphasis needs to be placed on the referral process as on the understanding of the processes of diagnosis and disease models from which TCM has sprung (although this should not be underestimated since TCM *is* what constitutes general practice in China.)

TCM can provide a highly acceptable, safe, and potentially inexpensive additional resource for the care of the patient, and, this analysis suggests, for the support of the general practitioner.

REFERENCES

Aldridge D, Pietroni P 1987 Clinical assessment of acupuncture in asthma therapy: discussion paper. Journal of the Royal Society of Medicine 80 pp. 222–224

Budd C, Fisher B, Parrinder D, Price L 1990 A model of cooperation between complementary and allopathic medicine in a primary care setting. British Journal of General Practice 40 pp. 376–378

Gerrard T J, Riddell J D 1988 Difficult patients in general practice. British Medical Journal 297 pp. 530–532

Jobst K, Chen J H, McPherson K, Arrowsmith J, Brown 1986 Controlled trial of acupuncture for disabling breathlessness. Lancet pp. 1416—1412

Lancet correspondence 1990 31/3/90 p. 795, 21/7/90 p. 177, 17/11/90 p. 1254

Lewith G T 1984 How effective is acupuncture in the management of pain? Journal of the Royal College of General Practitioners 34 pp. 275–278

O'Dowd T C 1988 Five years of heartsink patients in general practice. British Medical Journal 297 pp. 528–530

Prance S E, Desser A, Wood C, Fleming J, Aldridge D, Pietroni P 1988 Research on traditional Chinese acupuncture—science or myth? A review. Journal of the Royal Society of Medicine 81 pp. 588–590

Reason P 1991 Power and conflict in multidisciplinary collaboration. Complementary Medical Research 3 pp. 144–150

Reason P, Chase D, Desser A, Melhuish C, Morrison S, Peters D, Wallstein D, Webber V, Pietroni P 1992 Towards a clinical framework for collaboration between general practice and complementary practitioners: a discussion paper. Journal of the Royal Society of Medicine 85 pp. 161–164

Thomas K J, Carr J, Westlake L, Williams B T 1991 Use of non-orthodox and conventional health care in Great Britain. British Medical Journal 302 pp. 207–210

Wharton R, Lewith G 1986 Complementary medicine and the general practitioner. British Medical Journal 292 pp. 1498–1500

MASSAGE: A REVIEW OF ITS INTRODUCTION AS A THERAPEUTIC INTERVENTION IN GENERAL PRACTICE

Claire McCormack
Patrick Pietroni

This report reviews the introduction of massage into the Marylebone Health Centre general practice surgery, describing the referral procedure, treatment, types of patient seen, and the results of the treatment with emphasis on the patients' subjective responses. It examines some of the processes involved in eliciting these responses and discusses the therapeutic effects and possible applications of massage to general practice. It also gives recommendations for making the inclusion of massage effective in this clinical setting.

INTRODUCTION

Massage, the art of structured touch, is one of the oldest therapies in the repertory of healing skills and is found in some form in nearly all health care systems throughout the world. It is a complementary therapy in the most literal sense, working as an adjunctive treatment equally well alongside physical or psychological therapies. However, unlike some other complementary therapies, it is no stranger to orthodox medicine, its therapeutic properties being appreciated by the great physicians throughout the early history of Western medicine, from Hippocrates to Avicenna. From the late Middle Ages, there appears to have been a decline in its general use, at least as evinced by medical texts, but by the nineteenth century it was enjoying a revival of clinical interest in Europe, accompanied by a spate of scientific investigations into its effects (Kleen 1918, Cuthbertson 1933). At the turn of the century, it was regularly used in this country both by physicians and by trained 'nurse-masseuses' in the treatment of a wide variety of disorders (Goodall-Copestake 1919, Mennell 1945). There are now clear signs of a new resurgence in the therapeutic use of massage by the nursing profession in a variety of fields (Byass 1989, Turton

1989, Martin 1990). This paper examines its use as a clinical intervention within the context of general practice.

The Marylebone Health Centre provides patients with all the usual services of an NHS general practice and in addition offers a range of educational and community activities. It also has a complementary therapy unit which comprises acupuncture, homoeopathy, osteopathy, counselling, stress management and massage. Massage has been offered at the health centre since it first opened in 1987. Initially, massage sessions were offered one afternoon each week and the massage therapist worked on a voluntary basis. However, as the demand grew, from both doctors and patients, the sessions were increased to two days each week, and funding for this service was provided by a grant from the Wates Foundation.

REFERRAL AND TREATMENT

Patients are referred for massage by the doctors or other clinicians at the health centre, who give their reason(s) for referral. The masseuse also has access to patients' files and medical history. In addition to registered patients at the centre, a common source of referral in the first 2 years has been from the Joint Assessment Clinic. Here the complementary therapists and a doctor collaborate in assessing chronically ill patients referred from outside the practice. Self-referrals are not accepted, though patients may ask their doctor to give a referral.

At the first appointment, a course of treatment is established. The average course comprised six sessions initially and this was lowered to four sessions as the number of referrals increased. In the first 12-month period, 113 patients were seen (92 women and 21 men). These patients came from all socio-economic groups and ranged in age from 18 to 98 years.

The type of massage practised is a variation of what is known as Swedish massage, combined with techniques from other systems. It incorporates the basic massage strokes—stroking (effleurage), kneading (petrissage), percussion (tapotement), pressure (friction) and vibration—

with passive movements and forms the basis of most types of massage currently practised. 'Holistic', 'intuitive' or simply 'therapeutic' massage are some of the names given to it. The effects can be relaxing and sedating or stimulating and invigorating, depending on the rate, rhythm and pressure of the movements. In general, the massages at the health centre are of the relaxation type employing predominantly slow rhythmic movements, the primary aim being to relax and soothe the patient. *Arachis* oil is used as the base oil, with aromatic essential oils added. Each appointment is for an hour, allowing for a full body massage when appropriate.

In addition to the massage itself, diaphragmatic breathing exercises are often incorporated into the treatment. As a basic self-help tool in stress management this can be a very relevant technique for those referred for massage. In practical terms, it is easy for this to be included in the session because the patient is lying down and is generally in a state of mind conducive to learning a technique which, like massage, can afford a direct experience of the mind/body connection. Similarly, if the patient can begin the massage session by breathing deeply, the effects of the massage can be greatly enhanced. Simple physical exercises, involving stretching and rotation of joints, are also given where appropriate. The Marylebone Health Centre is fortunate in that it has several educational classes on offer. Many patients are referred to the yoga, relaxation, and stress management classes which once again complement the effects of the massage and enable patients to continue self-help once the sessions are over.

Notes on each session are recorded in the patient's file and the therapist keeps her own more detailed notes which include the patient's own comments and responses. A simple questionnaire was sent to all 61 patients who attended a course of four or more sessions in the first year to evaluate the effects of the treatment and to ask patients to give an appraisal of their course in their own words. 47 questionnaires were returned. The responses indicated that patients felt a high degree of satisfaction with their treatment. Some representative comments are quoted in the following section.

PATIENTS' PROBLEMS, NEEDS AND RESPONSES

Initially, the most common referrals were of patients complaining of physical pains, often chronic and often with an underlying stress factor. As massage became more established at the health centre, the main reason for referral was nearly always a stress-related problem which sometimes did not include any particular physical complaint.

In an attempt to draw up some rough categories for effective referral to massage, the two very general headings of stress and pain relief can be given. The pain-relieving properties of massage have been recognised for thousands of years and will always be one of the main reasons for its use, even if the precise mechanisms are not always fully understood (Jacobs 1960). Often pain relief results from the release of muscular tension and so is directly associated with the first category of stress relief, somatic pain in many cases being the result of chronically contracted muscles due to accumulated tension in the body.

The statistics for the first 12-month period at the Marylebone Health Centre highlight the two categories of stress and pain relief. 101 of the total of 113 patients had a stress factor included among the reason for their referral, of whom 14 were referred purely for 'stress' without physical complaints. 99 patients presented with a physical disorder, generally pain or its accompanying immobility, of whom 12 were referred solely for this reason, without an obvious stress factor. Patients' perception of their reason for referral, however, often differed initially to that of the referrer. Many were unaware of any stress factor, viewing the problem as a purely physical one and expecting the sessions to be similar to a physiotherapy treatment. By the end of the sessions their perception had often shifted, as one of the direct effects of massage is to put people back 'in touch' with their bodies and enable them to listen to the messages their bodies are sending.

Stress-related disorders

The patients with stress-related disorders can be further divided into groups of appropriate patients for referral to massage—accepting that these categories are to a great extent interdependent. The groups are described mainly in terms of the needs they have rather than of presenting symptoms. The quotations selected are typical of many of the responses from the questionnaire, comments given during the massage or letters written after the course. Emphasis is laid on these subjective responses as they offer a different perspective on some of the valuable therapeutic effects of massage to that of other research studies (McCormack & Pietroni 1990) which attempt to isolate specific effects by measuring selected physiological parameters. This perspective perhaps gives a fuller and more useful picture of the potential role of massage as a clinical intervention.

General symptoms of stress, relaxation needs and body/mind connection

One group includes those showing general symptoms of stress and for whom relaxation therapy could be appropriate. Many of the patients coming to see GPs are first and foremost 'suffering from life', but it is their lack of energy, sleeplessness, breathing difficulties, gastrointestinal symptoms, tension headaches and general aches and pains that they present to the doctor. They may interpret their problem as a purely physical one, but at the heart often lie, for example, problems at work, difficulties in family and other relationships, loneliness or money worries. The working mother struggling to hold together the conflicting demands of a career and children, or the exhausted carer at home, the long-term unemployed, the harrassed businessman, or the patient trying to adapt to life with a debilitating chronic illness, are some examples of patients in this group. Major changes in everyday routine or life-crises—divorce, the death of a loved one, redundancy, moving to a new job or town, or the 'empty nest' syndrome—are all events which can also bring people to the doctor complaining of general aches and pains and non-specific illnesses.

For both the chronic and acute 'life-sufferers' massage is an extremely effective relaxation therapy. Moreover, it can help lead patients to understand how their mental and emotional states directly affect their physical well-being. For this to occur, it is essential that patients are aware of the tension they hold in their bodies. Many patients commented that until the massage they did not realise how tense they actually were. This acknowledgement was one of the main benefits of massage for these patients, helping them to recognise the difference between feeling tense and feeling relaxed. All the respondents to the questionnaire replied affirmatively to the question 'did massage enable you to relax?' and their accounts of the treatment typically described it in terms of feeling 'relaxed', 'soothed', 'glowing'. These patients often remarked that they had forgotten what it was like to feel good in their bodies. More poetically they likened it to 'walking in a perfumed garden', 'entering a timeless space or trance', 'angels dancing on my back soothing away the pain', or 'a rhapsody playing on my back, hypnotising me'.

The direct physical quality of massage makes it different to other relaxation techniques. Meditation, for instance, can be contraindicated in cases of chronic depression (McLean 1986) yet massage at the health centre has benefited such patients often by putting them in touch with their bodies again or through the 'caring' touch involved. A 60-year old woman with chronic back pain and depression whose husband had left her a few years previously for a younger woman commented: 'My back's a lot better—it feels like it's connected to the rest of my body. I see my pain is related to my other pain, my feeling of soreness about what happened.' A young woman with cancer, recovering from a major operation, emphasised the importance of massage for her in increasing her body awareness and her body's needs in a positive fashion:

I feel that we don't give enough chance for the body to really relax in daily life and although relaxation techniques help a lot, massage seems to me to go very deeply into the skin, muscles, nerves etc, and at the same time it makes me so much more aware of the tensions in the body and so much more aware of the pleasant sensations that can be experienced by being 'in the body'—the warmth of the touch, the sweet smell of the oil and the soft feeling of hands over the skin—it makes the skin feel supple and alive and the body worth caring for, worth loving and treating with respect.

These considerations on the effects of massage can obviously play an important part in the treatment of patients with anxiety, particularly those with physical symptoms of tension (McKechnie et al 1983). One young woman suffering panic attacks had tried several relaxation techniques with limited success but found her fear always prevented her from relaxing completely: 'massage showed me that I can let go and nothing terrible will happen'.

Need support/can't cope alone

For many patients who are going though a bad phase in their lives or for whom perhaps no 'cure' is possible, the therapeutic value of massage can be seen in the 'support' element afforded by the close contact involved and in improving patients' coping skills. The following examples will illustrate this.

A 72-year old lady with a long history of serious illness and multiple pains (many of which she considered iatrogenic so that she was also trying to deal with a deep resentment against doctors), wrote:

It was an oasis at a time when I was in a very low state and it was a 'bridge' that supported me. When I came to the clinic, I was just dragging myself about. I was cold, depressed and miserable. Now, although I have had bad news about my eyes, I feel stronger, better able to cope, more limber and most of my aches have gone. I now have very much more energy and am able to get through the day without feeling completely exhausted. I have been helped to realise that it is possible to help myself.

An 85-year old woman with cancer, 'imprisoned' in a home she hated, had a longer course of massage than average—appointments were arranged every 4 to 6 weeks. She had rejected all orthodox medical approaches to her condition but felt she needed support to help her deal with her

problem. In the first half of most of these sessions this patient would vent her feelings of anger and frustration at the circumstances of her home and life, but she would then relax completely into the massage and would leave the room 'a different woman'. She commented:

Massage is life for me—it brings life into me and helps me go on—it's like a maintenance course. I feel the tension moving out of me—a release from the terrible tension. This is the only place where I feel I can let go. I surprise myself at my own anger, but I'm amazed how differently I feel afterwards—I so badly need that relaxation.

A 58-year old woman, a natural 'carer', who was anxiously approaching retirement age with an invalid husband at home, came to massage nervously, not knowing what to expect, but hoping the treatment would help with a cough that would not clear. The cough did clear, but by the end of the sessions she no longer considered this to be the main benefit of the massage:

As the sessions went on, I felt more able to cope, my tenseness disappeared, and the pain in my right shoulder cleared with the massage and the gentle exercises I was shown. The combination of massage, help and encouragement to be positive made me more confident and light-hearted. I thoroughly recommend massage as a method of treatment which I believe will help in the healing process of mind and body.

These are typical of many responses from the sessions and the questionnaires commenting on the ways in which the massage sessions helped people to cope at difficult and stressful times in their lives, both through relaxation and, often, simply as a result of sharing their problem(s).

Need for touch

The need for touch is a fundamental need that is often denied in this society. Touch is the first sense to become functional in the womb and from birth onwards it plays a vital role in both the physical and emotional growth and development of the baby and infant (Montagu 1971). Tactile stimulation involving gentle stroking has been shown to enhance weight gain in pre-term babies as well as heighten responsiveness (Field et al 1987). Throughout all stages of life the need for touch continues, but at times of illness or crisis this need becomes particularly strong, regardless of sex or age. As a basic form of communication, touch can convey nuances of feeling and reaction more effectively than verbal communication. It can therefore be a useful therapeutic tool in the care of patients. Many studies, particularly in psychology and nursing journals, have examined its effects and appropriate use (Aguilera 1967, Cashar & Dixson 1967, Silvermann et al 1973, McCorkle 1974, Jackson 1985, Berry 1986, Le May 1986, Woodmansey 1988).

A distinction is drawn between 'caring' or 'comforting' touch, which aims to help the patient cope with illness and its related stressors, and 'procedural' or 'task-oriented' touch, associated with the diagnosis, monitoring and treatment of the illness itself (Glick 1986, Weiss 1986). The beneficial effect of caring touch commonly noted is its ability to:

- calm and comfort
- convey care and interest in the patient
- increase self-esteem
- lower anxiety levels
- soothe pain
- facilitate communication
- establish a rapport between therapist and patient.

As Byass, writing of her work with terminally ill patients notes: 'For patients who create barriers to communication, touch through massage can be a means of bridging gaps without offence or invasion of personal space' (Byass 1989). Barnett, in an overview of the concept of touch as a means of non-verbal communication in relation to nursing care, suggests groups of patients whose needs for touch are great:

- the isolated and sensory-deprived who need to relate to others
- those with an altered body image who need acceptance from both others and themselves
- those suffering depersonalisation who need to regain a sense of identity, or regression who need to communicate (both common symptoms often caused by hospitalisation)
- those with low self-esteem who need confir-

mation and affirmation
- those suffering anxiety and those terminally ill and frightened of death who need contact with others and reassurance (Barnett 1972).

From this brief résumé of some of the considered therapeutic uses of touch, it is evident that these effects would be beneficial in the care of many patients, with relevance not only to general practice but to a wide range of clinical areas.

Many patients at the Marylebone Health Centre remarked on the perceived benefits of simply being touched in a soothing, caring way. A 26-year old, very intelligent, professional woman with a traumatic childhood history, suffering deep depression with wrist-slashing episodes and suicidal attempts, wrote:

Touch had never been common as a child in my family and part of my psychotherapy has been to work through the effects of the lack of that. Massage has been complementary in giving me a structured experience of touch. The main benefit though was purely the relaxation element, again as part of a learning, or relearning, to be at ease with my body and relax my mind, without being overcome with weeping or anxieties.

A 73-year old woman was referred with high blood pressure from an overactive thyroid and suffering from palpitations. She was in a very depressed state and had just confided to her GP that she had been abused over a long period in her childhood—this was the first time she had revealed this information to anyone. Although this was not mentioned in the referral, she spoke openly of it during the massage sessions and talked of her subsequent hatred of her body. The original violations of her body were followed by a series of major operations, the removal of both breasts and her womb, which confirmed her extremely negative self-image, reinforcing her discomfort in and vehement disgust of her own body. She tended to wear layers of vests and corsets to hide her body and admitted that she had never let even her husband see her undressed since her first operation 40 years ago. She was obviously very wary about the massage and missed the first appointments. However, as the sessions wore on she talked of the difficult and traumatic events in her life and began to reassess and understand her attitude to her body. Although she was prevented by her life circumstances from maintaining the change—she eventually returned to her former closed emotional state—she did at least come to accept her body, no longer feeling the need for an armour of clothing to hide her shape and allowing others to see her: 'I've never let anyone touch me till now—it makes me feel my body is not so bad.'

A 31-year old solicitor, survivor of a car crash in which her husband had been killed, and now a widow with two young children, one of whom her husband had not lived to see, commented: 'When I leave, I feel I can cope better with the day and I'm not absolutely burdened by his death and all the worries—I miss being touched.'

A final example is from an ex-patriate recently returned from South Africa who found it difficult to adapt to this country and her highly stressful job as a radio presenter. She was referred for massage primarily for her chronic back pain, for which she had found no relief through osteopathy. Her pain was eased though the main benefit of the massage was its ability to serve as a kind of informal counselling session through its use of touch:

The massage sessions provided a regular link with a 'helping agency' at a time of stress and depression which cannot be underestimated. If tense and distressed, you usually just curl up and want to be alone, not the best way out! This particular type of contact, reminiscent of mother/child communication, is often more valuable and certainly more immediate than spoken communication.

The elderly, particularly those living alone, are a group who often have an increased need for touch yet to whom touch is often denied. As already indicated, the need for touch is not restricted by age and younger people not involved in a relationship or perhaps getting over the break-up of a long-term relationship, remarked on how much they needed simply to be touched.

Need for caring/time for oneself

Although the need to be cared for is applicable to most people in each of the categories listed above, it is dealt with separately here as it is so commonly singled out as one of the main benefits of the massage sessions. It is perhaps an undervalued benefit. This group is formed mostly of women who are carers at home and/or in their professional lives. They have spent so long listening to and fulfilling the needs of others that their own needs have been forgotten or repressed. Typically they initially view the hour-long session as an indulgence, but by the end of the course they have come to recognise that 'spoiling' themselves and allowing time for themselves is nothing to feel guilty about, but is actually necessary for their well-being, enabling them to continue caring for others.

A 64-year old inveterate carer, a committed social worker with a large family, referred primarily for back pain and sciatica as a result of a severe scoliosis, wrote:

I had a lovely feeling of peace and well-being and a new awareness of pampering myself which I never did. I learned through the massage and talking, to be aware of myself and my needs and I found that this enabled me to be even more aware of the needs of other people.

An arthritic lady, divorced after a loveless marriage with an unfaithful husband, who had worked all her life to bring up her daughter alone, but with little apparent return in terms of affection, described the benefits she experienced from massage:

I find it relaxing and soothing. I am usually full of aches and pains when it is damp and now I feel fewer pains after having a few sessions. It also makes me feel I'm being spoilt—I've never been spoilt before—it gives me a feeling of being taken care of, which makes me feel so much better.

Need to talk

From the quotations already cited it is evident that an important effect of massage is its ability to make people feel relaxed and secure enough to talk and share their problems. Often doctors are aware that there is a hidden agenda behind the presenting complaint which the patient will not acknowledge or talk about—perhaps because of the limited time allowed in the consultation or because of a particular relationship to the doctor. The complaint cannot be fully dealt with until this agenda is addressed. For many people, though, a referral for counselling can appear threatening and the doctor has to try gradually and gently to prepare the patient to accept the idea of a referral. Massage can perhaps help pave the way for this referral.

Massage is obviously a very physical therapy with little or no verbal communication essential to it. Nevertheless, an important element in the massages at the health centre is the time spent talking. This can range from general discussion on a particular problem (e.g. self-help tips, better coping strategies, and perhaps reassessing the roots of the problem) to an exploration of wider personal issues associated, albeit on an unconscious level, with the specific complaint. This is always instigated by the patient who can equally well choose to concentrate on the experience of the massage itself—the way in which the massage hour is used is very much the patient's choice. This paper has already described the therapeutic effects of touch and how it helps facilitate communication between therapist and patient. Massage, through touch combined with relaxation, provokes an opening-up, a self-disclosure that can be expressed at the simple problem-sharing level or can reveal highly significant issues. As one client said 'when I bare my body it seems natural to bare my soul as well'. This quality is something remarked upon by many of the patients at the health centre who often showed surprise at the expression of these deep-rooted anxieties and the accompanying emotion. In other words, massage is different to the counselling or psychotherapy setting, where verbalisation and exploration of problems is expected. It is desirable that the massage therapist should be open to this aspect and, if not trained in counselling skills, have at least the ability to listen and 'be there' with the patient. This function of massage at the health centre distinguishes it from what is usual elsewhere. It is a commonly held precept of massage practitioners that talk should be limited, if not avoided completely, so that the effects of this non-verbal therapy can be experienced fully. Obviously in practice this is

not always the case, but in the work at the Marylebone Health Centre it was even less so.

The massage sessions, in the setting of their own health centre, offered patients a 'safe place' to open up; the treatment, with 'caring' touch at its heart and experienced as pleasurable and soothing, enhanced patients' readiness for self-disclosure; and the role of the massage therapist, similar perhaps to that of the nurse, was interpreted as non-threatening and friendly, making for an easy, informal rapport. These factors help to explain why so many of the patients remarked on how free they felt to 'grumble' and to share problems or discuss more fundamental issues which they had not expected to do, and how this affected their physical condition. A recently bereaved man of 77 wrote simply: 'I did not understand how long-standing pain could be helped by relieving tension through massage and conversation'.

The following is taken from a letter from a young, single woman, referred with acute neck pain, who was working long shift hours in a multinational agency under the constant fear of redundancy. A large section of it is quoted as it not only illustrates this aspect of opening-up but also deals with the general relaxation qualities of massage and the enhanced awareness of the body/mind link previously discussed:

To say the first massage was a discovery is not too strong. What is difficult is to find the right words to express my reaction. Simultaneously, with the physical sensation of well-being, I felt the need to talk about my problems: imminent loss of job and the feelings of fear, self-doubt and incessant self-questioning, feelings which are all painful and probably the cause of much physical discomfort. I was very surprised after the first massage that I had been able to bring into the open all these fears and feelings. I most certainly would have been far less forthcoming and far less 'frank' in a situation of psychotherapy i.e. sitting, fully-dressed, face to face with a counsellor. It was as if the actual massage of the body had touched deeper inner nerves.

That the physical relief lasted so long also surprised me. I became much more aware, in the days following the first treatment, of body movements, relaxing my shoulders when sitting behind a desk and writing, bringing down shoulders when walking and breathing. The second and third sessions helped to consolidate the 'discovery' in terms of awareness of body posture and trying to merge relaxation movements when the fear of unemployment or the feeling of bitterness at my employer's behaviour entered my mind. . . Massage seems so simple (to the non-initiated!) and yet produces such deep results of well-being and awareness, of being put in touch with oneself.

Pain relief

Massage helps to alleviate pain through the relaxation of both body and mind. A rough analysis of the figures for the 99 patients whose referral included one or more pains shows that:

- 48 suffered neck and shoulder pain
- 32 suffered lower back pain
- 11 complained of aches and pains throughout the body
- 6 had headaches
- 4 had spinal malformations
- 4 had digestive problems and abdominal pain
- the remainder presented with sciatica, tennis elbow, and joint problems.

(It was common for patients to have at least two problem areas, the most noticeable combination being neck and lower back pain or headaches and neck pain.) The majority of these were caused by acute muscle spasm or chronic muscle contraction and arthritis. Other physical disorders were mainly associated with circulatory problems, such as Raynaud's syndrome, and fluid retention.

Patient responses showed a high level of immediate relief, commonly describing the pain as being 'soothed, stroked away', with an associated increase in mobility. This relief, though, especially in chronic degenerative disease, tended to be temporary, generally varying in duration from a few hours to a few weeks. Chronic pain sufferers are, however, a common referral for massage not only because it helps to alleviate the pain, albeit perhaps temporarily, but also because of the additional benefits already referred to under 'Stress-related disorders'. For example, several patients indicated increased feelings of control over the pain and better coping. A woman in her late 50s with very severe widespread rheumatoid arthritis who could find the most gentle massage painful, noted: 'Although the arthritis did not get any better, emotionally I myself felt much better. It also got rid of the tension and I was able to relax more, which helped me to bear the pain.'

Typical patients

From these groups, a picture builds up of patients, commonly seen by GPs, who might benefit from massage treatment. These include:

- the exhausted or anxious
- those experiencing loneliness or isolation
- those who need simple support
- the chronic pain sufferers.

Many elderly patients fall into one or more of these groups and hence can be appropriate referrals for massage.

Another group, some of whose characteristics GPs might have recognised in the preceding sections, are the 'difficult' or 'heartsink' patients (Cohen 1987, Corney et al 1988). A recent editorial warns that the changes proposed in the White Paper on the NHS could deter doctors from providing 'chronic somatisers' with the service they need which is primarily time, patience, listening skills and appropriate support (Bass & Murphy 1990). The authors argue that the biomedical model of illness implicit in the White Paper excludes the psychosocial dimension of illness and so cannot reflect the medical realities faced by GPs. Massage can sometimes help these patients, being seen as a very physical therapy that also induces relaxation and which offers patients time, undivided attention and support. It can assist in influencing or shifting patients' perspectives of their illness by enabling them to directly experience their 'somatic reality', rather than being put through the whole range of diagnostic and treatment services which further emphasise the split between mind and body. When all other referrals have been tried, massage can offer a new approach, the patient can be reassured that 'something is being done', and, not to be underrated, referral to massage allows a 'holiday' to be taken by both patient and doctor.

CONTRAINDICATIONS AND OTHER PROBLEMS

The main contraindications to massage generally cited are fever, acute inflammation, phlebitis, thrombosis, skin infection and extensive bruising. Classically, heart disease patients were included in this list, but currently massage is frequently employed for its calming properties with these patients. At Charing Cross Hospital in London, for example, massage has been used in the cardiac wards by nurses and volunteers for the last 7 years. Nursing research on this subject indicates that, although a careful assessment of the individual patient's response to touch and massage should still be made, particularly while in intensive care, it is inappropriate for a gentle soothing massage to continue to be included in the list of coronary precautions (Dunbar & Redick 1986, Glick 1986, Weiss 1986, Bauer & Dracup 1987).

Cancer patients are another group for whom massage has been restricted and there is still some controversy amongst doctors and practitioners about any risk involved. However, several cancer care and support groups use the services of a massage therapist or nurse trained in massage to work with their patients, often teaching patients and their families to massage each other. In their experience it is one of the therapies found most useful by patients and their carers. One study examining the effects of massage on six women receiving radiotherapy treatment for breast cancer found that the subjects reported less symptom distress, higher degrees of tranquillity and vitality and less tension and tiredness than after the control intervention (Sims 1986). Massage has been introduced into hospices where nurses find it eases their patients' physical discomfort as well as their isolation and fear (Byass 1989, Turton 1989). At Marylebone, several cancer patients have been referred for massage, generally while recovering from the unpleasant physical effects of their hospital treatment, and for them massage offered physical and mental relaxation and an opportunity to feel and enjoy their body again. After the often aggressive and invasive treatments they had undergone, the patients found it a relief to have a treatment that they actually experienced as pleasurable and where they felt cared for on a simple human level.

One group of people who do not benefit from massage are the 'tactually defensive'—those who, mainly due to their early tactile experiences, interpret touch as threatening. They find touch disturbing and massage for such people, instead of lowering the autonomic activity, would be seen as another stressor, raising arousal levels. Tactually defensive people are fortunately rare. Many patients who show an apparent aversion to touch initially are won over after a session of massage.

Other possible problems

From the above it is evident that gentle relaxing massages such as were predominantly employed at the health centre can rarely do anything but good. There were no problems reported by patients other than an occasional bruised feeling for a short period after the massage. Sometimes patients discovered that they had more pains after than before the massage, but this could nearly always be attributed to the fact that it had made them aware of chronic muscle tension in their body whose pain signals they had learnt to ignore.

The dependency of patients, particularly those with chronic complaints, could however become a problem. The limited length of the course was emphasised at the first appointment and repeated at each following session to try and avoid expectations of an extension. However, with some patients in particular need, extra treatments at monthly or 2-monthly intervals were given as part of a 'maintenance' course.

This highlights a limitation of rather than a problem with massage, i.e. that massage's effects in terms of symptom relief are often temporary. This need not necessarily detract from the value of the treatment which can often be judged simply in terms of the experience itself. Ted Kaptchuk described the joint assessment process to the Boston Pain Clinic in which the new patient sees all the therapists including the physical therapist and then finally has a session with the masseuse. Kaptchuk perceived the massage as one of the most important times for the patient himself, where for one short space of time he can experience what it feels like to feel good in his body (Griggs). From the experience at the Marylebone Health Centre, the chief therapeutic effects of massage are seen in terms of caring for the person rather than curing the symptom. The support element in massage is valued, helping people through a difficult phase, as again is its ability to get patients literally to sense their bodies and increase their awareness of the ways in which their posture and movements, emotional responses and behavioural patterns can all directly influence their physical state. This awareness can be greatly enhanced when incorporated with other stress management techniques such as diaphragmatic breathing. Whenever possible, patients are encouraged to continue this work after the sessions are over. In this way the benefits gained from the massage need not stop at the end of the course. One of the values of massage can perhaps be seen as its offering patients an enticing introduction to the principles of self-care, adherence to which might offer a more permanent resolution to their problems. As Marylebone offers yoga, relaxation, meditation and stress management classes, it is relatively easy for patients to find an appropriate method of self-care.

However, many patients expressed a desire to continue specifically with massage. Indeed, all of the replies to the questionnaire asking patients if they would like to continue having massage if it were available were affirmative. As massage is easily accessible in the private sector, advice on suitable therapists was given to interested patients. This was naturally not appropriate in many cases and, to try and address this issue, a pilot 'massage assistant' scheme was set up. This involved training volunteers (other patients from the health centre) to give a simple massage and then to work with suitable patients. Although the trainees greatly enjoyed learning and practising a new skill and the patients with whom they worked expressed satisfaction with their treatment, the scheme unfortunately was never sustained, due to administrative problems and the

lack of a readily available treatment room for the trainees. It did raise interesting questions as to the accepted boundaries between patients and clinicians, and to the reality behind the much trumpeted phrase 'patient empowerment'. An easier and more successful way of enabling patients to continue with massage, and one that conferred many benefits, was to spend some of the session time teaching both patients and spouses how to give a simple massage.

For the doctors too, there appear to be few problems with the introduction of massage into general practice. Massage is a truly 'complementary' therapy that does not affect the treatment already being given by the doctor, except, hopefully, by reducing the consultation rate or drug bill. A certain rivalry with the GP could be experienced by other complementary therapists offering a complete and distinct therapeutic system, but this was rarely the case with massage. The only territorial problems tended to be literal, with room space at a premium in the health centre.

IMPLICATIONS AND REVIEW OF THE USE OF MASSAGE AS A CLINICAL INTERVENTION

Keywords

To summarise this review, the keywords in the use of massage would be: relaxation; stress relief and management; pain relief; awareness of body/mind link; increased feelings of control and better coping; support; being cared for; touch; and sense of well-being. 'Relaxation' and 'touch' are keywords common to all the categories.

Perhaps 'pleasure' should also be included in the keywords, as it is important to stress that this therapy is also a very enjoyable one, one that has an immediate effect of making the patient 'feel good'. Many studies indicate an association between subjective well-being and physical health (Zautra & Hempel 1984). Although it can be argued that improving an individual's appraisal and coping skills confers greater therapeutic gain than inducing an increase in subjective well-being (Wood 1987) massage can be an extremely effective tool in this regard, particularly when linked to a stress management or self-care programme.

An important influence behind both the promotion of well-being and the improvement of coping skills, is the experience of truly sensing and being aware of the body, its needs and responses. This can lead to an understanding of the psychosomatic nature of a patient's problem and can be one of the most far-reaching effects of massage. An interesting idea in this respect is quoted by Bernie Siegel from the physicist David Bohm. He considers that the word 'psychosomatic' perpetuates the split between soma and psyche and suggests replacing it with a new word 'somasignificance' to emphasise the unity of soma with significance and ultimately with meaning in all its implications and possiblities (Siegel 1990). Part of massage's role in the clinical setting is to give patients insight into the 'somasignificance' of their illness by helping them to start listening to the messages their bodies give them and to understand their meaning.

Impact of and suggestions for the use of massage in general practice

The primary aim of this report has been to describe the introduction of massage into the clinical setting of general practice, looking at the types of patients referred, patient responses to the treatment and some of the processes involved in achieving its therapeutic effects. Its simple, undramatic but subtle modus operandi would appear peculiarly appropriate as part of the treatment and management plan for many of a GP's patients. As an adjunctive therapy it does not attempt to offer a system of diagnosis and curative treatment in cases of serious illness as other complementary therapies are able to do. However, the majority of patients (two-thirds according to one estimate (Kellner 1985)), who take the decision to consult their GP have no serious organic pathology, the GP often explaining their presenting symptoms in psychosocial terms. So the potential for massage's inclusion in the routine clinical work of general practice is great, but finding an appropriate way of assessing its

success rate is difficult. As yet, no study has been made on its impact by measuring variables before, during and after the course of treatments, such as consultation or drug prescription rates, or formal questionnaires on patients' perception of health and well-being. This review is primarily a descriptive account illustrated by the subjective responses of the patients.

Patient satisfaction

In terms of patient satisfaction, however, massage is rated highly, as is consistently reported by patients during the sessions and in their questionnaire responses. To the question asking patients to rate their treatment on the scale 1–5, (no benefit–very beneficial), 70% gave it the top rating, with none reporting no benefit; all rated it as 'enjoyable' with 85% awarding it the top score. This high satisfaction rate for massage is reflected by an independent survey involving 2000 people, carried out in 1984 by Research Surveys of Great Britain (Tisserand 1988). From the list of alternative therapies, the results revealed that the treatments with which people were most satisfied were relaxation and massage. Massage was the second highest scorer in the satisfaction ratings (82%) after meditation/relaxation, and had the lowest 'dissatisfied' score (9%). In the health centre's questionnaire, all the respondents said they would like massage to be part of the regular services on offer at the health centre and judged it a very useful complementary therapy for general practice. Whilst appreciating that 'success rates', however measured, are different to satisfaction ratings, these findings could have a topical relevance to GPs. Many patients remarked on how massage enhanced their perception of the health centre as a 'caring' centre and considered it a representative part of the 'whole person' approach followed by the centre. As the image of the health centre benefits from massage, so the massage also benefits from the environment of the health centre, a recognised 'safe place' whose clinicians patients could expect to trust.

Simple and effective referral for doctors

With the doctors too, massage came out well in the satisfaction stakes. It was readily accepted into clinical work, offered an unproblematic referral with no consequent complications (other than the dependency problems spoken of) and was appropriate for many of the doctors' patients as confirmed by the very positive feedback after treatment. One of the doctors commented that if he were to have just one complementary therapy available in the centre he would choose massage as the most useful clinical intervention.

Development of the role of the practice nurse

Another important figure in the primary care team who could benefit from familiarity with massage is the practice nurse. Although practice nurses are interested in developing and extending their nursing role, in reality this often means a shift towards traditionally medical tasks such as preventive or screening procedures (Greenfield et al 1987). As nurses research and attempt to define their role, they are identifying skills unique to nursing. It is a matter for debate whether acquiring greater clinical expertise—enabling the nurse to take over medical tasks from the doctor—is extending the nursing role or merely retaining the 'handmaiden' role as assistant to the doctor (Molde & Diers 1985). In general practice as in all fields of nursing, a large part of the nursing role has gradually become a task-orientated one. There are now signs, however, of a wish to reclaim some of the traditional functions of the nursing role such as defined by Florence Nightingale. She noted that nursing should 'put the patient in the best condition for nature to act upon him' (Nightingale 1952). The treatment and cure of illness were the concerns of the doctor while the nurse cared for the patient as an individual, supporting his natural recuperative powers and heeding his psychological as well as physical needs. Current research on nursing skills stresses the caring and educational functions that lie at the heart of a practice nurse's work, rather than technical skills alone (Diers & Molde 1983).

Another important role of the practice nurse is that of listener and counsellor. For many reasons the relationship between nurse and patient is different to that between doctor and patient, and a frequent result of the relative informality of the relationship is to facilitate communication. In identifying the value of the nurse's role in general practice, the extension of this role in communication and interpersonal relationships should be considered.

Massage is one skill that meets these criteria. In many areas of nursing, massage is being introduced as a clinical intervention that expands the nurse's role and allows the emphasis of primary nursing to rest on individualised patient care (Bamford et al 1990). Nurses are in an eminently suitable position to learn the skill, trained in the theoretical background and with abundant practical experience. That the practice nurse is already a member of the primary care team, trusted by both patients and doctors, is a bonus. There are many training courses on offer where nurses can learn massage and then bring this skill into the practice. Depending on the current workload of the nurse, one session each week or fortnight could be assigned to massage, perhaps with the appointments being slightly shorter than one hour to enable more patients to be seen. This proposal could lead to increased job satisfaction for practice nurses.

CONCLUSION

For GPs and practice nurses wishing to extend the range of clinical services they can call upon, there is an array of complementary therapies available, one of the simplest being massage. Massage offers a genuine 'whole person' approach, working as it does on the physical body and directly influencing emotional and mental states. It is a very adaptable therapy with a multiplicity of possible applications and is readily acceptable to both doctors and patients. Appropriate referrals include many of the patients on the GP's daily consultation list—the elderly, lonely, anxious or stressed, and chronic pain sufferers. Massage can fit into clinical practice without upsetting conventional treatment or even posing territorial problems for doctors and therapists. Patients rate it highly and it enhances their image of the health centre.

If the practice nurse is trained in massage the feasibility of its inclusion is improved while potentially enhancing the nurse's role—this accords with the current movement in nursing towards nurses regaining their traditional caring role. At the heart of the success of any therapy lies the relationship between client and therapist—the nurse is in a natural position to create an appropriate therapeutic relationship and rapport conducive to realising the full effects of massage.

While modern medicine is often criticised for losing its 'human touch' with its 'high tech' treatments, reliance on prescription pads, consultation time restraints, etc, this ancient therapy can help restore the balance. Touch, relaxation and 'being there' can help self-healing to occur. Massage is, therefore, a therapy that could and should be considered in many aspects of the care of patients and in many different clinical areas.

REFERENCES

Aguilera D C 1967 The relationship between physical contact and verbal interaction between nurses and patients. Journal of Psychiatric Nursing 1 pp 5–20

Bamford O, Dineen L, Pritchard B, Smith 1990 Change for the better—nursing development units. Nursing Times 86 (23) pp 28–33

Barnett K 1972 A theoretical construct of the concepts of touch as they relate to nursing. Nursing Research 21 pp 102–110

Bass C, Murphy M 1990 The chronic somatizer and the Government White Paper—Editorial. Journal of the Royal Society of Medicine 83 pp 203–205

Bauer W C, Dracup K A 1987 Physiological effects of back massage in patients with acute myocardial infarction. Focus on Critical Care 14 (6) pp 42–46

Berry A 1986 Knowledge at one's fingertips. Nursing Times 82 (49) pp 56–57

Byass R 1989 Soothing body and soul. Nursing Times 84 (24) pp 39–41

Cashar L, Dixson B K 1967 The therapeutic use of touch. Journal of Psychiatric Nursing, September

Cohen J 1987 Diagnosis and management of problem patients in general practice. Journal of the Royal College of General Practitioners 38 pp 349–352

Cuthbertson D P 1933 The effect of massage on metabolism: a survey. Glasgow Medical Journal 120 pp 200–213

Diers D, Molde S 1983 Nurses in primary care: the new gatekeepers? American Journal of Nursing 83 pp 742–745

Dunbar S, Redick E 1986 Should patients with acute myocardial infarction receive back massage? Focus on Critical Care 13 (3) pp 42–46

Field T, Scafidi F, Schanberg S 1987 Massage of pre-term newborn to improve growth and development. Paediatric Nursing 13 pp 385–387

Glick M 1986 Caring touch and anxiety in myocardial infarction patients in the intermediate cardiac care unit. Int Care Nurs 2 pp 61–66

Goodall-Copestake B 1919 The theory and practice of massage. Lewis, London

Greenfield S, Stilwell B, Drury M 1987 Practice nurses: social and occupational characteristics. Journal of the Royal College of General Practitioners 37 pp 341–345

Griggs B The healing arts. London

Jackson S 1985 The touching process in rehabilitation. Australian Nurses' Journal 14 (11) pp 43–45

Jacobs M 1960 Massage for the relief of pain: anatomical and physiological considerations. Physical Therapy Review 40 (2) pp 93–98

Kellner R 1985 Functional somatic symptoms and hypochondriasis. Arch General Psychiatry 42 pp 821–833

Kleen E A G 1918 Massage and medical gymnastics. Churchill, London

Le May A 1986 The human connection. Nursing Times 82 (47) pp 28–30

McCorkle R 1974 Effects of touch on seriously ill patients. Nursing Research 23 pp 125–132

McCormack C, Pietroni P C 1990 Massage, relaxation and touch: a review paper of 14 research studies on the effects of massage. Marylebone Centre Trust internal paper.

McKechnie A, Wilson F, Watson N, Scott D 1983 Anxiety states: a preliminary report on the value of connective tissue massage. Journal of Psychosomatic Research 27 pp 125–129

McLean J 1986 The use of relaxation techniques in general practice. Practitioner 230 pp 1079–1084

Martin S 1990 Nurses take in alternatives. Here's Health, February pp 18–22

Mennell J B 1945 Physical treatment by movement and massage. (5th edn., 1st edn. 1917) Churchill, London

Molde S, Diers D 1985 Nurse practitioner research: selected literature review and research agenda. Nursing Research 34 pp 362–367

Montagu A 1971 Touching—the human significance of the skin. Columbia University Press, New York

Nightingale 1952 Notes on nursing (first published 1859). Duckworth

Siegel B 1990 Peace, love and healing. Rider, London p 39

Silvermann A F, Pressman M E, Bartel H W 1973 Self-esteem and tactile communication. Journal of Humanistic Psychology 13 pp 73–77

Sims S 1986 Slow stroke back massage for cancer patients. Nursing Times 82 (13) pp 47–50

Tisserand R 1988 Aromatherapy for everyone. Penguin Books, London

Turton P 1989 Touch me, feel me, heal me. Nursing Times 85 (19) pp 42–44

Weiss S J 1986 Psychophysiological effects of care-giver touch on incidence of cardiac dysrhythmia. Heart and Lung 15 pp 495–506

Wood C 1987 Are happy people healthier? Discussion paper. Journal of the Royal Society of Medicine 80 pp 354–356

Woodmansey A C 1988 Are psychotherapists out of touch? British Journal of Psychotherapy 2 pp 57–65

Zautra A, Hempel A 1984 Subjective well-being and physical health: a narrative literature review with suggestions for future research. International Journal of Ageing and Human Development 19 pp 95–110

COUNSELLING IN AN INNER CITY GENERAL PRACTICE: ANALYSIS OF ITS USE AND UPTAKE

Vivien Webber
Peter Davies
Patrick Pietroni

Background: In recognition of the emotional problems which frequently underlie somatic complaints, practices increasingly offer counselling as part of their services to patients. In an inner city practice, a combination of short-term counselling, volunteer befriending, community outreach and social work services is offered as a means of responding to the full range of patients' counselling needs.
Aim: This study set out to establish the use and uptake of these services.
Method: A retrospective analysis of patients referred for counselling over one year was carried out.
Results: The analysis identified a broad range of emotional problems among referred patients as well as problems of a practical nature. A quarter of the patients referred failed to keep their initial appointments or to complete their contracts. One-fifth of the patients were referred on for longer term counselling and/or psychotherapy. Subsequent feedback revealed that preparation of a patient before referral was an important factor affecting uptake of counselling.
Conclusion: Early assessment of the use and uptake of such services is essential if they are to be integrated successfully and a counsellor's individual skills employed effectively.
Keywords: Counselling; patient satisfaction; uptake; inner city general practice.

INTRODUCTION

The increasing number of counsellors working in general practice [1] has coincided with a change in the pattern of primary health care. Practitioners, by choice and necessity, now work in a multidisciplinary network [2]. Frequently, these networks link medical care with nursing care, social work and, more recently, complementary therapies [3]. Moreover, patients as well as practitioners now tend to perceive illness as the

Reprinted with permission from the British Journal of General Practice: 44 pp. 175–178 April 1994.

result of a complex interaction of social, psychological, physical and environmental factors [4, 5]. This change has taken place against a background of cultural and environmental changes, for instance, the fact that more varied social and ethnic class groupings now live in the same area [6]. As these changes have occurred, so the need for counsellors has become widely recognised [7].

The literature on counselling in primary health care emphasises the subjective, positive experiences of general practitioners and counsellors working together [8–10]. Research projects, in which the experiences of social workers with psychotherapeutic skills and psychotherapists in primary health care are described, also emphasise the importance of interdisciplinary collaboration [11, 12]. In addition, various studies have attempted to look at the effectiveness of different styles of counselling [13–15] while others have compared trained staff with non-trained helpers [16–18].

Although these studies have highlighted the value of counselling in general practice there is a pressing need for further evaluation of both the types of problems being referred and how they are being met [19]. At present, no standardised training guidelines exist for counsellors working in general practice [20] and only recently have general accepted standards of practice been set [21]. Furthermore, few studies have addressed how practices might respond more imaginatively to the full breadth of counselling need.

The aim of the present study was to analyse and assess how a range of counselling, volunteer befriending, community outreach and social work services was being employed in an inner city health centre, as well as how these services might be developed further.

METHOD
The Marylebone Health Centre

The Marylebone Health Centre is a National Health Service general practice which emphasises a multidisciplinary approach to patient care. In addition to a core team of one full-time and two part-time general practitioners, a practice nurse, and health visiting and district nursing staff, the centre provides counselling, complementary therapies (traditional Chinese medicine, massage, homoeopathy and osteopathy), a community care and outreach programme and stress management group activities.

At the time of this analysis, the practice had just under 3700 registered patients. The practice has an 'open door' policy towards new registrations. It is situated in an area of social extremes, and attracts a high proportion of underprivileged patients, as a result of the large number of local bed and breakfast hotels for homeless families [6]. The practice population generally reflects local demography, although it has relatively more patients in the 20–29 years age group (31% versus the mean for the family health services authority of 23%) and fewer patients over 65 years of age (8% versus 13%). The proportions of male and female patients are 42% and 58%, respectively; approximately a quarter of patients are from an ethnic minority background.

Counselling

The counsellor is trained as a social worker and psychoanalytic psychotherapist as well as having counselling, stress management and family therapy skills. She is employed for 9 hours per week. The usual channel of referral for counselling is directly from the general practitioner with the patient making an appointment to see the counsellor through reception. Occasionally, referrals are made by the complementary practitioners following discussion with the general practitioner and in one or two instances patients refer themselves. Details of the patient's problems are written in the patient's notes as well as on a separate referral form, with a comment on the type of help required. In some instances, either after the first assessment meeting or after several sessions, the counsellor may refer a patient for long-term psychotherapy or some other service, as appropriate.

Depending on the nature of the problem, patients are normally offered a counselling contract of a maximum of six to eight sessions at either the first or second appointment. This can be extended by mutual agreement as a result of on-going assessment. A focus for the work is agreed early on. Each session usually lasts 50 minutes, but can be shorter. At the end of each session, a summary is written in the patient's notes which are accessible to all members of the multidisciplinary team. Patients are made aware of this and if they wish information to remain confidential, this wish is normally respected.

A social work student, trainee counsellor and a group of volunteer befrienders, attached to the health centre, provide a wide range of resources for the counsellor to draw upon. They offer more flexibility in the amount of contact that is possible with patients and in the case of the trainee counsellor and social work student this flexibility also meets their training needs. It also means that home visiting is possible, an aspect of work not normally considered part of a trained counsellor's role. Feedback from homeless families staying in temporary hotel accommodation and from patients living on their own suggests they particularly value this extended length of involvement.

Analysis

A retrospective analysis was carried out of patients referred for counselling between September 1989 and August 1990, inclusive. The information compiled included patients' date of birth, sex, referring general practitioner, date of referral, reason(s) for referral (as corroborated by the counsellor), and uptake and length of treatment. General practitioner consultation and referral rates were calculated by reviewing the practice's appointment sheets and referral letters over this period.

RESULTS
Referrals

A total of 92 patients were referred by general practitioners for counselling over the study period and three further patients referred themselves. Of the total of 2260 patients who consulted a general practitioner over the analysis period 37.7% were male and 62.3% were female.

Table 4.5 Age distribution of patients on the practice list and of those referred for counselling, and the referral rate for each age group

| Age (years) | % of patients | | No. of referrals per 1000 GP consultations |
	On practice list (n = 3697)	Referred for counselling (n = 95[a])	
0–9	12.3	0	0
10–19	7.0	3	10.1
20–29	31.4	38	19.2
30–39	18.9	20	15.1
40–49	10.8	16	19.2
50–59	7.7	11	14.3
60–74	8.1	12	11.1
75+	3.8	1	1.8

n = total number of patients. [a]Includes three self-referrals.

The high number of referrals for counselling and the high referral rate in the 20–29 years age group reflected the high number of patients in this age group in the practice (Table 4.5). However, patients aged 40–49 years were also more likely to be referred to the counsellor than patients from other age groups. The mean referral rate for counselling was 13.5 referrals per 1000 general practitioner consultations and the rates of the three general practitioners ranged from 8.1 to 18.9. In comparison, the practice made 1.7 referrals per 1000 general practitioner consultations to psychiatric outpatient services over the same period.

Wait before first appointment

Of the 95 patients referred for counselling 60% were offered appointments within 1 week of referral (including three self-referrals) and 87% within 3 weeks. Of the 12 patients seen after this period four had delayed making an appointment with the counsellor following referral.

Reasons for referral

The primary and secondary reasons for referral were broken down into the following problem areas: alcoholism, bereavement, depression, financial problem, housing problem, refugee issue, relationship problem and general stress. Often, these

were defined by the general practitioner at the referral stage and then confirmed by the counsellor following assessment (Table 4.6). Patients were referred either with straightforward practical problems, such as housing, and/or with a single or combination of emotional problems. By far the largest numbers of referrals were for relationship problems (primary reason for 42 patients, 45%), followed by problems causing general stress (21 patients, 23%), such as the burden of caring for a handicapped child, mid-life crises or traumatic experiences. No families or patients with psychotic illness were referred. Of those for whom reasons for referral were known, 77% were women.

Table 4.6 Reasons for referral for 93 patients[a]

| Primary/secondary reason for referral | Number of patients | | |
	Men	Women	Total
Alcoholism	2	0	2
Alcoholism/relationship problem	0	1	1
Bereavement	2	10	12
Depression	3	5	8
Depression/bereavement	0	1	1
Financial/relationship problem	1	0	1
Housing problem	0	3	3
Housing problem/ bereavement	0	1	1
Refugee issue	1	0	1
Relationship problem	3	25	28
Relationship problem/ depression	0	3	3
Relationship/housing problem	0	1	1
Relationship problem/ bereavement	2	3	5
Relationship problem/ general stress	1	4	5
General stress	6	13	19
General stress/ bereavement	0	2	2
Total	21	72	93

[a]Reason for referral unavailable for two patients.

Table 4.7 Treatment provided to 83 patients

Treatment	Number of patients		
	Men	Women	Total
Assessment only	2	4	6
Assessment plus:			
Counselling	6	26	32
Counselling and practical advice[a]	2	8	10
Counselling and referral for further counselling/psychotherapy	2	17	19
Immediate referral to another resource	1	3	4
Practical advice[a]	3	7	10
Referral to befriender	2	0	2

[a]Self-help, such as breathing and relaxation techniques or information about local group resources.

Treatment

Of the 95 patients referred, 12 never attended, 12 terminated their contract prematurely (four missing the final session), three had their contract reassessed and shortened and the remaining 68 completed their contract. The treatment provided to the 83 patients attending is shown in Table 4.7. 11 patients were seen by the social work student, and two by befrienders and two by a trainee counsellor, all four following assessment by the counsellor. 19 patients were referred for longer term therapy following a period of counselling. Issues that could not be resolved by short-term counselling were usually related to long-standing problems and almost always concerned relationship problems.

Of the 83 patients who kept their first appointment, 28 were seen for one session only—these tended to be patients who wanted practical advice or for whom it was appropriate to make an immediate referral to another community resource. 38 patients were seen for between two and five sessions, 12 were seen for six to 10 sessions and five were seen for more than 10. Of those patients who were seen for between six and 10 sessions, two were referred on for longer term counselling and psychotherapy. Feedback from general practitioners suggested that for all those who were referred on, the initial short-term counselling often provided a 'safe space' to begin exploring their problems and the confidence to continue the exploration in another setting. Of the 68 patients who completed their contracts, 47 (69%) did so within a 13-week period.

DISCUSSION

The British Association for Counselling defines the counsellor's task as being 'to give the client an opportunity to explore, discover and clarify ways of living more resourcefully and towards greater well-being' [22]. This analysis highlighted the wide range of problems referred. It also showed that practical advice on self-help, such as breathing and relaxation techniques or information about local group resources, was often required. It was therefore important for the counsellor to use her skills flexibly.

The reasons for referral could only be categorised broadly since different general practitioners tended to emphasise different aspects of the patient's problems. For example, although a separate category of bereavement (following a death) was included, underlying themes of loss (the end of a relationship, mid-life crisis) were present in many of the referrals. These may not have been stated by the general practitioner as a reason for referral but they were identified during the initial counselling assessment.

A general practitioner would occasionally refer a patient in order to alleviate pressure on him/herself and gain extra support. Patients were also sometimes referred if a difficulty in communication between doctor and patient arose. Feedback both from the analysis and from individual counsellor/client contacts regarding the appropriateness of referrals refined the understanding and collaboration between the general practitioner and counsellor.

Given the demand for the counselling service and its limited resources, emphasis was placed on short-term work as a way of responding to the needs of as many patients as possible. The short-term counselling contracts were seen in the context of a primary health care philosophy of continuing general practitioner care of the patient. It was therefore accepted by all concerned that a patient could be referred again at a future date if further problems arose. However, more than one-fifth of patients were referred on for longer term counselling and/or psychotherapy. It should be recognised that, even if the counsellor had had additional skills in cognitive and behavioural therapy, a number of patients would require further referral.

The analysis showed that 24 of the 95 patients failed to keep the initial appointment or complete their contract. Although this group was not followed up specifically, feedback from general practitioners, the complementary practitioners and from patients themselves allowed some insight into the reasons for these failures. A lack of patient preparation by the general practitioners sometimes appeared to be a factor in patients not attending their first appointment. Patients were sometimes referred for counselling at a time when they did not feel confident enough to explore their attitudes, behaviour and feelings. Although they would respond positively to a general practitioner's invitation to see a counsellor, it was discovered during subsequent consultations with the general practitioner that they had not, in fact, wanted to be referred and so had experienced a sense of rejection.

For the 12 patients who failed to complete the counselling contract several factors are relevant. In some instances, patients commented that they felt better after two or three appointments and so simply did not return. For others, the style of counselling was different from what they were expecting. They came wanting advice or instant solutions to their problems, when this was neither appropriate nor possible. Others felt ambivalent about the opportunity to explore and understand their problems within the context of a short counselling contract—while they welcomed the opportunity, they felt unsafe about exploring very personal struggles, knowing that they might be referred to someone else at the conclusion of the contract. Four patients missed the final session. This may have been related to difficulty in facing the sense of loss associated with the ending of counselling, even though patients knew they could be re-referred at a future date.

Following up the patients who did not complete their contract would have given a better indication of the reasons for defaulting. It might also have enabled those individuals who missed the final session to face and contain feelings about the ending and helped them to deal with similar situations in the future. Since this analysis, a change in policy has meant that all patients who do not complete their contracts are contacted and offered the opportunity to complete the initial agreed number of sessions. Subsequent discussion has also resulted in better preparation of patients and a reduction in the number who default.

One aspect of the analysis was to look at the value of having a spectrum of resources available including a befriending service provided by patient volunteers [23]. The fact that only two referrals were made to befrienders by general practitioners via the counsellor prompted an appraisal of how this new service was being used. It transpired that the service's novelty, combined with a general uncertainty on the part of the general practitioners as to what it could offer, resulted in fewer referrals than expected being made. There is now greater understanding between befrienders and general practitioners, and this has meant referrals to befrienders of elderly and isolated patients, in particular, have increased and the service has become more integrated into the practice.

It is widely recognised that patients present to general practitioners with a wide range of psychological and social problems [7] and that emotional problems frequently underlie presenting somatic complaints [24]. In addition, the relevance of short-term counselling is now widely accepted in the primary health care field [21].

Patient analysis features centrally in the planning and monitoring of a number of primary health care services. The increased use of analysis of referrals to counsellors would not only help training organisations to 'fine tune' their training programmes but would also provide general practitioners with a better understanding of how best to meet their practice's counselling needs.

A similar analysis undertaken in another practice would be expected to highlight a different set of problems to those reported here. It is unlikely, however, that a single counsellor in an average size practice will have the time or expertise to respond to the full range of patients' counselling needs. Therefore, depending on what these needs are, general practitioners might consider taking on other team members, such as those with skills in social work and befriending, who have a good working knowledge of local support services and community facilities. This would ensure the provision of a more comprehensive range of counselling care and support which, with the current emphasis on care in the community, will almost certainly have an increasingly important role to play in the future [25].

ACKNOWLEDGEMENT

We thank Dr Derek Chase for his comments.

REFERENCES

1. Sibbald B, Addington-Hall J, Brenneman D, Freeling B. Counselling in English and Welsh general practices: their nature and distribution. BMJ 1993; 306: 29–33.
2. Kilcoyne A, Pietroni P C. The history of the primary health care team. In: Royal College of General Practitioners. 1990 members' reference book. London: Sabrecrown, 1990.
3. Reason P, Chase H D, Desser A, et al. Towards a clinical framework for collaboration between general and complementary practitioners: discussion paper. J R Soc Med 1992; 85: 161–164.
4. Helman C. Culture, health and illness: an introduction for health professionals. Bristol: Wright, 1984.
5. Pietroni P. The greening of medicine. London: Victor Gollancz, 1990.
6. Chase H D, Davies P R T. Calculation of the underprivileged area score for a practice in inner London. Br J Gen Pract 1991; 41: 63–66.
7. McLeod J. The work of counsellors in general practice. Occasional paper 37. London: Royal College of General Practitioners, 1988.
8. Gray D P. Counsellors in general practice [editorial]. J R Coll Gen Pract 1988; 38: 50–51.
9. Bhaduri R. A prescription for counselling—GP attached social work. Social Work Today 1989; 30: 16–17.
10. Rowland N, Irving J, Maynard A. Can general practitioners counsel? J R Coll Gen Pract 1989; 39: 118–120.
11. Graham H, Sher M. Social work and general practice. J R Coll Gen Pract 1976; 26: 95–105.
12. Brook A, Temperley J. The contribution of a psychotherapist to general practice. J R Coll Gen Pract 1976; 26: 86–94.
13. Waydenfeld D, Waydenfeld S W. Counselling in general practice. J R Coll Gen Pract 1980; 30: 671–677.
14. Brodaty H, Andrews G. Brief psychotherapy in family practice. A controlled prospective intervention trial. Br J Psychiatry 1983; 143: 11–19.
15. Martin E, Martin P M L. Changes in psychological diagnosis and prescription in a practice employing a counsellor. Fam Pract 1985; 2: 241–243.
16. Durlak J A. Comparative effectiveness of paraprofessional and professional helpers. Psychol Bull 1979; 86: 80–92.
17. Hattie J A, Sharpley C F, Rogers J H. Comparative effectiveness of professional and paraprofessional helpers. Psychol Bull 1984; 95: 534–541.
18. Berman J S, Norton N C. Does professional training make a therapist more effective? Psychol Bull 1985; 98: 401–407.
19. Corney R H. Counselling in general practice—does it work? J R Soc Med 1990; 83: 253–257.
20. Rowland N, Irving J. Towards a rationalisation of counselling in general practice. J R Coll Gen Pract 1984; 34: 685–687.
21. Working Party of British Association for Counselling. Counselling in medical settings. Guidelines for the employment of counsellors in general practice. Rugby: BAC, 1993.
22. Rowland H, Hurd J. Counselling in general practice: a guide for counsellors. Rugby: British Association for Counselling, 1989.
23. Webber V, Barry V, Davies P, Pietroni P. The impact of a volunteer community care project in a primary health care setting. J Soc Work Pract 1991; 5: 83–90.
24. Irving J, Heath V. Counselling in general practice: a guide for general practitioners. Rugby: British Association for Counselling, 1989.
25. Means R, Harrison L. Community care before and after the Griffiths report. Bristol: School for Advanced Urban Studies, University of Bristol, 1988.

THE MUSCULOSKELETAL CLINIC IN GENERAL PRACTICE: A STUDY OF ONE YEAR'S REFERRALS

David Peters
Peter Davies
Patrick Pietroni

Background: A musculoskeletal clinic, staffed by a general practitioner trained in osteopathy, medical acupuncture and intralesional injections, was set up in an inner London general practice in 1987.
Aim: A retrospective study was undertaken of one year's referrals to the clinic in 1989-90 to determine how general practitioners were using the clinic in terms of problems referred; consultation patterns of patients attending the clinic and 12 months after initially being seen; and how access to the clinic influenced referrals to relevant hospital departments.
Method: Daysheets were studied which recorded information on demographic characteristics of patients referred to the clinic and their problems, diagnoses made, duration of symptoms, number and range of treatments given, and recurrence of problems. Use of secondary referral sources was also examined.
Results: During the study year 154 of 3264 practice patients were referred to the musculoskeletal clinic, and attended a mean of 3.5 times each. Of all the attenders 64% were women and 52% were 30–54 years old. 81 patients (53%) presented with neck, back or sciatic pain. A specific traumatic, inflammatory or other pathological process could be ascribed to only 19% of patients. Regarding treatment, 88% of patients received osteopathic manual treatment or acupuncture, or a combination of these treatments and 4% received intralesional injections. Nine patients from the clinic (6%) were referred on to an orthopaedic specialist during the year, two with acute back pain. Referrals to orthopaedic specialists by the practice as a whole were not significantly lower than the national average, although the practice made fewer referrals to physiotherapy and rheumatology departments than national figures would have predicted. 17 patients (11%) returned to the clinic with a recurrence of their main complaint within a year of their initial appointment; second courses of treatment were usually brief.
Conclusion: The clinic encouraged a relatively low referral rate to musculoskeletal specialists outside the practice. However, a need was identified for better communication about the potential of the approaches used in order that referrals to secondary specialists, particularly orthopaedic specialists, could be further reduced.
Keywords: Musculoskeletal disorders; referral of patients; GP clinics; complementary medicine; orthopaedics.

Reprinted with permission from the British Journal of General Practice: 44 pp. 25–29 January 1994.

INTRODUCTION

Musculoskeletal disorders are a major cause of morbidity in the United Kingdom and an increasingly important reason for consultation in general practice. The number of patients consulting with musculoskeletal problems per 1000 at risk has risen from 91.2 in 1971–72 to 132.8 in 1981–82. The number of consultations for back pain over the same period rose from 17.6 to 32.8 per 1000, an increase of 86% [1].

Musculoskeletal disorders have a prevalence of approximately 190 per 1000 patients per year; an estimated 7.5 million people seek help from their general practitioners each year, about one in 10 of whom are referred to a specialist [1]. As well as accounting for 10–15% of all general practitioner consultations and more than 44 million working days lost (12%) [2], musculoskeletal disorders also cause a high proportion of chronic disability [3]. According to figures from the Department of Health and Social Security, in 1982–83 back pain was responsible for 33.3 million days of certified incapacity to work [4].

Manipulative therapies for musculoskeletal problems have a long history, and their use has been formalised in the osteopathic [5] and chiropractic disciplines whose methods, though somewhat different, are alike in their strong reliance on manual and tactile approaches to diagnosis and treatment. Although their use is better established in the private sector, in recent years they have become more widely available within the National Health Service. A number of controlled studies document the application of Maitland's manipulation and osteopathic manipulation in general practice [6, 7], and hospital settings [8, 9], Doran & Newell's study finding no support for the use of manipulative methods. In some cases, trial design had been problematic [10] and even a well-known trial of outpatient chiropractic treatment [11] has been widely criticised [12]. However, a rigorous study of primary care based manipulative therapy in the Netherlands has shown manipulative therapy to be significantly more effective than physiotherapy for back and neck pain [13]. A 1991 survey of all general practitioners in the UK showed that 29% of 23 865 respondents thought that, assuming adequate resources were made available, it would be appropriate to offer osteopathy at their surgeries [14].

The present study took place in an inner city general practice in London which, as well as offering orthodox medical care, also provides a range of complementary therapies through clinics staffed by part-time practitioners. A musculoskeletal clinic staffed by a general practitioner trained in osteopathy, medical acupuncture and intralesional injections was set up in 1987. Patients with musculoskeletal problems are usually referred by general practitioners in the practice although some refer themselves. Only NHS patients registered with the practice are seen. Clinic sessions last 3 hours and are held twice weekly with appointments at 20-minute intervals.

The aim of the study was to examine one year's referrals to the musculoskeletal clinic in 1989–90, and in particular the study aimed to investigate the number of patients referred and their demographic characteristics; the type of problems referred; the duration of symptoms; the diagnoses made; the number and range of treatments given; the frequency with which patients returned with their presenting problem within a year of initially being seen at the clinic; the clinic's referrals to secondary sources during the study year; and the practice's use of secondary referral sources.

METHOD

The study period covered new referrals to the musculoskeletal clinic between 15 September 1989 and 14 September 1990. During this time, the practice list size grew from 2831 to 3697 patients, a mean for the year of 3264 patients.

Daysheets noting date and source of referral, type of problem, chronicity, diagnoses made, treatment given, referral date and discharge date were filled in for each session by the practitioner running the clinic. Separate note sheets were kept in patients' files to ensure accurate record keeping and to facilitate final assessment of progress and any referral made.

Patients' notes were reviewed in September

1991, one year after the study period, to establish whether patients discharged from the clinic had returned within a year of initially being seen for further treatment or consulted their general practitioner subsequently with the same problem. A record was also kept of all referrals made to orthopaedic, physiotherapy and rheumatology departments during the study period. All practice referral letters were reviewed in September 1991, to calculate the practice referral rate to relevant specialties during this 2-year period.

RESULTS

Demographic characteristics

The practice population is comparatively young in relation to that of the local family health services authority as a whole. During the study period, 91.7% of patients in the practice were under 65 years old compared with 86.7% in the family health services authority. In the practice, 8.3% were aged 65 years and over and 30.7% were aged 20–29 years compared with 13.3% and 23.4% in the family health services authority, respectively.

Of the 154 patients who were seen in the musculoskeletal clinic, 56 were male (36.4%). During the study period 37.8% of patients who consulted a general practitioner were male. Of the 154 patients attending the musculoskeletal clinic, there was one patient in the 0–19 years ag group, 18.2% of patients were aged 20–29 years, 23.4% were aged 30–39 years, 28.6% were aged 40–54 years, 13.6% were aged 55–64 years, 13.0% were aged 65–74 years and four (2.6%) were aged 75 years and over.

Of the three general practitioners referring patients, two referred approximately two patients per 100 seen to the clinic, while the other referred one per 100 patients seen. When working as an occasional general practitioner locum in the practice, the musculoskeletal clinician referred four patients per 100 seen. 16 patients referred themselves.

Types of problems referred

Of the principal problems initially presented to the clinic, over half of the patients (81) reported neck (22), back (44) or sciatic pain (15), 33 presented with large joint pain (14 of whom had shoulder pain), 11 had limb pain (usually of the arm, eight patients), 10 had peripheral joint pain, six had head pain and four had thoracic pain. The other nine patients comprised four patients with paraesthesia, two with congenital deformity, two with stiffness and one with stress.

Diagnoses

The majority of patients seen (125, 81.2%) had musculoskeletal pain which could not be explained in terms of structural pathology (Table 4.8). 74 patients were classified as having spinal somatic dysfunction. Disc prolapse, root entrapment, trauma and inflammation did occur, but relatively rarely.

Table 4.8 Diagnoses for the 154 patients attending the musculoskeletal clinic

Diagnosis	Number of patients
Structural pathology	
Arthritis	2
Bursitis	1
Congenital kyphoscoliosis	2
Capsulitis	2
Carpal tunnel syndrome	1
Fasciitis	1
Osteoarthritis	10
Prolapsed intervertebral disc	3
Root entrapment syndrome	5
Tendinitis	2
Non-specific[a]	
Fibrositis	3
Pain arising from ligament	10
Stress related pain	5
Specific joint dysfunction	3
Specific muscle dysfunction	30
Spinal somatic dysfunction	74

[a]Classification based on model of primary somatic dysfunction.

Table 4.9 Duration of problem before presentation at the general practitioner, by sex, age and presenting complaint[a]

	Duration of problem before presentation			
	0–7 days	8–30 days	31–365 days	366+ days
No. of patients	26	28	53	44
No. of men	15	9	20	12
No. of women	11	19	33	32
Mean age of all patients (years)	40.5	42.2	47.8	46.6
No. of patients with:				
Back pain	11	9	14	10
Neck pain	8	4	3	6
Sciatica	2	6	3	4
Large joint pain	4	5	12	12
Limb pain	0	0	8	3
Peripheral joint pain	1	1	3	5
Head pain	0	1	2	3
Thoracic pain	0	1	3	0
Other	0	1	5	1

[a]Data missing for one patient with neck pain; two patients with kyphoscoliosis not included.

Symptom duration and length of time before appointment

In 54 of 151 cases (35.8%) the principal symptom had been present for less than 1 month (Table 4.9). Of the 26 who had acute symptoms of a week or less, 19 presented via their general practitioner and seven came directly to the clinic. Nine of these acute referrals from the general practitioner were seen in the clinic within 1 week (five on the same day as they presented), and the remainder within a fortnight. Of the 28 patients with symptoms of 8 to 30 days' duration four referred themselves and 24 came via their general practitioner. Half of these were seen within a week and 18 within a fortnight. 23 of the 54 patients reported that they had had similar episodes of pain over a number of years. 40 of the 54 patients (74%) attended with neck, back or sciatic pain.

53 patients (35.1%) attended the clinic with pain that had been present for between 1 month and 1 year before they had consulted the general practitioner. Although 13 patients presented with a recurrence of a longstanding musculoskeletal problem of more than 1 year, the remaining 40 denied any such previous history.

11 of this latter group (28%) complained of neck, back or sciatic pain.

44 patients (29.1%) complained of pain which had been present for more than 1 year. These patients consulted because of an intermittent or episodic chronic problem, for example, headache or large joint pain, rather than because of a clear recent exacerbation of symptoms. In terms of mean age, there was little to distinguish this group from the others. However, as with those who had had their symptoms for between 1 month and 1 year there was a greater proportion of large joint, limb and peripheral joint pain than in the acute groups.

Two patients with congenital kyphoscoliosis were referred to the clinic for advice about exercise.

Treatments

Among the 41 patients who were seen at the clinic only once, four patients had somatic symptoms related to stress so received no treatment and were referred back to their general practitioner. Five others (two with hyperlordosis, two with congenital kyphoscoliosis, and one with osteoarthritis) were assessed as unlikely to benefit from treatment in the musculoskeletal clinic and were given an exercise programme and referred back to their general practitioner to discuss other options for management. The remainder were given a single osteopathic treatment or acupuncture (often with advice for self-care and prevention) and asked to return only if they felt it necessary. The majority of patients (80) were treated between two and four times and 25 patients received between five and 10 treatments. Only six patients received courses of 11–15 treatments and two patients were treated more than 15 times. The patients requiring more than 10 treatments either had profound physical problems (such as acute trauma or chronic prolapsed intervertebral disc pain) or had chronic pain requiring regular support. In all, 539 appointments were kept (3.5 per patient) and 26 appointments were missed.

Different patterns of treatment were used. 43 patients received treatment by the osteopathic manipulative technique only, 11 had this treatment with musculoskeletal acupuncture and 12 had the manipulative treatment followed by acupuncture later. 14 patients had musculoskeletal acupuncture only, four had acupuncture followed by osteopathic manipulation later and two had acupuncture followed by injection of trigger points with local anaesthetic. Two patients had treatment by soft tissue articulation techniques (deep tissue massage, pressure techniques and stretching), 14 had this treatment followed by manipulation techniques later, 24 had soft tissue articulation with acupuncture and 10 had soft tissue articulation with specific self-care instructions. One patient was given an oral non-steroidal anti-inflammatory drug, three patients received an intralesional triamcinolone injection and one patient had only an injection of trigger points with local anaesthetic. Three patients received self-care advice only, six patients were given an exercise programme only and four patients were only assessed. In almost all cases, advice was given about self-care, especially about exercise and posture, and this was usually reinforced by appropriate leaflets.

Recurrence of symptoms

It was found that 27 of the 154 patients seen began a second course of treatment within 1 year of their initial appointment at the clinic; in all but four cases they returned to the clinic on their own initiative rather than seeing their general practitioner first. 10 patients presented with a different problem and of the 17 who returned with the same problem, 13 had back pain. 13 patients received a single second treatment and seven patients received more than four.

Referrals

During the study year, nine patients who had attended the clinic were referred to an orthopaedic outpatient department, five at the request of the doctor running the musculoskeletal clinic and four because their general practitioner referred them on for different complaints, subsequent to their attending the musculoskeletal clinic. Two patients were referred to the musculoskeletal clinic from physiotherapy while three others were referred from the clinic to physiotherapy. In one further case, physiotherapy and treatment in the clinic overlapped. One patient who had attended the musculoskeletal clinic was referred to a rheumatology clinic.

During the study period, the practice made a total of 32 other referrals to an orthopaedic outpatient department, 26 to physiotherapy and two to a rheumatology outpatient department. The 29 referrals in total to physiotherapy gave a referral rate of 8.9 per 1000 patients. 41 patients in total were referred to an orthopaedic specialist, giving a referral rate of 12.6 referrals per 1000 patients. Of these, 11 (27%) had non-specific back, joint and limb pain while the other patients had structural pathology (five patients had back pain). Four patients (two of whom were referred by the musculoskeletal clinician) had chronic non-specific back pain.

In the year following the study period the practice list size grew from a mean for the year of 3264 to 3957 patients, an increase of 21%. The practice as a whole made 49 referrals to an orthopaedic outpatient department, 30 to physiotherapy (referral rate of 7.6 per 1000 patients) and three to a rheumatology outpatient department. Six of the patients referred to an orthopaedic outpatient department had attended the musculoskeletal clinic during the study period. Three of these were referred by the doctor in the musculoskeletal clinic, two by the general practitioner for further management of osteoarthritis of the hip and one was referred with a new problem. One patient who had attended the musculoskeletal clinic was sent to a rheumatology outpatient department with polymyalgia rheumatica.

DISCUSSION

Of the patients referred to the clinic 52% were aged between 30 and 54 years, mirroring the peak incidence of back pain in the general community [1] as well as being in the age band most often referred for physiotherapy [15].

It is interesting that 81% of the patients in this study presented with mechanical pain and movement restriction in the absence of any obvious traumatic, inflammatory or degenerative cause. According to conventional methods, treatment for the majority of patients classified as suffering non-specific musculoskeletal pain would be either symptomatic or unsupported by published information on precise indications and efficacy. However, in this study a classification, consistent with a model of primary somatic dysfunction, provided a range of diagnostic categories encompassing most patient presentations [5]:

1. Pain, movement restriction and tenderness predominating at one spinal segmental level are referred to as spinal somatic dysfunction [16].
2. Where somatic dysfunction involves a single muscle or group of muscles this is referred to as specific muscle dysfunction [17].
3. In the case of non-spinal single joint involvement, this is referred to as specific joint dysfunction.

These dysfunction states produce their own distinct palpatory signs which include changes in local tissue tension and range of movement. Osteopathy aims to make clinical diagnoses based on these changes and to provide specific strategies for management and treatment.

The neurophysiological mechanisms that could cause somatic dysfunction are at an early stage of investigation. Slosberg has reviewed some experimental justifications for the concept [18] while Roland has reviewed evidence that cycles of pain–spasm–pain can be continually reinforced by a number of aggravating factors [19]. Such factors would include overloading, unaccustomed use, anxiety and intramuscular metabolite accumulation.

Manipulative approaches to treatment, for which osteopathy is renowned, predominated among this series of patients as the method used first (43% of patients). However, non-manipulative osteopathic techniques such as articulation, deep tissue massage, pressure techniques and stretching were also interventions of first choice (32% of patients). Dry needling of trigger points (musculoskeletal acupuncture) was less commonly used as a first line treatment (13% of patients). In some cases, additional methods were introduced at subsequent appointments, for instance, where a dysfunctional joint had become amenable to manipulation, or when trigger point pain unresponsive to soft tissue techniques called for more intensive treatment. Trigger point injections with local anaesthetic [17] were usually employed for specific muscle dysfunctions only after manual or needling techniques had failed. Triamcinalone was injected where a problem was clearly a result of an inflammatory lesion, such as bursitis or capsulitis.

Whatever the treatments given, efforts were made to ensure that patients did what they could to minimise factors that would reinforce any pain–spasm–pain cycle. Consequently, advice about posture, appropriate exercise, lifting techniques and patients' working environment was usually given and in some instances relaxation techniques were taught.

Estimates of national figures suggest a referral rate to an orthopaedic specialist of 4.2 per 1000 general practitioner consultations [20]. However, this figure conceals wide variation between practices [21]. In their Oxford study of 73 general practitioners Noone and colleagues found a three-fold variation in referral rates, with an overall figure of 13 referrals per 1000 patients per year to orthopaedic specialists [22]. In another study of 36 practices covering 480 000 patients in Oxford Regional Health Authority during 1990–1991 an overall referral rate was found of 15 per 1000 patients, with a broadly similar range of variation [23]. In the present study, the referral rate to an orthopaedic specialist was 12.6 referrals per 1000 patients over the study year. The majority of these patients had structural pathology which could be appropriately managed by an orthopaedic department; but the remaining 27% of these referrals were for non-specific back, joint and limb pain which could have been referred to the practice's musculoskeletal clinic. Five of these referrals (12%) were for back pain, compared with 14% in Bradlow and colleagues' study [23]. Perhaps surprisingly, in this study, access to an expert opinion in musculoskeletal treatments did not seem to have influenced the orthopaedic referral rate for back pain, relative to available national figures. However, four of the five referrals were for chronic non-specific back pain (two referrals having been made by the musculoskeletal clinician and two by general practitioners), and all five patients had long-term problems. Having failed to respond to treatment these patients had requested the reassurance of a further opinion. In none of these cases was a specific surgical intervention offered by the orthopaedic department.

This finding raises the question of how best to make use of an in-house musculoskeletal clinic. As well as being an opportunity to improve patient management such a service allows general practitioners to increase their knowledge and skills. The 21 patients with non-specific musculoskeletal pain whom it would have been appropriate to treat in the clinic were instead referred by the general practitioners to orthopaedic specialists or to physiotherapists. This suggests that communication had not, at this stage, been sufficiently developed for adequate learning [24]. Furthermore, few precedents exist for collaboration between general practitioners and osteopaths and both parties were having to learn a new style of interdisciplinary cooperation. When introducing a new in-house clinic, but especially one involving complementary medicine, time is needed for the new team member to establish credibility and confidence as a specialist resource in the practice [25].

A survey of 20 general practitioners in Liverpool found a referral rate to a physiotherapy department of 22 per 1000 patients [15]. By comparison, the practice referral rate was nine per 1000 patients for the study year and eight per 1000 patients in the following year. Referrals to rheumatology outpatient clinics were fewer. Whereas national average rates (0.8 per 1000 general practitioner consultations [20]) would have predicted 4.5 referrals in the study period, in fact only three were made and the same in the following year.

No comparable figures were available for referral rates prior to the clinic being established. However, it appears that, at least compared with national figures, the clinic influenced referral rates to physiotherapy and rheumatology more than it changed general practitioners' referrals to orthopaedic outpatient departments. Improving feedback between general practitioners and the musculoskeletal clinician, allowing more reflection on referrals made both to the clinic and externally, may lead to a more appropriate use of resources. A prospective study testing this hypothesis is currently under way.

Recurrences in the second year and referral on to musculoskeletal specialties of patients in the study group were unusual, indicating that the clinic was providing effective management. As acute musculoskeletal pain is often self limiting, [3] many patients may have recovered while on an outpatient waiting list. Almost two-thirds of those referred to the clinic had medium- to long-term problems and spontaneous improvement in this group would have been unlikely. Had these patients not been referred to the clinic, management might have been by the general practitioner prescribing drugs or giving advice about posture, home exercise and rest or by referral, especially to the physiotherapy department.

Several authors have suggested not only that referrals for musculoskeletal problems are increasing [26], but also that they could often be avoided if resources were available for practitioners to cope with the majority of complaints which are a result of non-inflammatory disorders [27, 28]. This study suggests that a general practice based musculoskeletal clinic can provide a specialist opinion coupled with readily available treatment, when indicated.

In this study, few patients returned to general practitioners for further help, the clinic was generally able to cope with those recurrences that did occur, and the practice had a relatively low level of referrals to physiotherapy and rheumatology. We suggest that similar musculoskeletal clinics could offer effective and appropriate resources for diagnosing and managing the majority of patients presenting with musculoskeletal problems in general practice.

ACKNOWLEDGEMENT

The authors gratefully acknowledge the helpful suggestions and insightful comments of Dr Roderic MacDonald.

REFERENCES

1. Royal College of General Practitioners, Office of Population Censuses and Survey, and Department of Health and Social Security. Morbidity statistics from general practice. Third national study, 1981–82. London: HMSO, 1986.
2. British League Against Rheumatism working party. The challenge of arthritis and rheumatism. London: BLAR, 1977.
3. Fry J. Common diseases. Lancaster: MTP Press, 1979.
4. Office of Health Economics. Back pain. Paper 78. London: OHE, 1985.
5. MacDonald R S, Peters D. Osteopathy. Practitioner 1986. 230: 1073–1076.
6. Sims-Williams H, Jayson M I V, Young S M S, et al. Controlled trial of mobilisation and manipulation for patients with low back pain in general practice. BMJ 1978; 2: 1338–1340.
7. MacDonald R S, Bell C M J. An open controlled assessment of osteopathic manipulation in non-specific low-back pain. Spine 1990; 15: 364–370.
8. Sims-Williams H, Jayson M I V, Young S M S, et al. Controlled trial of mobilisation and manipulation for low back pain: hospital patients. BMJ 1979; 2: 1318–1320.
9. Doran D M L, Newell D J. Manipulation in treatment of low back pain: a multicentre study. BMJ 1975; 2: 161–164.
10. Koes B W, Assendelft W J J, van der Heijden G J M G, et al. Spinal manipulation and mobilisation for back and neck pain; a blinded review. BMJ 1991; 303: 1298–1303.
11. Meade T W, Dyer S, Browne W, et al. Low back pain of mechanical origin: randomised comparison of chiropractic and hospital outpatient treatment. BMJ 1990; 300: 1431–1437.
12. Smidt G L, Andersson G B J, Paris S V, et al. Research study analysis. J Orthop Sports Phys Ther 1991; 13: 288–299.
13. Koes B W, Bouter L M, van Mameren H, et al. Randomised clinical trial of manipulative therapy and physiotherapy for persistent back and neck complaints: results of one year follow up. BMJ 1991; 304: 601–605.
14. General Medical Services Committee. Building your own future: an agenda for general practice. London: BMA, 1991.
15. Akpala C O, Currant A P. Physiotherapy in general practice: patterns of utilisation. Public Health 1988; 102: 262–268.
16. Bourdillon J F. Spinal manipulation. London: Heinemann, 1975.
17. Travell J, Simons D. Myofascial pain and dysfunction. London: Williams and Wilkins, 1983.
18. Slosberg M. Spinal learning: central modulation of pain processing and long-term alteration of interneuronal excitability as a result of nociceptive peripheral input. J Manipulative Physiol Ther 1990: 13: 326–336.
19. Roland M O. A critical review of the evidence for a pain–spasm–pain cycle in spinal disorders. J Clin Biomechanics 1986; 1: 102–109.
20. Fleming D. The European study of referrals from primary to secondary care. Occasional paper 56. London: Royal College of General Practitioners, 1992.

21. Wilkin D, Dornan C. General practitioner referrals to hospital. A review of research and its implications for policy and practice. Manchester: Centre for Primary Care Research, University of Manchester, 1990.
22. Noone A, Goldacre M, Coulter A, Seagroatt V. Do referral rates vary widely between practices and does supply of services affect demand? A study in Milton Keynes and the Oxford region. J R Coll Gen Pract 1989; 39: 404–407.
23. Bradlow J, Coulter A, Brookes P. Patterns of referral. University of Oxford: Health Services Research Unit, 1992.
24. Arnold C W B, Bain J, Brown R A, et al. Moving to audit. Dundee: University of Dundee Centre for Medical Education, 1992.
25. Reason R, Chase H D, Desser A, et al. Towards a clinical framework for collaboration between general and complementary practitioners: discussion paper. J R Soc Med 1991; 85: 161–164.
26. Somanta A, Roy S. Referrals from general practice to a rheumatology clinic. Br J Rheumatol 1988; 27: 74–76.
27. Helliwell P S, Eright V. Referrals to rheumatology. BMJ 1991; 302: 304–305.
28. Roland M O, Porter R W, Matthews J G, et al. Improving care: a study of orthopaedic outpatient referrals. BMJ 1991; 302: 1124–1128.

RELAXATION AND IMAGERY IN THE TREATMENT OF BREAST CANCER

Linda Bridge
Pauline Benson
Patrick Pietroni
Robert Priest

Objective: To see whether stress could be alleviated in patients being treated for early breast cancer.
Design: Controlled randomised trial lasting 6 weeks.
Setting: Outpatient radiotherapy department in a teaching hospital.
Patients: 154 women with breast cancer stage I or II after first session of 6-week course of radiotherapy, of whom 15 dropped out before end of study.
Intervention: Patients saw one of two researchers once a week for 6 weeks. Controls were encouraged to talk about themselves; relaxation group was taught to concentrate on individual muscle groups; relaxation and imagery group was also taught to imagine peaceful scene of own choice to enhance relaxation. Relaxation and relaxation plus imagery group were given a tape recording repeating instructions and told to practise at least 15 minutes a day.
End point: Improvement of mood and of depression and anxiety on self-rating scale.
Measurements and main results: Initial scores for profile of mood states and Leeds general scales for depression and anxiety were the same in all groups. At 6 weeks total mood disturbance score was significantly less in the intervention groups, women in the combined intervention group being more relaxed than those receiving relaxation training only; mood in the control group was worse. Women aged 55 and over benefited most. There was no difference in Leeds scores among the groups.
Conclusion: Patients with early breast cancer benefit from relaxation training.

INTRODUCTION

In an attempt to understand more about the aetiology of cancer several studies have investigated whether life stresses (often 'loss' events) are among the psychological risk factors for the disease. Though some significant links have been reported [1–3], other studies have failed to show this relation [4, 5]. Doubts have been cast on the validity of linking life events and cancer, as the variations in growth rates of tumours make it difficult to establish whether any particular stressful event antedates the 'biological' onset of cancer [6–8].

As yet there appears to be no consistent evidence of a causal relation between life stresses and cancer, but it seems reasonable to suppose that the procedures of being diagnosed and treated for cancer are themselves stressful [9–11]. Maguire suggested that:

Most of the mood disturbance which occurs in patients with cancer probably results from their inability to cope psychologically with the stresses caused by their disease and treatments. They face the threats that they may lose their health, role, and life. They also have to live with the uncertainty as to whether and when these losses will occur [12].

Patel and co-workers have shown that relaxation treatment reduces stress in hypertension [13, 14]. Fleming found that relaxation treatment offered to patients with far advanced cancer seemed to benefit most those who were seen on an individual basis [15]. Another study of patients with cancer showed that the systematic use of positive thought and imagery when patients were in a relaxed frame of mind helped prolong their lives [16].

This study investigated ways of alleviating psychological stress in patients with diagnosed breast cancer, which is the commonest cancer and chief cause of death in women aged 35–54 [17]. (In 1984 there were 13 000 deaths from breast cancer in England and Wales [18].) We hypothesised that patients given either of two relaxation treatments would show a more positive effect on their mood states than a control group of similar, untreated women and that the group given relaxation training with an imagery component would show more change than women given relaxation training alone.

PATIENTS AND METHOD

The sample was made up of a consecutive series of women who had been treated by either mastectomy or breast conservation for early breast cancer

Reprinted with permission from the British Medical Journal: 297 pp. 1169–1172 November 1988.

stages I and II—that is, as defined by the Union International Contra le Cancrum as tumours of 5 cm diameter or less with or without palpable axillary nodes and having no evidence of distant metastases [19]. All the women were outpatients having a 6-week course of radiotherapy at the Middlesex Hospital, London, were under age 70, and could understand English. (Because the study period covered the 6-week period of radiotherapy, to avoid possible confusion we refer to the 6-week study programme as treatment.)

Initially 183 women fulfilled the study criteria but 22 (12%) refused to participate. Informed consent was given by the remaining 161, who were then allocated by means of a random numbers table to either a treatment or control condition. Seven of these had to be excluded after staging tests detected metastases, leaving 154 women. Of these, 15 dropped out before the end of the study (five assigned to the relaxation plus imagery group, six to relaxation only, and four to the control group). Thus 139 women completed the full treatment package.

Selection of methods of assessment was determined by the need to be non-intrusive and cause minimum disruption to the routine of patients attending for radiotherapy. The profile of mood states questionnaire [20–22] and the Leeds general scales for the self-assessment of depression and anxiety [23] were chosen, as they are self-rating measures which have been used in patients with cancer [24]. The profile of mood states uses 65 items to yield scores on sub-scales for tension, depression, vigour, fatigue, anger, and confusion. A total mood disturbance score is calculated from these scores and used as a global measure of dysphoric mood. The Leeds general scales measure the severity of depressive and anxiety symptoms in patients who have not received a primary diagnosis of affective illness. The scales contain six items each for depression and anxiety, all self-rated on a four point scale. A score of 7 or more indicates the presence of either state. To minimise response set some items are scored negatively.

All the women had received at least one session of radiotherapy before being invited to join the study. They were told that a study was being carried out to investigate ways of alleviating stress during radiotherapy and that participants would be randomly allocated to one of three groups, about which full details were given. They would also be required to complete several questionnaires. We emphasised that agreement or refusal to join the study would not affect their course of radiotherapy, that no drugs would be given, that nothing would appear in their medical records, and that confidentiality would be maintained throughout.

Patients completed a profile of mood states and Leeds general scales questionnaire on entry to the study and again at the end of the 6-week treatment period. The 139 women in the study were seen individually by one of the two researchers once a week for the 6 weeks of their radiotherapy courses. The researchers were equally concerned in working with all three groups.

Both treatment groups (relaxation and relaxation plus imagery) were taught a relaxation technique which by a process of direct concentration focuses sensory awareness on a series of individual muscle groups [25]. These patients were also given instructions for diaphragmatic breathing, which slows respiration, induces a calmer state, and reduces tension [26]. In addition to the breathing and relaxation, each patient in the relaxation plus imagery group was taught to imagine a peaceful scene of her own choice as a means of enhancing the relaxation [27]. Sessions lasted about half an hour. During this time the exercises were practised by the treatment groups, whereas the women in the control group were encouraged simply to talk about themselves and their interests.

All patients in the treatment groups were given a tape which repeated the breathing instructions and contained the relaxation or relaxation and imaging exercise. It was suggested to them that this should be practised at home for at least 15 minutes each day. (If required, tape recorders were available on loan for the duration of the study.)

Table 4.10 Characteristics of patients in the three study groups. Except where stated otherwise figures are numbers of patients

	Relaxation group (n=47)	Relaxation plus imagery group (n=44)	Controls (n=48)
Mean age (SD) (years)	51 (10)	53 (11)	54 (10)
Marital state:			
Married/cohabiting	37	30	38
Widowed/divorced/ separated	4	9	4
Never married	6	5	6
Social class:			
I	1	6	3
II	20	5	13
IIIa	11	9	12
IIIb	6	4	8
IV	6	15	10
V	3	5	2
Mean total mood disturbance score on initial profile of mood states (SD)	61.7 (31.2)	59.6 (34.5)	54.4 (26.0)
Mean score on initial Leeds general depression scale (SD)	4.3 (2.9)	4.8 (3.5)	5.1 (3.2)
Mean score on initial Leeds general anxiety scale (SD)	6.0 (4.0)	5.7 (4.0)	6.4 (3.9)

Data analysis

Demographic variables were compared by the X^2 test. Initial scores on the profile of mood states and Leeds general scales were examined by analysis of variance. Relative changes in these scores were examined by analysis of covariance to control for the initial test score [28]. All the tests were two tailed except when indicated.

RESULTS

Table 4.10 gives details of the 139 women who completed the 6-week study programme. 47 were randomised to receive relaxation training, 44 to receive relaxation plus imagery training, and 48 to serve as controls. Demographic variables and initial questionnaire scores were compared across the groups; no significant differences were found at the 5% level.

25 women had received adjuvant chemotherapy at the time of or after operation before being recruited to the study. Their initial scores on the profile of mood states and Leeds general scales were compared with the scores of the 114 women who did not have adjuvant chemotherapy; no significant differences were found at the 5% level.

Of the 139 patients studied, only 19 had had a mastectomy (reflecting the current shift towards breast conservation). When the sample was divided by type of surgery initial scores on the profile of mood states and Leeds general scales were similar for mood state and psychiatric morbidity.

The initial and 6-week scores on the profile of mood states and Leeds general scales were compared by analysis of covariance (controlling for initial scores) to test for the effects of treatment. Because it had been predicted that relaxation treatment would be better than no treatment (control) and that relaxation plus imagery would be better than relaxation alone the linear polynomial trend for treatment effects was calculated. There were no significant differences on the Leeds general scales but the total mood disturbance score on the profile of mood states differed significantly in the predicted way (p<0.05, one tailed; Table 4.11).

Table 4.11 Mean scores on profile of mood states at beginning and end of treatment (SD in parentheses)

Profile of mood states	Relaxation group (n=39)	Relaxation plus imagery group (n=43)	Controls (n=46)	p Value* (one tailed)
Tension:				
Initial	11·2 (7·0)	11·3 (7·9)	10·6 (7·0)	
6 weeks	9·5 (7·7)	8·8 (5·0)	10·7 (8·1)	0·043
Depression:				
Initial	7·4 (7·2)	8·3 (9·2)	5·5 (6·5)	
6 weeks	6·9 (8·5)	5·8 (5·2)	7·5 (10·8)	0·023
Vigour:				
Initial	18·5 (7·5)	16·6 (7·7)	17·3 (6·6)	
6 weeks	18·5 (6·3)	17·4 (8·3)	18·9 (7·9)	0·254
Fatigue:				
Initial	9·2 (8·1)	8·7 (7·1)	8·7 (6·5)	
6 weeks	11·9 (8·5)	10·4 (8·0)	11·9 (8·0)	0·152
Anger:				
Initial	7·9 (6·0)	7·8 (6·9)	5·6 (5·2)	
6 weeks	7·8 (8·3)	5·9 (4·4)	5·5 (6·4)	0·149
Confusion:				
Initial	7·5 (4·9)	6·8 (5·4)	6·8 (4·2)	
6 weeks	7·3 (5·0)	5·7 (4·1)	7·0 (5·2)	0·066
Total mood disturbance:				
Initial	61·7 (31·2)	59·6 (34·5)	54·4 (26·0)	
6 weeks	61·9 (34·8)	53·9 (27·4)	61·4 (38·7)	0·036

*For linear trend in analysis of covariance, controlling for initial scores.

This indicated that relaxation positively affected mood state and that this positive effect was further enhanced when relaxation was combined with imagery.

Though none of the sub-scales of the profile of mood states showed a statistically significant difference among the three groups of patients, all the relative changes over the treatment period were in the predicted direction (except for the vigour sub-scale, where relaxation was superior to relaxation plus imagery).

The item 'relaxed' is part of the sub-scale for tension in the profile of mood states, and relaxation training was a main component of the treatment package. Interestingly, therefore, at the end of the study period analysis of covariance showed that the women trained in relaxation plus imagery were more relaxed than those trained in relaxation only, who in turn were more relaxed than the controls (p<0.025, one tailed) as judged by scores for this item.

Before examining the data we had decide to divide the sample by age and compare the effect of treatment in younger and older women. The cut point was the median age—that is, 54. On the divided sample the interaction between age and treatment was found to be significant in the profile of mood states for tension (p<0.025), depression (p<0.005), and total mood disturbance (p<0.005) (Table 4.12). This showed that relaxation and relaxation plus imagery particularly helped the overall mood state of the older women by reducing tension and depression relative to that of the controls and that the relaxation plus imagery treatment group showed the most effect. Another finding was that women aged 55 and older were less likely to work during the 6 weeks of radiotherapy than the younger women (X^2=12.62; df=1; p<0.001). No differences were found in the Leeds general scales when the sample was divided by age.

To see whether anger and treatment were related those women with initial scores for anger in the lower quartile in the profile of mood states (n=30; scores 0–2, mean 0.93) were compared with the rest of the sample (n=98; scores 3–31, mean 9.20). There were no significant differences in scores on the profile of mood states or Leeds general scales at the end of the treatment period. Those women with initial anger scores in the upper quartile in the profile of mood states (n=35; scores 10–31, mean 15.29) were compared with the others in the sample (n=93; scores 0–9, mean 4.24). Analysis of covariance showed that the women with high scores for anger who were in the relaxation and relaxation plus imagery groups were less vigorous (p<0.05), more fatigued (p<0.05), and, with exclusion of the anger component, had greater total mood disturbance (p<0.025).

DISCUSSION

The question that we set out to answer was whether relaxation and relaxation plus imagery

Table 4.12 Mean scores on profile of mood states at end of treatment in the three study groups stratified by age

Profile of mood states	Relaxation group		Relaxation plus imagery group		Controls		p Value*
	Age<55 (n=29)	Age≥55 (n=15)	Age<55 (n=17)	Age≥55 (n=23)	Age<55 (n=22)	Age≥55 (n=24)	
Tension	9·1	10·3	9·4	8·4	7·9	13·2	0·018
Depression	6·6	7·6	6·6	5·2	4·1	10·8	0·002
Vigour	18·0	19·4	20·5	15·0	17·7	20·0	0·068
Fatigue	12·6	10·6	13·7	7·9	10·9	12·8	0·095
Anger	8·8	5·9	6·9	5·1	4·9	6·0	0·391
Confusion	7·3	7·1	6·1	5·4	5·6	8·3	0·105
Total mood disturbance	62·3	60·9	63·1	47·0	51·0	71·0	0·005

*Analysis of covariance, controlling for initial scores.

were effective ways of reducing stress in a group of patients with early breast cancer who were attending as hospital outpatients for radiotherapy. When mood state and morbidity during radiation treatment were studied by Peck and Boland they found that anxiety increased at the end of a course of radiotherapy [29]. They suggested that this was because reactions to radiation, both systemic and local, were then at their peak, adding to the distress which existed before treatment. Forester et al claimed that people may experience a decrease in dysphoric mood during radiotherapy because this is when they feel that something is being done about their illness and they are receiving attention [30].

In view of these suggestions we should have expected increased scores at the end of radiotherapy for all the patients in our study. In fact, our results on the profile of mood states scale showed that at the end of the treatment period for the cohort as a whole not only had overall mood state improved most in the relaxation plus imagery group, followed by the relaxation group, but also that the overall mood state of the women in the untreated group had become worse. As hypothesised, relaxation plus imagery had a more positive effect on mood state than relaxation only, and both treatment programmes were more effective than no treatment. On examining the characteristics of the groups we doubt that the results of treatment can be explained on the basis of the initial selection.

Why was relaxation plus imagery more effective than relaxation alone? The simplicity of the imagery, suggesting a peaceful, pleasant scene of the patient's choice, meant that it was within everyone's grasp. Often the image made the patient smile, at a time when smiles were perhaps few and far between. The pleasant scene could be recalled easily at any time, and the researchers emphasised that it was a resource which every person had within her. By contrast, the more aggressive style of imaging, which aims at strengthening the immune system by visualising the symbolic destruction of cancer cells [31], may bring about a sense of failure and helplessness if this desired result does not subsequently occur.

Both types of treatment used in this study were shown to be more effective in women aged 55 or over, who showed less tension and depression at the end of the 6 weeks as well as more improvement on overall mood state. Why did the older women respond better to treatment? As mentioned above, substantially fewer of these women worked during their course of radiotherapy. Because of their age they would be less likely to have children to care for and possibly led less busy lives than the younger women. Thus it may be that the older women had more time to practise our treatment programme.

Several studies of cancer have focused on abnormal release of anger, suggesting that both extreme suppression and extreme expression of anger may be characteristic of patients with cancer [32, 33]. In this study we found no differences in the profile of mood states or Leeds general scales at the end of the treatment period for women with low anger scores—that is, extreme suppression—but we found that women with high anger scores who received relaxation or relaxation plus imagery treatment showed more fatigue, less vigour, and greater total mood disturbance than the controls. It may be that some women are so angry that they are unable to derive any benefit from relaxation treatment. We do not know whether before diagnosis those women with high scores for anger had always expressed their anger. Possibly they had been accustomed to suppressing anger and the knowledge that they had cancer gave them a legitimate reason for displaying it. Peck found that almost half of his sample of 50 patients displayed extreme anger in response to their cancer [9]. We hope that future work will clarify this point.

Other studies have found a high prevalence of psychiatric morbidity in patients with mastectomy given adjuvant chemotherapy [24, 34]. We cannot address this issue, as only one of the 19 patients with mastectomy in our study had received adjuvant chemotherapy.

The Leeds general scales for anxiety and depression showed no significant changes over the 6 weeks of treatment. This may be because the scales contain certain somatic items—for example, disturbed sleep and appetite—which may have a physical cause and be less sensitive than psychological items to change in response to relaxation treatment. The hospital anxiety and depression scale [35], which omits somatic items, is currently being used to assess psychiatric morbidity in patients with cancer [36] and may prove to be a better measure for use in work on this subject.

Sims, in her review of published work relating to relaxation techniques and patients with cancer, criticised studies which did not identify the sample population, had insufficient numbers, groups all patients with cancer together as if they were a homogeneous group, and failed to control for attention by instructors [37]. Our study addressed these issues and showed that easily learnt relaxation treatments significantly improved the mood state of patients receiving a course of radiotherapy for early breast cancer, that relaxation plus imagery was the most effective treatment, and that women aged 55 and over benefited most.

This study was conceived and initiated by Betsy Little and funded by the Cancer Research Campaign. We thank Professor M Baum, of the Cancer Research Campaign Clinical Trials Centre, for monitoring clinical state. We are also indebted to Charlie Owen for statistical advice, Dawn Beaumont for computer programming, Lucy Albu for clerical work, and the staff and patients of the Middlesex Hospital's radiotherapy department for their support and cooperation.

REFERENCES

1. Snow H. Cancer and the cancer process. London: J and A Churchill, 1893.
2. LeShan L, Worthington R E. Personality as a factor in the pathogenesis of cancer, Br J Med Psychol 1956; 29: 49–56.
3. Jacobs T J, Charles E. Life events and the occurrence of cancer in children. Psychosom Med 1980; 42: 11–24.
4. Schonfield J. Psychological and life-experience differences between Israeli women with benign and cancerous breast lesions. J Psychosom Res 1975; 19: 229–234.
5. Greer S, Morris T. The study of psychological factors in breast cancer: problems of method. Soc Sci Med 1978; 12: 129–134.
6. Cox T, Mackay C. Psychosocial factors and psychophysiological mechanisms in the aetiology and development of cancer. Soc Sci Med 1982; 16: 381–396.
7. Greer S. Cancer and the mind. Br J Psychiatry 1983; 143: 535–543.
8. Hughes J. Cancer and emotion. Chichester: John Wiley and Sons, 1987.
9. Peck A. Emotional reactions to having cancer. American Journal of Roentgenology, Radium Therapy, and Nuclear Medicine 1972; 114: 591–599.
10. Greer S, Silberfarb P M. Psychological concomitants of cancer. Psychol Med 1982; 12: 563–573.
11. Maguire P. Psychological reactions to breast cancer and its treatment. In: Bonadonne G, ed. Breast cancer: diagnosis and management. Chichester: John Wiley and Sons, 1984; 303–318.
12. Maguire P. Psychological and social consequences of cancer. In: Williams C J, Whitehouse J W A, eds. Recent advances in clinical oncology. London: Churchill Livingstone, 1981: 376.
13. Patel C, Marmot M G, Terry D J. Controlled trial of biofeedback-aided behavioural methods in reducing mild hypertension. Br Med J 1981; 282: 2005–2008.
14. Patel C. Trial of relaxation in reducing coronary risk: 4 year follow up. Br Med J 1985; 290: 1103–6.
15. Fleming U. Relaxation therapy for far-advanced cancer. Practitioner 1985; 229: 471–475.
16. Simonton O, Simonton S. Belief systems and management of the emotional aspects of malignancy. Transpersonal Psychology 1975; 7: 29–47.
17. Consensus Development Conference Panel. Treatment of primary breast cancer. Br Med J 1986; 293: 946–947.
18. Office of Population Censuses and Surveys. Mortality statistics, 1984. Ser DH2 No 11. London: HMSO, 1985.
19. Union International Contra le Cancrum. TNM classification of malignant tumours. Geneva: UICC, 1974.
20. McNair D M, Lorr M, Droppleman L F. Profile of mood states manual. California: Educational and Industrial Testing Service, 1971. (Available from NFER-Nelson, Windsor, Berkshire.)
21. Worden J W, Sobel H J. Ego strength and psychosocial adaptation to cancer. Psychosom Med 1978; 40: 85–92.
22. Spiegel D, Bloom J R, Yalom I. Group support for patients with metastatic cancer. Arch Gen Psychiatry 1981; 38: 527–533.
23. Snaith R F, Bridge G W K, Hamilton M. The Leeds scales for the self-assessment of anxiety and depression. Br J Psychiatry 1976; 128: 156–65.
24. Cooper A F, McArdle C S, Russel A R, Smith D C. Psychiatric morbidity associated with adjuvant chemotherapy following mastectomy for breast cancer. Br J Surg 1979; 66: 362.
25. McLean J. The use of relaxation techniques in general practice. Practitioner 1986; 230: 1079–1084.
26. Everly G S, Rosenfeld R. The nature and treatment of the stress response. New York: Plenum, 1981: 131–141.
27. Lyles J N, Burish T G, Krozely M G, Oldham R K. Efficacy of relaxation training and guided imagery in reducing the aversiveness of cancer chemotherapy. J Consult Clin Psychol 1982; 50: 509–524.
28. Plewis I Analysing change. London: John Wiley and Sons, 1985.
29. Peck A, Boland J. Emotional reactions to radiation treatment. Cancer 1977; 40: 180–184.
30. Forester B M, Kornfeld D S, Fleiss J. Psychiatric aspects of radiotherapy. Am J Psychiatry 1978; 135: 960–963.
31. Simonton O, Simonton S, Creighton J. Getting well again. Los Angeles: JP Tarcher, 1978.

32. Greer S, Morris T. Psychological attributes of women who develop breast cancer: a controlled study. J Psychosom Res 1975; 19: 147–153.

33. Jansen M A, Muenz L R. A retrospective study of personality variables associated with fibrocystic disease and breast cancer. J Psychosom Res 1984; 28: 35–42.

34. Maguire G P, Tait A, Brooke M, Thomas C, Howat J M T, Sellwood R A. Psychiatric morbidity and physical toxicity associated with adjuvant chemotherapy after mastectomy. Br Med J 1980; 281: 1179–1180.

35. Zigmund A S, Snaith R P. The hospital anxiety and depression scale. Acta Psychiatr Scand 1983; 67: 361–370.

36. Fallowfield L J, Baum M, Maguire G P. Effects of breast conservation on psychological morbidity associated with diagnosis and treatment of early breast cancer. Br Med J 1986; 293: 1331–1334.

37. Sims S E R. Relaxation training as a technique for helping patients cope with the experience of cancer: a selective review of the literature. J Adv Nurs 1987; 12: 583–591.

THE EXPECTATIONS, HEALTH BELIEFS AND BEHAVIOUR OF PATIENTS SEEKING HOMOEOPATHIC AND CONVENTIONAL MEDICINE

Clare Harrison
Jenny Hewison
Peter Davies
Patrick Pietroni

Research was carried out to determine whether or not there was a difference in the health beliefs, expectations and behaviour of a sample of 92 patients attending a dermatological or rheumatological outpatient clinic which offered either homoeopathic treatment (N=47) or conventional treatment (N=45).

Self-administered questionnaires were used which examined patients' pathways to care, expectations, beliefs, behaviour and multidimensional health locus of control.

The two key differences between those seeking homoeopathic and those seeking conventional medicine were in terms of:

- their reasons for attending a homoeopathic or conventional clinic
- their beliefs about their presenting dermatological or rheumatological condition.

Keywords: Expectations, health beliefs, health behaviour.

INTRODUCTION

There has been considerable debate over the characteristics of people who are attracted to complementary medicine and whether or not they are in any way different from those who opt for orthodox medicine (Fulder & Munro 1985, Lewith 1985, *Which?* 1986). In particular, such differences have been suggested as having a major effect on the outcome of treatment.

The aim of the present study was to determine whether patients attending dermatological or

Reprinted with permission from the British Homoeopathic Journal: 78 pp. 210–218 October 1989.

rheumatological outpatient clinics at a homoeopathic hospital had different health beliefs, expectations and behaviour from those attending hospitals offering conventional treatment.

METHOD

92 out of a total of 107 consecutive patients attending four outpatient clinics at three different London NHS hospitals completed questionnaires. Questionnaires were self-administered, with a researcher on hand to help with any queries or difficulties. Of the total sample, 47 of the patients (group 1) were regularly attending a homoeopathic clinic, with the remaining 45 patients (group 2) attending orthodox clinics. The two groups had near equal numbers of patients attending dermatology clinics (24 in both groups) and rheumatology clinics (23 in group 1; 21 in group 2).

The characteristics of the group were as follows:

1. The mean age of the sample was 46 years.
2. 62% were from the UK or Ireland.
3. 54% were married.
4. 52% were in professional/managerial and non-manual employment.
5. 79% had had their condition for more than one year.

In terms of these characteristics there was no significant difference between the two groups, although there were significantly more females than males seeking homoeopathy (group 1) and significantly more females than males in the sample as a whole.

Questions were divided into five main sections:

1. A *Pathways to Care* section sought to identify previous treatments and the reasons for the patient coming to the present outpatient clinic.
2. Questions in an *Expectations* section sought to identify what patients were expecting from the consultations they were receiving.
3. A section on *Beliefs* sought to identify the patients' beliefs with respect to:

i. the meaning of his/her present dermatological or rheumatological condition

ii. the meaning of illness in general (Pietroni 1987).

4. The fourth section of the questionnaire sought to establish whether or not a patient was doing anything to keep him/herself mentally, physically or spiritually healthy both before and since the onset of his/her present condition.

5. The final section was a multidimensional health locus of control scale based on a questionnaire devised by Wallston, Wallston, and deVellis (1978). This sought to measure three distinct dimensions:

i. *Internality*—the degree to which the patients perceived their health outcomes to be contingent on their own decisions and actions.

ii. *Powerful others externality*—the degree to which the patients perceived their health to be determined by powerful other people (e.g. doctors, family).

iii. *Chance externality*—the degree to which the patients believed that health/illness was a matter of fate, luck or chance.

Data was analysed using chi-square tests or two-sample t-tests as appropriate.

RESULTS

Pathways to care

About one-third of each group had sought 'complementary' treatment prior to coming to the present outpatient clinic. However, significantly more of group 1, the homoeopathic group, had previously sought conventional medicine: 91% as compared with 73% of group 2 (X^2=5.27; df=1; p<.05).

As illustrated in Table 4.13, responses indicated that there was a significant difference between the two groups in terms of their reasons for attending the present outpatient clinic. More patients in group 1 were seeking homoeopathy because they were unhappy with the approach and/or treatment their previous doctor/therapist had offered, than patients in group 2. In addi-

Table 4.13 Reasons for attending the present outpatient clinic (group 1—patients seeking homoeopathic treatment; group 2—patients seeking orthodox treatment)

	Group 1 N	Group 1 %	Group 2 N	Group 2 %	X^2 (df=1)
Unhappy with their previous doctor/therapist's approach	11	23	3	6	4.99
Unhappy with the treatment the previous doctor/therapist was offering	24	51	1	2	27.71
Own decision to see the doctor at present outpatient clinic	29	62	10	22	14.67

The X2 values reported above are significant at the 0.05 level.

tion, significantly more patients in group 1 were taking action as a result of their own decisions and will.

Expectations

Of nine different expectations portrayed in the questionnaire, there was a significant difference between the two groups in terms of only one. A significantly higher proportion of those seeking homoeopathic medicine were hoping to understand what their dermatological or rheumatological condition was saying to them about their lifestyle (i.e. its meaning)—26% as compared with 9% of those seeking conventional medicine (X^2=4.43; df=1; p<.05).

Beliefs

Of the seven questions concerning patients' beliefs about their present condition there was a significant difference in the responses to three questions. Namely, a significantly higher proportion of those attending the homoeopathic hospital believed their condition could be partly psychological or that if they changed something in their life/lifestyle they could improve their condition. Conversely, a significantly lower proportion of this group believed that their condition was caused by something over which they had no control. Details of these results are given in Table 4.14.

Table 4.14 Patients' beliefs about their present condition (group 1—patients seeking homoeopathic treatment; group 2—patients seeking orthodox treatment)

| | Group 1 | | Group 2 | | X^2 |
	N	%	N	%	(df=2)
That their condition could be partly psychological	17	36	4	9	13.22
That by changing something in their life/lifestyle they could improve their condition	22	47	10	22	11.48
That their condition was caused by something over which they had no control	18	38	29	64	6.70

The X^2 values reported above are significant at the 0.05 level.

Although the trend evident in patients' beliefs about their present illness was still there when asked to describe their beliefs about health and illness in general, there were no significant differences between the two groups.

Behaviour

Similarly, there were no significant differences between the two groups in terms of their behaviours either before or since the onset of their present condition

Multidimensional health locus of control

Results for this section showed those who were seeking homoeopathic medicine to have significantly higher internality scores than those who were seeking conventional medicine (t=2.13; df=81; p=.036). No group differences were found on either of the other two dimensions.

DISCUSSION

The present study clearly indicates that the two key differences between those seeking homoeopathic and those seeking conventional medicine were in terms of:

1. their reasons for attending a homoeopathic or conventional outpatient clinic

2. their beliefs about their presenting condition—namely a dermatological or rheumatological condition.

Those who were attending the homoeopathic hospital were doing so predominantly as a result of their dissatisfaction with the treatment they had been offered and/or approaches they had experienced elsewhere. Furthermore, 62% of those attending the hospital offering homoeopathic medicine were doing so as a direct result of their own will and actions. Certainly in the instance of the present study—especially in the light of the long-term nature of most of the patients' conditions—it would seem that those seeking homoeopathy were reflecting dissatisfaction with conventional medicine and were actively seeking alternative solutions to their long-term condition. It is interesting to consider this in relation to Lewith's (1985) study in which in answer to his question 'why do people seek treatment by alternative medicine?' he concluded that such people were not 'cranks', but were well-informed individuals seeking a solution to unresolved long-term problems (Lewith 1985).

In the present study, although patients expressed some dissatisfaction with conventional medicine in terms of the treatment and approach experienced in relation to their present condition, this dissatisfaction was not as noticeably extended into patients' beliefs about health and illness in general. Thus although those currently seeking homoeopathic medicine may have been doing so as a result of dissatisfaction with the treatment and approach of conventional doctors concerning their present condition, they were not necessarily dissatisfied with conventional medicine generally, and may well still think first of seeking conventional medicine in the case of any other symptoms or illnesses.

The present study also indicated that in terms of patients' beliefs, significantly more of those seeking homoeopathy indicated a greater sense of responsibility for and control over the cause, course and future of their condition, than did those seeking conventional medicine. This is clearly supported by the additional finding that those seeking homoeopathic treatment had significantly higher internal health locus of control scores than did those seeking conventional treatment—indicating that they perceive their health outcomes to be contingent on their own decisions and actions.

It is interesting that there were no significant differences between the two groups in terms of their behaviour either before or since the onset of their present condition. Furthermore, there were no differences between the two groups in the nature of the changes made by patients who had altered their behaviour patterns since the onset of their present condition. This finding may be attributable to a number of factors. For example, it could suggest that, contrary to what one might expect, the advice given by homoeopathic and conventional doctors to their patients concerning behaviour patterns may not differ to any large extent. Conversely, it could reflect a lack of compliance of patients to doctors' advice concerning behaviour patterns. It is important to note that the results obtained in this section may solely reflect the behaviours of people with dermatological or rheumatological conditions. This gains support from specific comments made by several patients that, for example, although they would like to continue regular exercise, their condition physically prevented them from doing so.

This latter point is relevant to the study as a whole in that the results may not be generalisable to all people seeking homoeopathy or conventional medicine. It is also likely that the results reflect most accurately people with chronic rather than acute conditions.

REFERENCES

Fulder S, Munro R 1985 Complementary medicine in the United Kingdon: patients, practitioners and consultation. Lancet II pp. 542–545
Lewith G 1985 Why do people seek treatment by alternative medicine? British Medical Journal 290 pp. 28–29
Pietroni P 1987 The meaning of illness. Journal of the Royal Society of Medicine 80 pp. 357–360
Wallston K A, Wallston B S, deVellis R 1978 Development of the multidimensional health locus of control scales. Health and Education Monographs 6 pp. 160–170
Which? October 1986 Magic or medicine?

'SPIRITUAL' INTERVENTIONS IN A GENERAL PRACTICE SETTING

Patrick Pietroni

Summary: The similarity between some spiritual practices present in many of the world's religions and their secular counterparts is described. How these practices are incorporated within the work of a general practitioner is outlined and the pitfalls and problems are outlined.
Keywords: Spiritual intervention, rites of passage, medication, touch.

INTRODUCTION

Holism espouses an awareness of the links between body, mind and spirit. Much is written about the first two, and the ever expanding field of psychoneuroimmunology has allowed us to follow the pathways of how unhappiness enters a cell [1]. For many it is difficult to separate 'spirit' from mind. Yet 'spirit' implies more than emotional and psychological well-being. The divide between mind and spirit is not helped by the fact that psychoanalysis has incorporated the Greek word 'psyche', meaning soul, to describe mental structure. Without therefore defining spirit it would become increasingly difficult, if not impossible, to discuss whether such an entity as spiritual disease exists or not. Box 4.2 lists some of the many definitions that are used by theologians, the lay public and the dictionaries. The word 'spirit' is often linked with religious beliefs, be they Christian, Muslim or Buddhist. It is also associated with an experience, a sense of harmony or peace, a knowing from within. For others, 'spirit' is linked with the life-force, the will to live and in Eastern philosophies this life-force (Chi-Prana) is closely linked with the breath or energy which helps to explain our own words, 'inspired' and 'expired'.

Reprinted with permission from Holistic Medicine 1: pp. 253–262 1986 published by John Wiley & Sons.

Box 4.2   What is spirit?

Immaterial part of man
Religion/beliefs/conviction
Soul—vitality
Quintessence of various forms
Life-force
Breath of life
A possession
Something higher
Inspired
Emotional calmness
Everyday ecstasy
Sense of harmony
Sense of belonging
Knowing sure from within
Transcendent force
Mystical experience

Michael Balint, who wrote extensively on the psychological aspects of medicine, makes no direct mention of the interplay between spirit, mind and body. However, in his analytic articles, he comes close to a description of the spiritual dimension:

The aim of all human striving is to establish or probably re-establish an all-embracing harmony with one's environment—to be able to love in peace.
The unio-mystica, the re-establishment of the harmonious interpenetrating mix-up between the individual and the most important parts of his environment, his love objects is the desire of all humanity [2].

Balint's 'interpenetrating mix-up' is one of his most delightful phrases and captures the true nature of the best of general practice. Balint refers to two kinds of medicine, one where illness is seen as an accident arising from causes outside the patient and where the basis of rational therapy arises out of a theory about the causation of illness and the control of the presumed cause. The second is where illness is seen as a lack of integration between the individual and the environment and a meaningful phase in the patient's life. Here meaning is used to imply purpose as opposed to cause. Finding a purpose and meaning to one's life has always formed part of the 'spiritual journey' and is well described in all the world's great religions. The *Book of Job, Pilgrim's Progress, Canterbury Tales, Siddhartha, Heart of Darkness, Don Quixote, Epic of*

Box 4.3 Spiritual practice and the general practice counterpart

Spiritual practice	General practice counterpart
1. Providing a sanctuary	Consulting room as a 'safe space'
2. Confessional	Active listening
3. Interpret tribulation	Give meaning to stressful life events
4. Source of ritual and ceremony	Repeat prescription
5. Provide support and comfort	Teamwork
6. Increase spiritual awareness	Give permission for spiritual discussion
7. Laying on of hands Prayer and meditation	Use of touch Relaxation and quiet time
8. Communion	Self-help groups/patient participation

Gilgamesh, are all stories of journeys where answers are sought to the perennial questions.

However, it may be more helpful for the general practitioner to avoid the complex and difficult world of theology and start from a very pragmatic base. What are the spiritual interventions associated with a priest or rabbi's work and are any of these relevant to the needs of patients coming to see a doctor? And, more importantly, are these interventions practical within the context of general practice? Box 4.3 includes a list of spiritual practices common to many religions and the possible counterpart in a general practice setting.

SANCTUARY/SAFE SPACE

Churches were built not only as places of worship but also to serve as sanctuaries from invading forces. They were seen as sanctified territory providing the itinerant traveller with shelter and warmth. Spence describes the unit of medical practice as 'the occasion when in the intimacy of the consulting room a person who is ill or believes himself to be ill seeks the advice of a doctor whom he trusts' [3]. The words 'intimacy' and 'trust' invoke the notion of the consulting room as a 'safe space'. The necessity for the 'space' to feel 'safe' applies equally well to the physical and psy-

chological aspects of a general practitioner's work. The atmosphere created by the architecture, the furniture, lighting, position of the desk, those personal possessions displayed, all help to create a sense of peace, or conversely, 'business' and dis-ease. The chairs provided for patients to sit on can often ensure the patient feels anything but safe. Similarly, the 'space' of the consulting room needs to have its boundaries reasonably intact. Quality time is as important as quantity time, and interruptions by telephones, receptionists or partners will all help to create a feeling of 'invasion'. One need only reflect on the different quality of interaction that occurs when seeing a patient in his or her own home to appreciate the effects that atmosphere and safety have on communication. Certainly the next six interventions are facilitated by ensuring that the consulting room feels safe for the patient.

CONFESSIONAL/ACTIVE LISTENING

The act of unburdening oneself of troubled thoughts, feelings and resentments is an act that is as old as man. Since the notion of sin has been replaced with the notion of repression, the drama has moved from the confessional to the analytic couch. The general practitioner is neither a priest nor a psychoanalyst, yet possibly we are told more secrets during the course of our work than either of those two professions. The Greek word 'catharsis' or cleansing may be more useful to the doctor than the word confessional. 'Give up what thou hast and then they will receive', 'Confession is good for the soul', 'A burden shared is a burden halved': many psychotherapeutic techniques have been developed for aiding this process of unburdening, from the early use of hypnosis to free association. As Jung says though, 'The goal of the cathartic method is full confessional—not merely the intellectual recognition of the facts with the head, but their confirmation by the heart and the actual release of suppressed emotion' [4]. Heron provides an excellent overview of this process as it is utilised in many of the humanistic psychotherapies [5]. For the general practitioner, however, the ability of helping the patient to unburden himself needs to be carefully balanced by the realisation that emotional curiosity does not always indicate caring. As Balint has well documented, knowing 'when and how to stop' a patient is even more important than knowing 'how to start'. Nevertheless the skill required by the general practitioner for this aspect of his work is the ability to listen actively. This involves listening with the eyes as well as the ears. It involves indicating to the patient that you are present with him and requires the ability to communicate an empathic understanding. 'It is important for the doctor to free himself from trying to discover *why*, so that he can observe *how* the patient talks, thinks, feels and behaves the way he does.' [6] From time to time it may be necessary to *give meaning* or *interpret tribulation* but equally important is the ability to share, be with and avoid trying to find a solution. In hospital medicine, we are often told 'Don't just stand there, do something'. In general practice it is often necessary to remember 'Don't just do something, stand there'.

Example 1

Mrs G., aged 45—series of repeated consultations for minor sore throats, coughs and 'feeling tired'. On the fourth visit she was asked about her homelife and this provided the stimulus for a long discussion about a long-standing affair and the fact that her partner was leaving London to change jobs. No attempt was made to give advice or suggest counselling and she volunteered 1 year later that she had 'sorted her life out' and was feeling a lot better.

Example 2

A 27-year-old Spanish man presented with the classical symptoms and signs of duodenal ulcer, subsequently proved on X-ray. He had left his native country because of some misdemeanour and was much troubled and guilt-ridden. Even after unburdening himself he felt ill at ease. It transpired that he was a church-going Roman Catholic and felt he needed 'absolution' before his mind could rest in peace. He was referred to his local church.

PROVIDE SUPPORT AND COMFORT/TEAMWORK

The burden of caring for many isolated, lonely and distressed patients is not one that doctors are able to handle on their own any longer. The move towards teamwork is not only a recognition of the need to share this burden amongst several health-care practitioners, but also a recognition of the need of all health-care practitioners to be themselves supported in this work. The general practitioner's role, much like that of the priest, is to catalyse the family support, welfare services and community as well as the health-care team. Knowing how to make the system work for the patient and acting as his or her advocate is often more beneficial and less strenuous than taking on the burden of caring for the patient directly.

ORCHESTRATOR OF RITUAL RITES AND CEREMONY/GIVING MEANING TO STRESSFUL LIFE EVENTS

Going to see the doctor or the monthly 'chronic' visit can on occasions serve as important a function as the ritual of going to church every Sunday. The importance lies in the act itself, its repetitive nature and above all, its constancy. Balint's work on the nature of repeat prescription well illustrated the need to see these meetings, not in purely medical terms, but serving a much more basic need of the human condition. Ceremonials, rituals and rites have traditionally formed the mode by which a culture aids individuals across the transition of important life events. Some of these transitions have been endowed with important religious significance (births, marriages, deaths). Yet others almost as common do not attract the attention of the pastor, rabbi or priest and often present themselves to the doctor in some form or other. Such transitions have been labelled 'rites of passage' and as Holmes & Rahe have shown, whether happy or unhappy, these life events are points of stress [7]. Whether these life events lead to a breakdown and break-up or breakthrough and 'growth' can depend on how they are managed by the individual, his family and his advisers, including his doctor.

The doctor may choose to medicalise the problem and revert to the first sort of medical practice as described by Balint. He may, however, choose to raise the discussion between himself and the patient to explore the meaning of the problem.

Example 1

Miss C., aged 25, came in for medical examination, applying for a university place in America, mentioned many minor complaints. Parents from Syria—she was brought up in England. During the course of the consultation she was asked 'Can you see a purpose to your life?' which brought about an immediate discussion of the conflict of cultures she experienced and her wish to 'run away from home', her fear of intercourse with her boyfriend and a sense of panic she felt when faced with decisions. This young lady presented the doctor with many different problems:

- Physical—headaches, tiredness, vaginismus.
- Psychological—depression, poor self-esteem, lack of identity.
- Spiritual—lack of purpose, sense of alienation, loss of belief in system ('I don't know what is right or wrong any more').

Many similar examples could be given from every general practitioner's daily workload and it is clear that a spiritual dimension could be included, if the doctor so wishes, in many consultations. It is only with a few, however, that the opportunity arises and the right 'interpenetration harmonious mix-up' will result in a shift from the ordinary consultation to the extraordinary. Other possible 'rites of passage' are outlined in Box 4.4 and other forms of 'spiritual' questions in Box 4.5.

Box 4.4 Rites of passage (stressful life events)

New patient	Bereavement
Birth	Adoption
Death	Going on the pill
Infertility	Fitness medical
Termination	Retirement
Marriage	New employment
Divorce	Unemployment
Attempted suicide	Entering accommodation
Leaving home	Entering or leaving prison

Box 4.5 Spiritual questions

Are you a religious person?
Do you pray?
Is prayer important to you?
Do you believe in God?
Does your life have a purpose?
Are you a church-going person?
Do you believe in an after-life?
Have you thought about your death?

Example 2

54-year old Bangladeshi man complaining of painful knees, for which no obvious physical cause could be found. He was asked whether he prayed and whether his pain interfered with his prayer. This caused an immediate 'deepening' of the consultation and he talked about the 'cold weather' in England and the difficulty he experienced kneeling down. He also acknowledged his isolation and loneliness (his wife died soon after they had arrived in England).

COMMUNION/GROUPWORK/CLINICS

For most Christians, the act of going to Church not only serves as a reminder of the Trinity but is also an act of coming together to receive a blessing or sacrament. This coming together of people can be seen as a 'healing ceremony' and is to be witnessed in both secular and sacred forms. We have tended to individualise our encounters between doctor and patient and have forgotten the importance, power and significance of a group. One of the benefits of ante-natal clinics, and mother and toddler groups, lies in the sharing that occurs between the people attending. Similarly, the explosion of self-help groups could be seen as serving the need to bring people together in 'communion'. The need for a collective experience is often made possible through a shared illness. It would be interesting to ponder whether we could be more effective seeing our 10 patients together for 1 hour as opposed to giving them 6 minutes each. The two groups of patients that require most attention from the general practitioner are the elderly, isolated and the anxious, neurotic (usually young). Organising a method by which these two groups could come together would be a fascinating project. Our own efforts

Table 4.15 Psychophysiological changes in meditation

Pulse rate	↑	10/min
Blood pressure	↓	20%
Blood lactate	↑	
Gas exchange	↓	O_2 consumption
	↑	CO_2 elimination
Prolactin	↓	
Cortisol	↓	
EEG alpha wave	↑	
Carry-over effects	↑	Psychological stability
	↑	Internal locus of control

have been in the organisation of 'stress classes' where simple coping skills are taught to a group of patients. These groups have developed to the extent that 'ex-patients' are now able to take new groups through the six sessions.

PRAYER AND MEDITATION/ RELAXATION AND QUIET TIME

The last 20 years have seen an explosion of interest in the use of breathing and relaxation techniques and their application to medical conditions (asthma, hypertension, migraine). Meditation, as a secular act, can be described as a state of relaxed non-aroused physiological functioning which can help to liberate the mind from disturbing and distracting emotions. Table 4.15 details some of the alterations that occur both during and after meditation.

Teaching patients the importance of a 'quiet time' or meditation through the use of an audio-cassette or classes can provide them with the 'breathing space' that so many people need in their lives. The 10-minute appointment slot is perfectly suited for a joint meditation and I have at least one or two patients each day who come in solely to meditate in the consulting room. It is an activity that is as beneficial to the doctor as it is to the patient.

LAYING ON OF HANDS/TOUCH

Touching, laying on of hands and blessing have always formed part of spiritual practices and their therapeutic effects have been recognised through such terms as 'the King's touch', 'the healing touch', etc. Citing many examples from animal and human behaviour, Montagu points out how the skin and touching form an essential psychological and physiological first step in the proper development of the other sensory systems of the body [8]. Deprivation dwarfism is a well-recognised condition that occurs in institutions where children, in spite of good food and medical care, fail to thrive because they are not petted and cossetted. As doctors we are a specially privileged group allowed to touch more people in more places than almost every other profession bar one. However, as we have become more scientific, we have tended to reject this powerful gift to the detriment of our patients. Amongst the many reasons why people are turning to alternative medicine is the fact that many of these therapies are contact-based (osteopathy, massage, reflexology, acupuncture, etc).

There is now good laboratory and clinical evidence to indicate the therapeutic use of touch and we can, if required, quote numerous scientific studies in support. By the simple act of touching, the doctor can reaffirm to the patient that he, the patient, is a unique person and their interaction is altogether human. This can be achieved simply through a sincere handshake. A cold limp hand held out reluctantly induces the opposite effect. We do not hesitate to touch, hold or even sit a child on our knee when talking to him. There is no risk involved in the misinterpretation of this act. There is indeed a risk if we were to do this with our adult patients. For touching to be effective it must:

1. be acceptable to the patient
2. be acceptable to the doctor
3. be recognised that it has a unique meaning for each patient.

Touch as a method of communication differs according to culture as well as age and sex. Within each culture there are enormous variables and we may instinctively recognise this. Children usually have no say—wrongly so—as to whether they are touched or not. Adults may well feel uneasy and threatened by touch.

Touch should be used in a supportive way—meeting the patient's unsatisfied needs whilst allowing him to remain as independent as possible. Doctors approaching patients on whom they have to do an internal examination often start by introducing the speculum. A few seconds spent holding the patients' hands or placing the hand on the abdomen makes the examination easier for both the doctor and the patient. When examining a patient not only can one's hands be used as scientific probes for underlying disease, they can at the same time reassure and comfort the patient that there is a human being guiding those probes. Too often doctors poke instead of touch—and the sexual comparison is more than apt—with the subsequent unsatisfactory intercourse and frigidity. It is because of this sexual conflict that touching in the medical consultation has been so restricted. This may on occasions be justified. When examining a woman's breasts, a male doctor may well be aware that she is conscious of them as sexual objects, as indeed may the woman doctor. Asking about dyspareunia, however, is often best left till the pelvic examination. Not only does this appear sensible from a purely factual point of view, it also indicates to the patient that the doctor is really interested as to precisely where it hurts.

Kathryn Barnet [9], in an excellent paper on the concept of touch as it relates to nursing, summarises her propositions and suggestions for further research as follows:

1. The greater the patient's sense of isolation and sensory deprivation, the greater his need for relatedness to others through touch.
2. The greater the patient's altered body image, the greater his need for acceptance through touch.
3. The greater the patient's feeling of depersonalisation, the greater his need for identity through touch.
4. The greater the patient's regression, the greater his need for communication through touch.
5. The greater the patient's anxiety, the greater the nurse's responsibility regarding the appropriateness of the use of touch.
6. The greater the patient's dependency, the greater the nurse's responsibility regarding the appropriateness of the use of touch.
7. The greater the patient's self-concealment, the greater his need for communication through touch.
8. The greater the patient's need for privacy, the lesser his need for touch.
9. The greater the patient's need for territorial imperative, the lesser his need for touch.
10. The lesser the patient's self-esteem, the greater his need for confirmation through touch.
11. The greater the patient's sense of rejection, the greater his need for acceptance through touch.
12. The greater the patient's fear of death, the greater his need for relatedness to others through touch.

DISCUSSION

There are many omissions to this descriptive account of 'spiritual practices in general practice' and little attempt has been made to describe the pitfalls and problems involved for the general practitioner, least of which is the need to ensure that 'spiritual' enquiry is not a cover for physical and psychological incompetence. In addition, the separation of the 'religious' element from the secular is artificial and may lead to the loss of the importance of awe, wonder and mystery. The practitioner's own spiritual beliefs and spiritual practices will inform his/her approach, and the necessity for maintaining and tolerating an appropriate level of uncertainty seems even more necessary than in the physical and psychological domains. It may indeed be that:

the touch of the healer although it may be like the touch of the masseur is probably quite different. The touch of the mystic, the touch of the religious man, may have a special quality and it is this elusive and spiritual aspect that guides and fires the dimension which may give it power that what one might call the 'secular touch' does not have. [10]

This paper illustrates that doctors have a lot to learn from the other caring disciplines. Hopefully it will provide a stimulus for others to continue in this area of enquiry.

REFERENCES

1. Locke, Hornig-Rohan. Mind and immunology. Institute for Advancement of Health, 1985.
2. Balint M. The basic fault. Tavistock, 1984.
3. Horder, J, RCGP. The future general practitioner: learning and teaching. British Medical Journal, 1972.
4. Jung, C. J. Collected works, vol. 16, Routledge & Kegan Paul, 1981, p. 59.
5. Heron, J. Catharsis in human development. British Postgraduate Medical Federation, 1977.
6. Balint, M. Six minutes for the patient. Tavistock, 1973.
7. Holmes, T, Rahe, R. H. The social readjustment scale. J. Psychosom, Res. 1967 11: 213
8. Montagu, A. Touching: the human significance of the skin. Harper & Row, 1971.
9. Barnet, K. A. Theoretical constructs of the concept of touch
10. Fry, A. (Personal communication).

5

Issues in research and methodology

INTRODUCTION

The need for research and investigation into all aspects of an holistic approach to health care is widely accepted and has formed a central part of the work undertaken by the Marylebone Centre Trust and the Marylebone Health Centre. Yet, the very nature of the fields being subjected to research means that traditional methodologies are often inappropriate. Indeed it might be argued that the traditional nature of research within the medical establishment reflects an attitude towards health and illness which is itself limited and should be subject to scrutiny on these grounds alone. If the accepted 'truths' of medicine are being questioned, and by 'truths' I mean those which deny an holistic approach in favour of one which sees patients as groups of organs in need of treatment, then the means by which these 'truths' are obtained and substantiated must themselves be rigorously examined. It is this kind of examination which Aldridge & Pietroni undertake (Research trials in general practice: towards a focus on clinical practice, p. 168). They suggest, for example, that the randomised trial, the principal means accepted for medical investigation, is a misnomer. A trial can never be truly random, on the contrary it will always draw its subjects from a highly selected and atypical population. They also criticise much research for its lack of breadth. By adopting an 'elitist paper chase' approach, which ignores social and cultural aspects of ill-health, research may be not only inaccurate but positively unhelpful since illness is never a purely physical condition.

The notion that knowledge is something that can be objectively reached by the use of particular research methodologies is at the root of many of the problems with traditional studies and trials. Aldridge & Pietroni suggest that this should be dropped in favour of a recognition that all knowledge is subjective. This should not depress the clinician but rather it opens up new fields of inquiry and allows for 'truths' which do not fit neatly within randomised testing. It also brings to clinical research an approach which is more akin to real life. People, after all, 'know' many things about their bodies and their health without ever having undertaken or read a piece of research. In many cases 'belief' and 'knowledge' will be interchangeable and to reject this is to reject one of the central factors in health and illness. Researchers should come to terms with the fact that all knowledge and all truths are subjective constructs affected by context and circumstance. For as long as the medical profession persists in fooling itself that it can only discover 'truth' through the randomised test it will persist in providing only a limited service to its patients. 'Scientific' approaches are only one form of knowledge and should not be assumed to be superior to all others.

This critique of modern research practices is controversial. There are those who would argue that it rejects rational inquiry for an approach based on supposition and anecdote. Kottow argues this case forcefully (Classical medicine v alternative medical practices, p. 173) insisting that the approaches of classical medicine are superior and, indeed, that an holistic approach practised by doctors is unethical. He does not deny that modern medicine fails to meet many of the non-organic needs of its patients but insists that this is for sociological reasons, arising from the development of medicine as a science, and not because of the 'rational' methods it adopts. More than this, he denies that research grants should be given to projects investigating alternative therapies since they are unscientific and therefore unethical. The resources which might be diverted to these areas could and should be better spent on classical medicine since this is the only field in which rational methods can and

will be implemented. In his response, Pietroni (Alternative medicine: methinks the doctor protests too much and incidentally befuddles the debate, p. 179) points out that the assumptions Kottow makes about the nature of scientific knowledge are not in fact universally held. Far from making diagnoses on the basis of rational and inductive methods, as Kottow suggests, clinicians will use a whole host of approaches when arriving at a particular diagnosis. Moreover, the single definition of causality which Kottow uses has come to be questioned by 'pure scientists' the world over. As to the question of research funding, Pietroni notes that Kottow has presented a circular argument; untested therapies are unethical and therefore should not be funded, yet if unfunded these therapies will never be tested and therefore will never become 'ethical'.

This conundrum was also highlighted by Fleming et al (The trouble with research about acupuncture, p. 183). The research team undertook a study designed to look at the effect of acupuncture on patients with chronic asthma. They rejected as unethical a methodological approach incorporating a placebo control group, which in this case would have meant the use of 'sham' acupuncture. Instead they chose to use two control groups, one receiving their usual drugs as well as counselling and the other receiving only their usual drugs. They found that many of the Hospital Ethics Committees asked to approve this study for funding presented exactly the same objections as Kottow. It was argued by these committees that the only acceptable form of research was to use a control group who were given 'sham' acupuncture as this was the only methodology which conformed to a traditional and 'rational' approach. This was the only approach considered by the committee to be 'scientific' and therefore 'ethical'.

Not all ethics committees shared these reservations about the ethical basis of the study. It is suggested by the authors of the report that these differences in opinion are in part the result of the poor direction given to ethics committees but are also the result of a split in attitude towards different research methodologies within clinical settings. An 'explanatory' study, close in method to laboratory conditions, may be favoured by some, while others, especially those working in primary health, will favour a 'pragmatic' approach where the emphasis is on optimising treatment.

This is a gap that needs to be bridged. New ways of thinking about research and an acceptance of the many ways in which both knowledge and truth can be constructed appear to be the way in which this might be achieved. A range of research approaches are needed, just as a range of therapies are needed, if patients are to receive the best possible treatment. Randomised tests should not be rejected out of hand, but neither should they be held up as the only means by which knowledge may be furthered or acquired. As Aldridge & Pietroni (p. 168) suggest, the way forward is to accept a new way of evaluating research. It should be based not on whether a piece of research formally proves a point, but on whether it adds to the available evidence on a given issue.

RESEARCH TRIALS IN GENERAL PRACTICE: TOWARDS A FOCUS ON CLINICAL PRACTICE

David Aldridge
Patrick Pietroni

With current moves towards an emphasis on the 'whole' patient rather than fragmenting the person into organ systems, we need to develop research methods which reflect that emphasis and direct us in our endeavours as clinicians. It is possible to have a descriptive science of human behaviour which can be based upon clinical consultations. In this way the clinician is required to act as a clinical anthropologist as well as a clinical epidemiologist.

INTRODUCTION

Hart's vision of general practice calls for a major innovation in research (Hart 1984). A significant factor of that innovation is a growing awareness by the doctor of the patient's social and cultural milieu, and an understanding of health beliefs (Gregg 1985, Underwood et al 1985, Wilkin 1986). In this form of approach our research ceases to become an elitist paper chase but prompts the emergence of a discipline which seeks to discover what the practitioner does, why people come to the doctor, what appears to be effective and what can be taught.

METHODOLOGICAL ISSUES

While controlled trial methodology may appear to be scientifically sound, a number of articles have questioned the scientific premises of such methods.

The first of these criticisms is that a random selection of trial subjects cannot be achieved because any group of patients comprises a highly selected non-random group (Burkhardt & Kienle 1980, Anonymous 1983). Any results concerning this trial group cannot be generalised to other trial groups. These inductive generalisations, it is argued, are no more respectable than those made from anecdotal experiences.

Secondly, group generalisations from research findings raise problems for the clinician who is faced with the individual person in his or her consulting room. Individual variations are mocked by the group average (Barlow et al 1973). If a group of 50 patients in a treatment group does statistically better than a control group of 50 patients then such a difference could be due to a small number of patients in the treatment group showing a larger change while the majority of patients show no change or deteriorate slightly. It is the patients who change significantly who are of interest to us as clinicians and we would want to know the significant factors involved in that change. These factors however are lost within the group average.

Thirdly, there are issues of reliability which are linked to the practice of scientific research. As we have seen (Dudley 1983) the reliability of our knowledge is only as good as the underpinning hypothesis. An hypothesis by definition is capable of being disproved. Inevitably the reliability of a trial when extended to a broader population is an act of induction (Burkhardt & Kienle 1983).

It must be noted here that validity has to be conferred by a person or group of persons on the work or actions of another group. This is a 'political' process. With the obsession for 'objective truths' in the scientific community, other 'truths' are ignored. As clinicians we have many ways of knowing; by intuition, through experience and by observation. If we disregard these 'knowings' then we promote the idea that there is an objective, definitive, external truth which exists as a 'tablet of stone' and to which only we have access.

Observational awareness is an important precursor to clinical trials yet is all too easy to ignore. Yet the risk of doing so is to fail to ask the correct questions of the research. While clinical research may be easy to set up technically in that methodological guidelines are readily available,

Reprinted from Family Practice: 4 (4) pp. 311–315 with the permission of Oxford University Press.

the creative process of posing the right questions and formulating hypotheses is far more difficult.

Finally, there is no such thing as a purely 'physical' treatment (Heron 1984). Treatment always occurs in a psychosocial context. Medicine is a social as well as a natural science (Kleinman 1973, Mechanic 1986). The way people respond in situations is sometimes determined by the way in which they have understood the meaning of that situation (Harre & Secord 1971). By studying the accounts people give of their symptoms in the context of their intimate relationships we can glean valuable understanding of illness behaviour. The meaning of a headache in the context of a doctor/patient relationship may be a far cry from the meaning of a headache in a husband/wife relationship.

This reflects one of two fundamentally differing approaches to science. One is to develop precise and fixed procedures that yield a stable and definite empirical content. We have this in controlled trial methodology. The other approach to investigation depends upon careful and imaginative life studies which although lacking some of the precision of technical instruments have the virtue of continuing a close relationship with the natural social world of people.

ETHICAL AND POLITICAL ISSUES

The subject matter of our research endeavours and the way we carry out those endeavours reflect our views of the society in which we wish to live, the ways in which we wish to deal with our fellow human beings and the ways in which we wish to be dealt with by them (Burkhardt & Kienle 1983).

As clinicians the concern for the subject prevails over the interest of society at large and scientific medicine as an institution. Individual persons are not treated as a means to some collective end in clinical practice, although we may subscibe to a notion of community health. Furthermore, we discover a dilemma for research in that scientific standards of acceptability are juxtaposed with the ordinary therapeutic standards of the doctor. The standards of probability necessary for scientific statistical validity

may be more exacting than the standards of probability acceptable to either the patient or the doctor. Such standards can vary according to the context in which they are applied. For the dying person the rigour of the clinical trial and the level of probability in terms of treatment efficacy may be quite different to that of the 'healthy' person, a woman in mid-term or an infant.

The rejection of the null hypothesis—that there is no difference between treatment and control—is not only an end of trial decision. There are times when it is possible to discern a 'trend' which becomes clear. It is at these times that the clinician as researcher must ask the question 'If faced with "this trend" as a father, husband or patient, would I accept evidence of a less rigorous standard than a scientist?' (Anonymous 1983). This too begs the further question of whether or not scientific standards should prevail.

These dilemmas can be seen in the trials of periconceptional multi-vitamin supplementation for women who had previously given birth to one or more infants with a neural tube defect (Frei 1982). Mothers were not prepared to volunteer for trials where they faced the possibility of not being given folic acid. Medical teams also declined to take part in such trials. This example demonstrates that decisions can be made on the basis of observational awareness and the application of a common clinical sense. Rather than carry out a controlled trial using folic acid it was possible to offer vitamin supplementation to all women at risk to see if the level of incidence of neural tube defect fell.

There are also similar problems for clinical researchers who want to research a treatment method for a seriously ill patient, and who believe, on the basis of the clinical evidence they accrue, that the treatment is effective. They will find it unacceptable to withhold the treatment for some of their patients by assigning them to a non-treatment control group or a group using conventional but ineffective treatment. As the reader will see, this is the reverse process of the clinician withdrawing a patient from a trial because the trend indicates that there is no difference between treatment and control.

A further difficulty of accepting levels of probability is that trials of treatment are often scrutinised or judged by practitioners and scientists whose epistemology is different to that of those carrying out the trial. While it is necessary to have questions posed by 'outsiders' it is important that trials of homoeopathy, acupuncture and psychotherapy are assessed by panels which have representatives of these other therapeutic directions. By incorporating experts from differing disciplines it is possible to design procedures whereby any prevailing dogma is not granted a monopoly status as a compulsory 'current status of scientific knowledge' and minority groups representing other forms of medical practice are not suppressed by the majority vote. This plurality of opinion will enliven research endeavours and offer a broad platform of clinical practice (Pietroni & Aldridge 1986).

CLINICAL OR EXPERIMENTAL?

While trials within general practice may be set up to conform to an experimental methodology, those practising within the trial invariably approach their work from a clinical viewpoint. For the subjects of the trial the agenda is also likely to be 'clinical' in so far as their expectations are of treatment. Similarly the results of a trial need to be interpreted and applied by clinicians. Perhaps what we have failed to ask are the questions:

1. What is the nature of clinical judgement?
2. What is it capable of?
3. What realms of information are used to make that judgement?.

When controlled trials are carried out in a clinical setting then the benefit for the individual is set against the benefit for the group. The Declaration of Helsinki (1964) states: 'In any medical study, every patient—including those of the control group, if any—should be assured of the best proven diagnostic and therapeutic method.'

The clinical judgement of the doctor is on the side of the individual patient even if it means the corruption of a research project. When clinicians, who are bound by contracts for treatment, take part in clinical trials then the dilemma is revealed. Either they fulfil their individual contract for treatment with the patient, or they abdicate that contract and fulfil their obligations to the research contract which are concerned with group benefit. This raises two further conceptual issues for health care—is 'health' an individual or societal concept? Are we as clinicians committed to improving the health of the individuals we see, or are we directed to improving the health of the communities we serve?

These arguments are not new. Rychlak (1970) pointed out the difficulty of trying to account for human behaviour in 'only demonstrative terms, relying upon efficient and material cause description, when in fact man needs both demonstrative and dialectical conceptualisations'. It is these dialectical considerations we will debate in the next section.

'HARD' OR 'SOFT' DATA?

A social science explanation of human behaviour has emphasised that persons are not solely organisms responding to stimuli from the environment, or simply the sum of their interacting organ systems. The very difficulty of studying such behaviour is that people make sense of what they do (Dallos & Aldridge 1987), impose different meanings onto reality and alter their behaviour accordingly. When we try to understand social action we have to take into account that there are different available interpretations of that action. Furthermore, these actions take place as processes in natural settings and belong to social contexts (Tomson et al 1986).

When a person consults a doctor and presents a problem then that problem can be seen in varying ways according to the perspectives of the patient and the doctor. The presentation of that problem will have occurred after previous discussions with other family members, and previously attempted health care activities (Aldridge 1984, Aldridge & Rossiter 1985). Similarly the choice of healer and the available treatment is also part of a cultural context which embraces the doctor and the patient (Kleinman & Sung 1985).

Scientific medicine emphasises one particular way of knowing and this seems to maintain the myth that to know anything we must be scientists. If we consider people who live in vast desert areas, they find their way across those trackless terrains without any understanding of scientific geography. They also know the pattern of the weather without recourse to what we know as the science of meteorology. In a similar way people know about their own bodies and have understandings about their own lives. They may not confer the same meanings as we do, yet it is those meanings and particular beliefs about health to which we might best be guiding our research endeavours (Hasler 1985). While as clinicians we may help to bring about a change in behaviour by technical means, it is the person who we have to rely upon to describe the meanings and implications of that change. This also leaves out the problem for us as scientists of explaining how a change in meaning can bring about a change in behaviour (Baker 1987).

The practical difficulty of researching subjective variables is that they are not accessible to quantitative methods, nor are they generalisable; they are indeed subjective. To combat this difficulty and potential disruption of our knowledge we tend to ignore such data and reduce our variables to those which are easily manipulated. To do so reduces the person to simply being a vessel for the containment of a disease. When we include subjective variables such as emotion, we treat them as if they could be weighted like ballast (Porter 1986).

When we intervene or treat persons in our research studies then we are engaging in an activity which is not stable. Our intention is to bring about change. This too poses a problem for generalisability beyond that seen in the earlier section. Not only do we have to extrapolate from one group to another, we have also to induce meanings from a situation which is in a state of flux.

In natural science studies objectivity is sought by separating the subject from interfering with the experiment. Some authors state that by doing this the person is alienated from the study (Heron 1981, Reason & Rowan 1981). Yet we know that the attitudes and beliefs of the experimenter and the subject are important, and that the experimenter and the subject interact with each other. When we study health then we have to take into account biological, psychological and social factors (Engel 1977, Schwab & Schwab 1978).

For example, in reporting the impact of acupuncture for the treatment of asthma, patients said subjectively that they 'felt better' but there was no objective change in airway impedance (Berger & Nolte 1977, Dias et al 1982). These factors represent varying levels of understanding and are measured in varying ways which may be quite incompatible. They are not independent factors but interact with each other. As researchers we separate the world into discrete categories for our own purposes, yet social life occurs in natural settings quite different from the artificial ones created for research. The people whom we see in our practices make sense of their lives in many different ways. It is our task to understand their way of seeing the world and not to impose our categories upon their experience.

CONCLUSION

This all sounds rather difficult and leaves us wondering how health care researchers can ever make sense of anything. There is a way of reconciling these difficulties and that is to move to a position whereby we judge our research on 'whether it makes a powerful and important contribution to the cumulative evidence on a particular issue' (Holman 1990) rather than whether or not it formally proves a point.

It is this cumulative knowledge which Pringle (1984) directs us to. He suggests that the general practitioner is in a unique position to look at the total health of the person and to take part in comparative studies. Ironically, he suggests that journals are becoming more willing to accept the 'soft' data that these studies elicit compared with the 'hard' data of random trials. The main implication is that such data will increase the core knowledge of general practice.

This recognition of subjective data is occurring at a time when an emphasis is being placed on the 'whole' patient rather than fragmenting the person into organ systems (Pietroni 1984). Balint showed us that it is not solely scientific skills which help us to fully understand the patient. It is possible to have a descriptive science of human behaviour which can be based upon clinical consultations. In this way the clinician is required to act as a clinical anthropologist as well as a clinical epidemiologist (Shepherd 1982).

REFERENCES

Aldridge D 1984 Suicidal behaviour and family interaction: a brief review. Journal of Family Therapy 6 pp. 309–322

Aldridge D, Rossiter J 1985 Difficult patients, intractable symptoms and spontaneous recovery in suicidal behaviour. Journal of Systemic Strategic Therapies 4 pp. 66–76

Anonymous 1983 Ethics, philosophy and clinical trials. Journal of Medical Ethics 9 pp. 59–60

Baker G H 1987 Inquiry review: Psychological factors and immunity. Journal of Psychosomatic Research 31 pp. 1–10

Barlow D H, Hersen M, Jackson M 1973 Single-case experimental designs. Archives of General Psychiatry 29 pp. 319–325

Berger D, Nolte D 1977 Acupuncture in bronchial asthma: body plethysomographic measurements of acute bronchospasmolytic effects. Complementary Medicine East and West 5 pp. 265–269

Burkhardt R, Kienle G 1980 Controlled clinical trials and drug regulations. Controlled Clinical Trials 1 pp. 151–164

Burkhardt R, Kienle G 1983 Basic problems in controlled trials. Journal of Medical Ethics 9 pp. 80–84

Dallos R, Aldridge D 1987 Handing it on: family constructs, symptoms and choice. Journal of Family Therapy

Declaration of Helsinki 1964 Recommendations guiding doctors in biomedical research involving human subjects. Adopted by the 18th World Medical Assembly, Helsinki, Finland and as revised by the 29th World Medical Assembly, Tokyo, Japan, 1975

Dias P L, Subraniam S, Lionel N D 1982 Effects of acupuncture in bronchial asthma: a preliminary communication. Journal of the Royal Society of Medicine 75 pp. 245–248

Dudley H A F 1983 The controlled clinical trial and the advance of reliable knowledge: an outsider looks in. British Medical Journal 287 pp. 957–960

Engel G 1977 The need for a new medical model: a challenge for biomedicine. Science 196 pp. 129–136

Frei 1982 Ethical dilemmas in evaluation—a correspondence. Science 217 pp. 600–606

Gregg I 1985 The quality of asthma in general practice—a challenge for the future. Family Practice 2 pp. 94–100

Harre R, Secord P F 1971 The explanation of social behaviour. Blackwell, London

Hart J T 1984 Where is general practice going? New Doctor 33 pp. 8–10

Hasler J C 1985 The very stuff of general practice. Journal of the Royal College of General Practitioners 35 pp. 121–127

Heron J 1981 Experimental research methodology. In: Reason P, Rowan J (eds) Human inquiry. John Wiley, Chichester

Heron J 1984 Position paper on research methods. London Research Council for Complementary Medicine

Holman C G 1990 Culture and health and illness. Butterworth-Heinemann, Oxford

Kleinman A M 1973 Medicine's symbolic reality. On a central problem in the philosophy of medicine. Inquiry 16 pp. 206–213

Kleinman A, Sung L H 1985 Why do indigenous practitioners successfully heal? Social Science and Medicine 13 pp. 7–26

Mechanic D 1986 The concept of illness behaviour: culture situation and personal disposition. Psychological Medicine 16 pp. 1–7

Pietroni P 1984 New map, old territory. British Journal of Holistic Medicine 1 pp. 3–13

Pietroni P C, Aldridge D 1986 Summary of discussion on BMA report. Holistic Medicine 1

Porter R 1986 Psychotherapy research: physiological measures and intrapsychic events. Journal of the Royal Society of Medicine 79 pp. 257–261

Pringle M 1984 A minority interest: why? British Medical Journal 289 pp. 163–164

Reason P, Rowan J (eds) 1981 Human inquiry. John Wiley, Chichester

Rychlak J F 1970 The human person in modern psychological medicine. British Journal of Medical Psychology 43 pp. 233–240

Schwab J J, Schwab M E 1978 Sociocultural roots of mental illness. Plenum Medical Books, London

Shepherd M 1982 Psychiatric research and primary care in Britain—past, present and future. Psychological Medicine 12 pp. 493–499

Tomson P, Ineson N, Milton J 1986 Feasibility and usefulness of family record cards in general practice. Journal of the Royal College of General Practitioners 36 pp. 506–509

Underwood P, Gray D, Winkler R 1985 Cutting open Newton's apple to find the cause of gravity: a reply to Julian Tudor Hart on the future of general practice. British Medical Journal 291 pp. 1322–1324

Wilkin D 1986 Outcomes of research in general practice. Journal of the Royal College of General Practitioners 36 pp. 4–5

CLASSICAL MEDICINE V ALTERNATIVE MEDICAL PRACTICES

Michael Kottow

Classical medicine operates in a climate of rational discourse, scientific knowledge accretion and the acceptance of ethical standards that regulate its activities. Criticism has centred on the excessive technological emphasis of modern medicine and on its social strategy aimed at defending exclusiveness and the privileges of professional status.

Alternative therapeutic approaches have taken advantage of the eroded public image of medicine, offering treatments based on holistic philosophies that stress the non-rational, non-technical and non-scientific approach to the unwell, disregarding traditional diagnostic categories and concentrating on enhancing subjective comfort and well-being, but remaining oblivious to the organic substrate of disease. This leads to questionable ethics in terms of false hopes and lost opportunities for effective therapy.

Keywords: Alternative therapies, holism, placebos, traditional medicine.

INTRODUCTION

Contrary to widespread belief, medicine only began to achieve the social status of a profession in the Middle Ages, when it became a fundamentally intellectual discipline that did not fully develop its therapeutic and counselling functions until the nineteenth century. Consequently, so-called traditional or classical medicine has always co-existed with alternative therapies, both paradigms sharing the social functions of palliating suffering, healing, and controlling biological disorders and the vagaries of the deviant [1].

Discrepancy mounted and expectations became somewhat frustrated as medicine increasingly stressed the scientific and highly technical aspects of its methods; hopes were

Reprinted with permission from the Journal of Medical Ethics: 18 pp. 18–22 1992 published by BMJ Publishing Group.

nourished that often remained unfulfilled and were then rechannelled towards alternative therapeutic offers, leading to acrid sociological, medical and ethical controversies between traditional and alternative therapeutic approaches. There is hardly any aspect of medicine that is not profoundly affected by the differences between medical and alternative therapies, and it appears of some urgency that medicine establish its position in the debate, in order adequately to meet the rhetorical and dialectic challenges it faces in such multifarious areas as allocation of resources, research priorities, hubris and nemesis, criteria of efficiency, areas of relevancy, and right to the exclusive practice of medicine.

THE SOCIOLOGICAL ISSUES

Medicine has been able to convince society that it holds unique qualifications, exclusive competence and undoubted efficacy in matters concerning health and disease. By any standards that define disease as some sort of disruption or revolution of an established order, be it organic, cultural or social, medicine has managed to monopolise the management of a substantial number of such derangements, gaining the economic and strategic support of the social system of which it is part. Such a process has been criticised as medicalisation [2, 3], but a more exact analysis shows a generalised process that goes beyond a mere take-over, where medicine and society enter a mutually beneficial symbiosis.

Originally, religion monopolised medical and many other social functions, as is exemplified by numerous hygienic and civic regulations to be found in the Old Testament. Religion has yielded social power to medicine as well as to other institutions, at the same time willingly surrendering supra-natural areas of competence to these more profane and visibly effective systems of compensation for everyday misfortunes. From its inception medicine has competed with the traditional healing functions of religious institutions (as shown by the common etymology of the words 'heal' and 'holy'). To achieve its privileged and respected status, medicine had to show a convincing record of therapeutic effectiveness, usually gaining territory at the expense of religion and other social institutions. Thus, medicalisation seems to be a secular invasion of areas that traditionally had been managed in transcendent terms [4].

A gap seems to have developed between the interests of medicine as a social system and the patient's need for comfort and support; a gap that is exploited by opponents of the medical establishment and that provides an easy bonus for alternative approaches [5]. A number of reasons make scientific medicine pursue interests that do not always cover the non-organic needs of its beneficiaries. In this macroscopic view, criticism is easy to come by, for not all that is good for medicine as a social system is good for the individual patient.

This kind of insight goes a long way to explaining why scientific medicine, being rational and mundane, has been unable to fulfil certain yearnings that religion no longer attends to. Alternative therapies are for the most part immersed in a theoretical framework with clear metaphysical undertones that seem to offer a new form of gratifying sacralisation [6, 7]. Seen in this social perspective, medicine appears to fail in its task of providing an emotional environment of meaning and direction, and alternative therapies can hardly be blamed if they manage to convey a sense of existential protection which operates not on the basis of some truth, but by means of its soothing and comforting effects.

THE MEDICAL ISSUES

Scientific aspects

Medicine is a rational enterprise built on a scientific tradition that operates with logical arguments, the laws of causality and the epistemic strategies of observation and experimentation. The scientific community rejects the intellectual elements used by alternative disciplines, dismissing them as charlatanry, but it is easier to attack the epistemic claims of alternative therapies, than to counter criticism that both these therapies and public opinion have directed at medicine, accusing it of being an ineffectual, impotent, expensive, blindfolded and unimaginative enterprise [8].

Medicine is ineffectual, it is said, because whatever progress mankind has achieved in its capacity to survive, has been obtained independently of medical progress [9]. Economic growth and sanitary developments have been major factors in improving health standards, far beyond the minute engineering of medical interventions. Medicine is impotent, for it is unable to solve most biological problems that afflict mankind, such as degenerative diseases, senescence, death or, more recently, AIDS. Medicine is expensive, for where it does help, it also creates enormous social and economic expenses, thus operating with unacceptable high cost–benefit ratios. Medicine is blindfolded in that it cherishes its own scientific bias but will not see truth in any testimony rendered by people dealing with or being treated by alternative forms of therapy. Finally, medicine is unimaginative because it is incapable of conceiving explanations beyond the realm of the scientific paradigm [8].

How much of all this is true and valid criticism? Much, and yet very little. Much, because it is true that the practice of medicine is fraught with failures, mistakes, risks, complications and side-effects. But very little, for the critics of medicine are using the same language and comparable reasoning to try and show that this language and this reasoning are inadequate [3, 10]. Alternative schools are inconsistent in their use of empirical data, presenting anecdotal pieces of experience as convincing evidence that consciousness, for example, can have telepathic and telekinetic influences. Strong claims are present in vague language, where terms remain undefined, observations are not clarified, causality is treated lightly, testimonies receive no validation and conclusions are not demonstrated. After all, whoever asserts postulates that do not fit accepted paradigms is under obligation to buttress his or her claims and make them plausible. Rejecting and replacing accepted ways of thinking is a rational enterprise, not an act of faith, and must therefore abide by the laws of rational thinking. In point of fact, alternative therapies employ rational language with the explicit purpose of clouding issues or letting unclear arguments emerge and compete for validity. Concepts like health, well-being, the natural, responsibility for moral weakness of dysfunctional lifestyles, and many more are very hard to pinpoint as to their intention—what they designate—and their extension—which entities they apply to. Terms used in this way become ubiquitous, useful for ill-defined propositions and elusive to serious analysis and criticism.

Ever since Descartes created a formidable chiasm between the material and the mental, the history of thought has battled to explain the interaction of these two apparently distinct worlds. Traditional medicine, even psychiatric and psychosomatic approaches, have decidedly taken sides with materialism, considering the body to be a machine, subject to deterministic explanation and causal intervention. This has been the strength of medical diagnosis and the weakness of its therapy. The main stumbling-block of a scientific approach has been that science operates with generalities whereas medicine has to act on sick individuals. Science is inductive, but induction is probabilistic and does not work for the individual [11]. As science progresses, the individual *qua* individual appears to be side-tracked from its benefits. It is hardly surprising that patients feel neglected by 'high-tech' medicine and turn towards alternative approaches. Surely it is here where alternative therapies find their most plausible justification, stressing as they do the personal approach, while medicine becomes increasingly technical, aloof to any non-quantifiable aspects of disease and disengaged from the individuality of patients. Alternative approaches do concentrate on the individual, but they disparage personal values by reducing the patient to the metaphysical and administrative order of their holistic perspective, where he becomes an acquiescing appendage.

Clinical aspects

The most powerful tool of medicine is diagnosis. It serves to specify and at times aetiologically to explain the disease state; it helps establish prognosis and it outlines a therapeutic approach. It has been pointed out that diagnosis is of no heuristic value in itself, but that it increases the chances of rational and effective therapy [12]. Clinicians will probably disagree, for innumerable diagnostic efforts are carried out in good faith in spite of lacking therapeutic consequences, but it remains true that diagnosis is not a labelling process but rather an orientation aimed at directing medical action.

Not only is diagnosis based on scientific data, it is a rational process in its own right, although coloured by strong institutional components; diagnosis utilises the scientific tools of controlled observation, exploration and experimentation (as in provocation tests). Additionally, diagnosis is indispensable for adequate control and evaluation of therapy, for the efficacy of treatment can only be gauged by permanently reverting to comparisons with the initially diagnosed condition. A disease is cured when the mosaic of initially observed derangements disappears, signs and symptoms fade away and lab tests normalise. The diagnostic process is thus therapeutically normative, for it establishes the parameters that must be changed in order to gauge the efficacy of treatment and the elimination of disease. Medicine must therefore be scientific in its diagnostic approach both to establish and to evaluate therapeutic courses.

In contradistinction, alternative medicine has little use for standardised diagnostics. The diagnosis of clinical entities is neglected, only the elimination of symptoms is of interest [13]. The diagnostic evaluation of therapeutic success is replaced by a subjective process that remains refractive to any parameters of comparison.

Traditional medicine is more consistent in its loyalty to diagnosis than is alternative medicine in disregarding it. Even though holistic therapies deny diagnostic procedures, they often purport to reach diagnostic levels of knowledge through finely honed, at times esoteric-sounding, explorations such as feeling the pulse, mapping the iris or detecting microenergetic channels along the body. A further inconsistency is seen when alternative medicine decides to employ the diagnostic labels of allopathic medicine, albeit distorting or remodelling them at will [14].

The primary purpose of medicine is to bring a disease-diminished human organism to its best possible state of adaptation to its environment. This goal is best reached by removing disease, a second-best strategy being to enhance well-being by improving the individual's attitude towards his infirmity when the disease cannot be eradicated. Traditional medicine pursues knowledge about morbid entities for the purpose of offering disease-eradicating therapy, while alternative therapy appears unconcerned with the underlying processes and seeks to remove the disturbing facts of disease by attacking symptoms and increasing patients' well-being, often restricting its actions to dysfunctional states and preferring to leave the management of anatomical derangements to traditional medicine, or to disregard them completely. In other words, alternative medicine does not cure but rather peripherally changes patients' attitudes towards the natural event of their disease. Records of therapeutic accomplishments remain anecdotal and testimonial, leading to unwarranted extrapolations and generalisations.

By stressing the patient/therapist relation, alternative approaches fulfil the second objective of medical intervention, namely to change the patient's attitude towards his disease, despite the fact that the disease process has not been removed. Needless to say, this change in attitude may coincide with, or even be instrumental to actual cure, so that it is hardly surprising that the therapeutic claims of alternative medicine appear at times justified, although they will just as often create false confidence and hinder opportune medical help.

THE ETHICAL ISSUES

Possibly the strongest issues dividing alternative and traditional therapies lie in the ethical arena. The history of therapeutics is richly spiced with charlatanry and quacksalvery, practised both by licensed doctors and by self-appointed healers. Also, both traditional and alternative therapies rely heavily on the healer/patient relationship, employing psychological props, placebos and rituals to gain therapeutic efficiency even at the cost of disrupting the laws of causality. The ethical aspects of such fringe-therapies as placebos can be reduced to two fundamental attitudes. Favouring their use is the utilitarian argument that any relief obtained by the patient will justify them. The argument against placebos claims that deceitful manipulation of the patient is not permissible and that ineffective medication tends to nourish excessively high and unwarranted expectations in the powers of medicine [15].

The point to be made is that, independent of the ethical stance one may take regarding placebos, they are conceptually embedded in the scientific matrix of clinical medicine. Without a clearly outlined diagnosis, the therapeutic possibilities of specific, non-specific or placebo intervention cannot be accurately appraised. This cluster of clinical judgements, although perhaps in itself not an act of science, derives from a scientifically gained pool of knowledge. Thus, although the use of placebos may possibly be the most marginal activity of medicine, it is, independently of its ethical status, coherent with the scientific environment of clinical judgement.

The vice of falsehood lies not necessarily in the discipline but in its practitioners. Medicine has defended the professional privilege of inner control, thus assuming the responsibility of ethical practice and surveillance, but at the same time serving as a tolerant and often blind refuge for misconduct. Alternative therapies have also been practised in good as well as bad faith, so the black-sheep argument will hardly serve to settle this issue.

More relevance in gauging the ethical stance of therapeutic efforts must go to the three other issues: allocation of resources, comparability of competing therapies and vulnerability to criticisms.

Medicine is plagued by insufficient funding because of increasing costs, ever-growing expectations and the expansively competing needs of other social services. Much of what organised medicine spends is superfluous and yet, in absolute terms, resources are insufficient. An ethical allocation policy requires plausible and well-grounded requests for funds, presented on the basis of empirical knowledge, state-of-the-art appraisals and rational argument. Alternative therapies shun this kind of exposé, being unwilling and unable to negotiate in technically acceptable terms. Any resources diverted to non-medical therapies are therefore unethical, be they to subsidise benefits and material implementation, or to support official accreditation and public approval.

The damages of therapeutic courses of action lie not only in their side-effects, mistakes and shortcomings, but more importantly in the opportunities lost for other possible actions that might prove more beneficial or less harmful. Within the realm of orthodox medicine, the course of disease and the effects of medical management are permanently being subjected to evaluation: antibiotics are replaced, dosages are adjusted, expectancy v intervention is under permanent comparison, additional opinions are culled. Alternative treatment lacks any comparative apparatus and is much less flexible in adjusting its therapeutic strategies and treatments, basically because it does not operate with a cause/effect rationale, but also because alternative therapies are usually monothematic and exclusive of any supplementary forms of management which appear foreign to their theoretical premises. If the alternative therapy fails, much opportunity will have been lost and by the time the patient reaches traditional medical advice he may be in a state of irreversibility or chronicity, and be developing sequelae and complications that could, perhaps, have been avoided. It is for these reasons that the denomination 'alternative medicine' is a misnomer; for if it actually is effective therapy, it becomes incorporated into current medical practice and ceases to be alternative, whereas, if it remains alternative it can no longer claim to be medicine. To insist on representing a valid therapeutic option becomes, under the circumstances, a case of dubious morality.

Finally, whereas both orthodox medicine and alternative therapies partake of the epistemic hiatus that exists between experts and lay-people, there is an important ethical difference in the way they deal with this knowledge gap. Medicine, like any scientific or highly technical discipline, functions within a theoretical framework that is in principle open to everyone. Medicine has often and validly been criticised for artificially keeping its knowledge from being universally accessible. In fact, much of what has been written about themes like the doctor/patient relationship, informed consent (rather, informed decision) and the autonomy of patients, has aimed at reducing the difference between what the doctor knows and what the patient ought to know. The medical knowledge gap can in principle be bridged, and it has become a standard of ethical excellence to reach the patient with as much information as it necessary for him to decide about the management of his disease.

Alternative medicine operates with a holistic concept of health/disease which necessarily buttresses its theoretical grounds and diminishes the individual [16]. Holism believes that a sound biological system depends upon physical, mental, social and spiritual well-being. Thus, being healthy means living a well-rounded existence and being sick is a demonstration of one's incompetence in some aspect of one's way of life. The ascribed nature of disease is buttressed by the responsibility that holistic movements require individuals to take for their health or disease states. Having thus diminished the sick individual, holistic movements see therapists as teachers more than health providers, thus emphasising the distance between the initiated, knowledgeable and presumably overall healthy therapist and the diseased, deficient, uninformed and untrained patient. Out of this predicament comes a yoke of two additional holistic tenets, namely:

1. the insufficient scope and lack of behavioural, social and environmental dimensions imputed to traditional medicine
2. the preferability of natural (= non-invasive) means in lieu of artificial (= interventionist) medicine.

These non-technical therapeutics might at first glance seem to be amenable to unsophisticated usage and self-application, but it must be remembered that they are embedded in esoteric and transcendent world-views which the initiated has reached through long years of discipline, whereas the sick person has become deranged precisely because he does not partake of this insight. Being by definition refractive to and ignorant of the philosophical perspective of the healthy, the patient must become dependent on the enlightened therapist, to which purpose the healing theory is clad in metaphysics that stress an overwhelmingly optimistic valuation of man and nature. This is exemplified by the harmony of Yang/Yin, the outstanding gifts ascribed to man by anthroposophy, the benign healing powers attributed to nature by naturopathy, the wholesomeness of macrobiotics or the presence of Life's Universal Healing Force as maintained by so-called healers. Consequently, therapeutic failures constitute the demonstration that the patient lacks the necessary armamentarium fully to subscribe to and benefit from the healing powers of the therapeutic school of thought he has chosen, so that alternative approaches can bathe themselves in the self-fulfilling prophecy that only he who believes in his own cure will actually get better.

The ethical problems of alternative medicine do not, therefore, rest in its lack of efficacy, nor can its strength be seen in the occasional therapeutic successes it achieves, for medical ethics do not comfortably operate on a merely utilitarian evaluation of medical acts. Placebos are useful, yet they are ethically vulnerable to criticism because they mislead the patient and leave him uninformed. Research on insufficiently informed subjects may be very enlightening; it nevertheless remains unethical. By the same stringent standards, alternative medicine cannot gain moral status on the mere argument of efficacy, especially if it is unwilling to abide by scientific gauging standards.

Non-rational arguments, as employed by alternative practices, are rejected by the scientific-minded community. In addition, there is no reason to believe that such irrational methods will always be employed for a good purpose [14]. If paranormal healing powers really exist, they might just as well be used intentionally to harm people, for if there is no commitment to abide by scientific medicine, there will also be no valid rea-

son to respect culturally accepted forms of ethical discourse.

In sum, critics of medicine and alternative therapies share an understandable negative view of modern scientific medicine. The medical establishment is certainly slow to accept and act upon such criticism, but this reluctance is merely sociological and not intrinsic to its rationality, whereas so-called paranormal therapies depend on scientific incoherence, esoterism and intolerance towards both traditional medicine as well as competing alternative stances operating on premises equally based on faith or assertions that are not amenable to validation.

REFERENCES

1. King L S. Medical thinking. Princeton: Princeton University Press, 1982.
2. Aries P. Geschichte des todes. Munich and Vienna: Hanser, 1980.
3. Illich I. Medical nemesis. Toronto/New York/London: Bantam, 1977.
4. Bull M. Secularisation and medicalisation. British Journal of Sociology 1990; 41, 2: 245–262.
5. Brewin T B. 'Orthodox' and 'alternative' medicine. Scottish Medical Journal 1985; 30: 203–205.
6. Frank J D. Persuasion and healing—a comparative study of psychotherapy. Baltimore and London: The Johns Hopkins University Press, 1961.
7. Allander E. Holistic medicine as a method of causal explanation, treatment, and prevention in clinical work: obstacles or opportunity for development. In: Nordenfeld L, Lindahl B I B, eds. Health, disease and causal explanation in medicine. Dordrecht: Reidel, 1984: 215–224.
8. Stanway A. Alternative medicine. Harmondsworth: Penguin, 1982.
9. McKeown T. The role of medicine. Oxford: Blackwell, 1979.
10. Dossey L. Space, time and medicine. Bouldex: Shambhala, 1982.
11. Gorovitz S, MacIntyre A. Towards a theory of medical fallibility. The Journal of Medicine and Philosophy. 1976; 1, 1: 51–71.
12. Whitbeck C. What is diagnosis? Some critical reflections. Metamedicine 1981; 2, 3: 319–330.
13. McQueen D V. Nordamerika als beispiel heilkundlicher pluralitaet. In: Schipperges H, Seidel E, Unschuld P U, eds. Krankheit, heilkunst, heilung. Freiburg/Muenchen: Alber, 1978; 343–395.
14. Skrabanek P. Paranormal health claims. Experientia 1988; 44: 303–309.
15. Simmons B. Problems in deceptive medical procedures: an ethical and legal analysis of the administration of placebos. Journal of Medical Ethics 1978; 4: 172–181.
16. Kopelman L, Moskop J. The holistic health movement: a survey and critique. Journal of Medicine and Philosophy 1981; 6: 209–235.

ALTERNATIVE MEDICINE: METHINKS THE DOCTOR PROTESTS TOO MUCH AND INCIDENTALLY BEFUDDLES THE DEBATE

Patrick Pietroni

Dr. Kottow in his paper Classical medicine v alternative medical practices (Kottow 1992) places the alternative/orthodox medical debate within an historical context of anti-quackery literature. My paper explores the nature of science as it is applied to clinical practice and the narrow view of the diagnostic process as outlined by Dr. Kottow. Research methodologies more appropriate to 'whole person' medicine are suggested as having more ethical value than those based on the clinical trial.

INTRODUCTION

Alternative medicine has had a good press in the last 10 years, so it is not surprising to begin reading critiques on this topic from the medical community. Dr. Kottow, like several of the previous contestants in the centuries-old battle, chooses to define the terms 'scientific medicine' and 'alternative medicine' himself, and thus falls into the elementary trap of many who venture into this field. He equates alternative medicine with holism, confuses concerns for patients' emotional well-being and therapies that have 'clear metaphysical undertones' and implies that 'truth' is something that can be objectively measured by the application of the rational technical science which he claims is the basis of modern medicine. He thus has written an out-of-date critique using out-of-date notions of science, which is a pity because he makes some valid and perceptive points.

It is almost impossible to have a reasoned debate on the subject of alternative medicine unless a serious attempt to define terms is made at the outset. The term 'alternative medicine' is used as a 'catch all' definition for 'anything that is not taught in Western-based undergraduate medical school'. It is as useless a term as the word 'foreign'. An Englishman setting out to comment on 'foreignness' would be as accurate in his descriptions of foreigners as Dr. Kottow is of alternative medicine. His commentary, like Dr. Kottow's, would end up telling us about the prejudices of being English rather than forming the basis for an informed discussion. Dr. Kottow rightly asserts that 'traditional or classical medicine has always co-existed with alternative therapies'. However, he does not advance the debate much further than an early seventeenth-century anti-quack author who wrote:

> But our Empirics and Imposters, as they are too ignorant either to teach or to practise Physic. . . and too insolent, and too arrogant to learn of the Masters of that Faculty, or to be reduced into order: so are they most dangerous and pernicious unto the Weale public. . . . These Crocodiles, disguised with the vizard of feigned knowledge and masking under the specious titles of Physicians and Doctors, not attained in Schools, but imposed by the common people, do with their Absolonicall Salutations steal away the affections of the inconstant multitude from the Learned Professors of that Faculty, with their Loablike Imbracings, stab to the heart their poor and silly patients, ere they be aware or once suspect such uncouth Treachery (Beier 1987).

To take the arguments Dr. Kottow makes in turn:

SCIENTIFIC ASPECTS

I am not sure how many doctors would agree with Dr. Kottow's one-sided definition of medicine—that it is a rational science based on the laws of causality and the strategies of observation and experimentation. The practice of medicine is indeed all of those but fortunately it is also much more. The need to be seen as 'scientific' is so great amongst doctors that it is difficult to prise them away, as is evidenced by Dr. Kottow's article, from an outmoded view of science. Confusion abounds between science as a method of inquiry and science as a body of knowledge. This narrow and inaccurate conception of science within medicine has led to a promulgation of measurement and measuring instrumentation, the

Reprinted with permission from the Journal of Medical Ethics: 18 pp. 23–25 1992 published by BMJ Publishing Group.

consequences of which are as yet not fully recognised. Dr. Kottow identifies alternative medicine as persuing a paranormal, telepathic and telekinetic understanding of the human universe, which may indeed be true of some alternative therapies but by no means all. He seems to be unaware that different theories of causality exist in the philosophy of scientific thought and are much debated by 'pure' scientists all over the world. Modern science is no longer wedded to the inductive model any more than it accepts the Newtonian theory of causality as the only explanation for events 'out there'. Joseph Needham's description of the nature of 'co-relative and co-ordinative relationships' has found much acceptance amongst modern systems analysts:

Things behave in particular ways, not necessarily bcause of prior actions or impulsions of other things but because their position in the ever-moving cyclical universe was such that they were endowed with intrinsic natures which made their behaviour inevitable for them.

The idea of correspondence has greater significance and replaces the idea of causality because things are *connected* not caused (Needham 1956).

Dr. Kottow allows his prejudices to emerge when he comments on the terms 'health', 'well-being' and 'life-style'. He says terms used in this way become ubiquitous, useful for ill-defined propositions and elusive to *serious* [my italics] analysis and criticism. By serious I assume that he means that such terms cannot be accurately measured. Schön, who has written most accurately on the problem of rigour or relevance in professional practice, writes of Kottow's position:

Many practitioners, locked into a view of themselves as technical experts, find little in the world of practice to occasion reflection—for them uncertainty is a threat, its admission a sign of weakness. They have become proficient at techniques of selective inattention and the use of junk categories to dismiss anomalous data, procrustean treatment of troublesome situations all aimed at preserving the constancy of their knowing in action (Schön 1984).

CLINICAL ASPECTS

If some doctors would find Dr. Kottow's first section debatable, I believe that most experi-

enced practitioners would view his second as somewhat tendentious, especially those doctors in primary health care.

A diagnostic model that bases itself on inductive reasoning—doctors beginning 'from scratch' to obtain all the data before deciding on the diagnosis, or, as Bacon said: 'We must put the patient on the rack to make him reveal his secrets'—is indeed the preferred method taught at medical school. However, numerous studies indicate that experienced clinicians fortunately no longer operate that way and have adopted a 'hypothetico-deductive' mode of diagnostic formulation. Thus Crombie found that in over 300 consecutive consultations, a specific medical diagnosis was arrived at in only 150 and that treatment was commenced even though the problem presented would not fit any of the classical medical diagnoses (Crombie 1963). Elstein, in his own survey of the diagnostic process, found that 'expert clinicians' formulated a tentative hypothesis within the first few seconds of a consultation, used a form of 'pattern recognition' in obtaining information and relied on a series of highly discriminative questions to test their original hypothesis (Elstein et al 1978). The problem with the diagnostic model described by Kottow is that it leads to a diagnostic bias towards illness, never better illustrated than by the study undertaken in New York. This study revealed that of 1000 11-year-old children in New York, 61% had had their tonsils removed. The remaining 39% were examined by a new panel of doctors and 45% of these were recommended to have a tonsillectomy. The rejected group were re-examined by another panel of doctors and and a further 46% were recommended to have surgery (American Child Health Association 1934)!

ETHICAL ISSUES

Dr. Kottow acknowledges that both traditional and alternative medicine put a heavy reliance on the 'placebo effect' and describes the ethical problems regarding its use. I disagree with his view that the placebo effect 'may possibly be the most marginal activity of medicine', but accept that both traditional and alternative practitioners practise in good as well as bad faith. His ethical arguments focus on the three issues of allocation of resources, comparability of competing therapies and vulnerability to criticisms. The argument, as I understand it, goes something like this:

Alternative therapies can not be accepted as effective approaches because they have not been subjected to rigorous study, clinical trials etc. If alternative practitioners are willing to undertake such trials and studies then we as doctors would have no difficulty in accepting them as valid, for we are an objective, rational, scientific-based group of professionals. Let them research their approaches like we do, *but* when they do put forward protocols and grant applications, it is unethical to grant them money and support because their methods are unscientific and unproven!

The need to ascertain which of two treatments is superior is clearly an important ethical question. If the method used to obtain such knowledge is itself unethical, then the knowledge acquired will almost certainly be only partially valid and not generalisable to patients as whole people. Put another way:

If morality and methodology conflict it seems to us that the onus is upon us to develop methodologies that harmonise with our morality rather than compromise with morality on the probably false assumption that we are dealing with an immaculate methodology (Metroff & Kilman 1978).

For scientific medicine, the accepted method since Bradford-Hill has been the randomised controlled clinical trial. Yet the ethics surrounding this approved method are themselves dubious and have been much debated.

It could be argued that grant-giving bodies that fund research using dubious methodologies are themselves colluding in unethical behaviour. It has been suggested that the pursuit of an analytic and scientific mode of thinking in problem-solving makes it much more difficult to tolerate the confusion and messiness of complex moral, legal and ethical problems. Indeed it may result in the doctor being peculiarly unqualified in arriving at such decisions:

Once the complexity of these judgements is appreciated and once their evaluative character is understood, it is impossible to hold that the doctor is in a better position to make them than the patient or his family. The failure to ask what sort of harm/benefit judge-

ments may properly be made by the doctor in his capacity as a doctor is a fundamental feature of medical paternalism (Gillon 1986).

Therapists whio claim to treat the 'whole person' will require methodologies which allow for comparability of results which at the same time respect the uniqueness of every human being. The nature of scientific inquiry and its limitations has been a point of debate and exploration among 'pure' scientists and 'social' scientists for several decades. The medical profession, which is so well-placed between both extremes has, for the most part, not entered the debate, and has attempted to resolve the conflict by identifying with the 'pure' form of analytic science, which strives to reject the indeterminate, relies on Aristotelian logic and considers the nature of scientific knowledge to be impersonal, value free, precise and reliable. The analytic scientist's approach to 'knowledge' can be contrasted to that led by the Particular Humanist:

The Particular Humanist naturally treats every human being as though he or she were unique, not to be compared with anyone or anything else. Thus the Particular Humanist is not interested in formulating general theories of human behaviour at all—not so much because this is impossible (although the Particular Humanist agrees that it is impossible) but because it is not desirable. To study people in general, even from a humanistic perspective, is for the Particular Humanist inevitably to lose sight of the unique humanity of an individual—to fail to capture precisely this person. The Particular Humanist takes to heart Kant's dictum to treat everyone as a unique means rather than as an abstract theoretical end (Metroff & Kilman 1978).

The Particular Humanist's view of scientific knowledge is that it is personal, value constituted, partisan, non-rational and political.

The debate regarding the ethical nature of research and the inquiry method is far more complex and far less clear than suggested by Dr. Kottow. Unfortunately, as long as critiques of alternative medicine remain at the level of Dr. Kottow's article, then the long-overdue discussion will be delayed and patients will continue to seek alternative treatments of doubtful value. These therapies should be properly studied by doctors and scientists willing to enter into an honest debate in which the high ground of 'rigour' is eschewed for the messy swamp of relevance.

REFERENCES

American Child Health Association 1934 Physical defects— the pathway to correction. ch. 8 pp. 80–96. New York
Beier L 1987 Sufferers and healers—the experience of illness in seventeenth-century England. Routledge and Kegan Paul, London
Crombie D L 1963 Diagnostic process. Journal of the Royal College of General Practitioners 6 pp. 579–589
Elstein A et al 1978 An analysis of clinical reasoning. Harvard Press, Harvard
Gillon R 1986 Philosophical medical ethics. Wiley, Chichester
Kottow M H 1992 Classical medicine v alternative medical practices. Journal of Medical Ethics 18 pp. 18–22
Metroff I, Kilman R 1978 Methodological approaches to social science. Jossey Bass, Chicago
Needham J 1956 The history of scientific thought. Cambridge University Press, Cambridge
Schön D 1984 The crisis of professional knowledge and the pursuit of an epistemology of practice. Massachusetts Institute of Technology, Massachusetts

THE TROUBLE WITH RESEARCH ABOUT ACUPUNCTURE

J Fleming
Arnold Desser
David Aldridge
Patrick Pietroni

This article describes problems which arose in setting up a trial of acupuncture for asthma; they proved insurmountable but also threw light on the work of hospital ethics committees.

The Marylebone Health Centre is a general practice which is examining the use of complementary medicine as an adjunct to routine therapies. As part of that project it was planned to carry out a controlled trial of the effects of acupuncture when used as an adjunct to the routine therapy of patients with chronic asthma. Several problems were encountered in the planning and implementing of this study. This paper describes and discusses problems encountered with ethics and grants committees who became involved with the trial.

BACKGROUND

The number of asthmatics in the UK is estimated to be about 2 million persons. Such a number is too great for hospital services alone and the general practitioner is in an excellent position to provide adequate continuing care.

Many persons seen in hospital outpatient departments could be managed just as easily in the context of a general practice [1]. The proposed trial would investigate the management of chronic asthma in such a context using acupuncture (within the context of traditional Chinese medical diagnosis) as an additional form of treatment, along with conventional drug treatment.

From a literature search eight studies were identified which reported a controlled trial of acupuncture for asthma [2]. They showed that acupuncture may provide minor improvement in expiratory flow rates, airways conductance and thoracic gas volumes, but greater improvement in the perception of symptom relief. However, these studies, by virtue of being controlled, were reduced to testing the insertion of needles at particular points instead of varying the treatment according to presenting symptoms.

Jobst et al in a pilot study of traditional Chinese medicine for disabling breathlessness in asthma showed encouraging improvements in subjective assessment scores of disability and breathlessness [3]. They point out that acupuncturists cannot give treatment blind and that finding truly 'dead' areas where placebo or 'sham' needling might be totally ineffective is not possible. They also suggest that the use of a placebo control in the context of traditional Chinese medicine may present ethical problems for the practitioner.

DESIGN

A number of possible designs were discussed, including crossover trials and double blind placebo. With the help of a Scientific Advisory Group a study containing three treatment groups was proposed.

Suitable patients, referred from one of two hospital chest clinics, would be randomly allocated to a group receiving acupuncture plus their normal drugs, a group receiving counselling plus their normal drugs or a group receiving normal drugs alone. All patients would keep a diary of their symptoms, drug intake and peak expiratory flow rates during a treatment period.

It was decided that the acupuncturist should be free to give an adequate number of treatments without artificial restrictions as to which needle sites to use. Measurable improvement, it was felt, could be produced in patients receiving treatment once a week for 8 weeks. Patients can be treated indefinitely with acupuncture and treatment for chronic conditions often continues for many weeks. It was planned to follow up patients at 8 weeks, 6 months and 1 year. This was to see if the benefits lasted over a short- or long-term period.

The difficulties of assessing acupuncture and finding a suitable control for the treatment have previously been acknowledged [4]. We decided that it would be unethical to use 'sham' acupuncture or the random insertion of needles into non-acupuncture points. We felt that it was unfair to needle patients without expecting some therapeutic benefit. A control group using no other therapeutic intervention than that already received from the patient's doctor was not considered to be sufficient to control for time and attention received by the acupuncture group.

It was decided to use two control groups, one receiving individual counselling from a nurse practitioner, receiving the same time and attention as the acupuncture group, but without needles, and a group receiving no other therapeutic intervention. All patients were to be cared for by their general practitioner and/or hospital doctor and their routine drug therapy would continue. Any changes to that therapy were to be recorded (see Fig. 5.1).

The sample size, for the study to have statistical power, was calculated to be 150 patients. Two outpatient chest clinics at London teaching hospitals agreed to take part. This required protocols of the study to be sent to two hospital ethics committees. A grant application was submitted to gain additional funding to employ the nurse counsellor.

ETHICAL PROBLEMS

The different ways in which these ethics committees worked soon became apparent. The first ethics committee sent three separate letters over a 3-month period querying various aspects of the trial. All enquiries were answered and after a minor change to our consent form approval was finally obtained for the trial to begin.

The second ethics committee had our application for over 7 months during which time we received no communication as to its progress. A letter was finally received which stated that the ethics committee was unhappy with the *scientific* content of the study, so had referred it to their own Scientific Advisory Committee. They turned down our application on grounds that the project was 'unscientific, therefore unethical'. (The protocol had already been considered

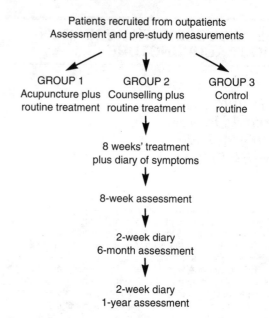

Figure 5.1 Plan of the study.

and approved by our own independent Scientific Advisory Committee—senior academics in General Practice, Community Health and Research Methodology.)

The grants committee sent a list of comments from its meeting. Some of the remarks were very positive and, although our application was turned down, it was suggested we should re-apply. All comments and queries were answered in our second application, although we did not change the protocol significantly. But this application was also turned down.

No explanation was given, only the statement that we were unsuccessful on this occasion. The whole process took 6 months.

A number of different trial designs were suggested by the various ethical and scientific committees involved and their comments are summarised in Table 5.1.

The difference of opinion about whether the trial was ethical left us confused. Of the two hospitals from which we were to recruit patients, the committee of one had accepted our application; the other had turned it down. We wondered whether this variation would occur with other ethics committees.

In order to obtain more feedback about the

Table 5.1 Summary of responses from participating groups in research trial

	Latin Square design	Control with counselling	2 limb crossover	Sham acupuncture
Scientific Steering Committee	Too complex	Agreed	Carry over effect of acupuncture	Unethical
Grant Committee 1		Did not consider it a placebo double blind trial		
Ethics Committee 1 Teaching Hospital		Queried a number of points Approved as ethical	Suggested crossover design would be better	
Ethics Committee 2 Teaching Hospital		Unscientific therefore unethical		Only satisfactory control
BMA		Project is reasonable and acceptable		Ethically dubious to practise invasive technique which has no therapeutic benefit

trial, a number of copies of the protocol were sent to other committees around the country. A copy was also sent to the British Medical Association's ethics committee. The British Medical Association's reply, among others, is summarised in Table 5.1.

The other committees took between 4 weeks and 6 months to reply. Three committees kindly sent detailed replies. All of the committees which replied approved the study. It was interesting to see that different committees focused their comments on different aspects of the trial, and these comments are illustrated in Table 5.2.

PRACTICAL PROBLEMS

As soon as ethical approval was received from one of the committees, we began to recruit patients from the chest clinic. Patients were keen to try acupuncture, but were unwilling to enter one of the other groups and we experienced some difficulties in recruiting them. Some patients refused to take part in the study when randomised to the counselling and control groups.

With those patients who did receive acupuncture, another problem arose at the end of the 8-week treatment period. Many of them felt

benefit and wanted to continue. For the patients to continue treatment would have been detrimental to the project as their progress without it was to be followed over the next 10 months.

DISCUSSION

Many ethics committees were created in Britain after the publication of a report by the Royal College of Physicians [5]. No specific guidance was given in the report on their structure or functioning. A study in Scotland [6] showed that the way ethics committees were formed and coordinated varied considerably. This would seem to be the case for the committees we approached. Their structures and their processes of operation varied, as did their opinions as to what was 'ethical'.

A possible reason for this variation of opinion may stem from a confusion by the ethics committees between the ethical demands of clinical practice and the ethical demands of experimental science [9]. This dilemma between the ethical demands of the clinician and the ethical demands of the scientific researcher is not easily reconciled in the clinical practice of scientific medicine. Furthermore, within clinical trials

Table 5.2 Summary of responses from non-participating groups in research trials

	Project in general	Acupuncture	Counselling
Grant Committee 2	One external referee was impressed with the study Apparent freedom of therapeutic action allowed to GPs will produce large variation in treatment results	The variation allowed to the acupuncturist may render his treatment results unrepeatable by other acupuncturists	Group will not act only as control, they will receive a therapeutic component from counselling
Ethics Committee 3		Lay member felt acupuncture would be a last resort tactic originating in Eastern mysticism Patient would be thrown open to spiritual forces of doubtful origin	What is the role of the nurse practitioner and what would be her qualifications to carry out counselling?
Ethics Committee 4	No adverse comments Excellent protocol from an ethical viewpoint, satisfactory on all counts		
Ethics Committee 5	Happy with protocol and felt it would achieve its aim Applauded the freedom of clinicians to adjust treatment during study but felt it may make assessment difficult	Felt consent form weighted in favour of acupuncture and suggested minor change	Felt unclear about how the patients would be counselled i.e. in groups, individually and by whom?

there are different procedures for *explanatory* studies, where the emphasis is closer to laboratory conditions, and *pragmatic* trials, where the emphasis is on optimising treatment in clinical practice.

A major difference of opinion concerning the proposed trial was about adequate control for acupuncture. One committee stated that 'sham' acupuncture was the only adequate means of control. The BMA Board of Science Working Party on Alternative Therapy Report [7], however, suggested that ethics committees may refuse permission for an invasive sham treatment such as random needling. Our experience shows that the opposite was true. The study was rejected on the grounds that we were not using sham acupuncture. This study was considered 'unscientific' for that reason.

Our experience was that there was some confusion among the committees about the nature of the treatment we were studying. Acupuncture has

a rationale different to that of orthodox medicine [8]. We have written elsewhere about the need for assessment of trials using complementary medicine by scrutinising panels which have some knowledge of medical alternatives [9].

It is vitally important that trials of acupuncture and other forms of complementary practice are considered by ethics committees [9]. The acceptance of complementary medicine is dependent upon clinical research for validity. If such research is denied on the a priori grounds that complementary medicine, in this case acupuncture, is not scientifically valid because there is no research, then we have a circular argument which excludes the opportunity for complementary medicine ever to be investigated in clinical practice.

The procedure of designing and implementing the trial took over a year. We acknowledge that it is important for ethics committees to exist, and that some of their comments have been helpful in creating a more precise study. However, there are serious inconsistencies between committees in practice. These inconsistencies may be relieved by structural guidelines which indicate some necessity for expertise in clinical research methodologies, procedural guidelines for reporting and ethical guidelines concerning the clinical practice of complementary medicine. It may be necessary for future research endeavours that a series of such guidelines be formulated for ethics committees so that those committees, and those submitting to those committees, have some idea of what is required of them both.

REFERENCES

1. Arnold A G, Lane D J, Zapata E. Acute severe asthma: factors that influence hospital referral by the general practitioner and self-referral by the patient. Br J Dis Chest. 1983. 77: 51–59
2. Aldridge D, Pietroni P C. Clinical assessment of acupuncture in asthma therapy: discussion paper. J of the Royal Society of Med. 1987. 80: 222–224
3. Jobst K, Chen J H, McPherson K et al. Controlled trial of acupuncture for disabling breathlessness. Lancet. 1986. ii: 1416–1419
4. Lewith G. Can we assess the effects of acupuncture? Br Med J. 1984. 288: 1475–1476
5. Denham M J, Foster A, Tyrrell D A J. Work of a district ethical committee, Br Med J. 1979. ii: 1042–1045
6. Thompson I A, French K, Melia K et al. Research ethical committees in Scotland. Br Med J. 1981. 282: 718–720
7. BMA Report of the Board of Science Working Party on Alternative Therapy. 1986. Appendix I, 2. 4: 97
8. Pietroni P C, Aldridge D. Summary of discussion on BMA Report of Board of Science Working Party on Alternative Therapy. Holistic Medicine. 1987. 2: 95–102
9. Aldridge D, Pietroni P C. Research trials in general practice: towards a focus on clinical practice. Family Practice. 1987. 4(4): 311–315

6

From conflict to creativity: interprofessional collaboration, education and training

INTRODUCTION

The discussion about the nature and aims of interprofessional collaboration, education and training is extremely wide and at times diffuse. This is no surprise since interprofessional work is itself hard to pin down and define. It cuts across boundaries and disciplines; the arts, sciences and social sciences; politics, social administration and clinical practice. This is its strength—its raison d'etre—but it can also help to make the debates and issues hard to follow. For this reason it is worth taking the unorthodox step of stating the main conclusion of all the work in this chapter at the outset. It is a conclusion arrived at in different ways and sometimes stated in different terms, but the point is invariably the same; health and social care professionals need an education which enables them to be 'reflective'. This term, associated with the work of Professor Donald Schön of the Massachusetts Institute of Technology and Janet Mattinson of the Tavistock Clinic (1992), implies an approach to care by individual professionals which 'recognises that others have important and relevant knowledge to contribute and that allowing this to emerge is a a source of learning for everyone' (Schön 1983). Crucially the professional will also 'look for a sense of freedom and real connection with, rather than distance from, the client' (Schön 1983). This concept has come to infuse much of the work of the Marylebone Centre Trust and the Marylebone Health Centre, and is the touchstone for this chapter.

The growing recognition of the importance of interprofessional education for professionals and carers in the broad fields of health and social services, which emerges in this chapter, has developed within a context. In part the preceding chapters of this book have aimed to present that context and also its development. For the Marylebone Centre Trust the development was a natural one since an holistic approach to health and social care naturally encourages a multidisciplinary and interprofessional stance. The experience of the Marylebone Health Centre, with its extended range of clinical interventions and community outreach programme, was interprofessional from its inception and hence the focus on interprofessional issues and interprofessional education followed naturally thereto.

There is, however, a much broader context of social change which has led to the growing recognition of the importance of interprofessional collaboration. The impetus for this change came, in part, from public and professional responses to now notorious failures of interprofessional collaboration particularly in the field of child protection, for example in Cleveland (The Cleveland Report, DHSS 1988). In part the impetus was political. As Spratley & Pietroni point out (Creative Collaboration: interprofessional learning priorities in primary health and community care, p. 254) good interprofessional and interagency care can no longer be regarded as a theoretical possibility that can be left to local inclination; it is now a matter of law. The changes in notions of health and social care legislated for in The Children Act (1989) and the NHS and Community Care Act (1990), were a clear break with traditional practice. The purchaser–provider split, creating the 'internal market of care', the growing emphasis on the importance of audit and the altered relations between the health and social care professions have meant that interprofessional and interagency collaboration are a necessity if care is to be provided with any degree of competence.

Yet successful interprofessional collaboration cannot become a reality without successful interprofessional education. As Kilcoyne & Pietroni point out, (The history of the primary health care team, p. 194) current difficulties in interprofessional work have their roots in the piecemeal development of the health and social services and their educational structures. The authors make the point that these structures mirror social structures and their conventions, for example in relation to gender, class and race. Traditionally doctors, and thus in a primary care setting GPs, would have a de facto position of leadership in most, if not all, interprofessional collaborations. Now, in a climate which holds up interprofessional work as the most desirable structure for the delivery of health and social care, but which is also questioning the definitions of traditional roles, such a legacy can be difficult to deal with. New management structures and obligations have meant that power relationships have shifted and the result has often been confusion and dislocation. Kilcoyne & Pietroni suggest that such a state of affairs needs remedying and that interprofessional education of a particular kind is the way forward. They criticise successive government reports, and especially the Griffiths report, for failing to put sufficient emphasis on interprofessional education as a priority within health and social services which increasingly call for interprofessional collaboration.

Hey et al (Interprofessional and interagency work: theory, practice and training for the nineties, p. 199) look more specifically at the history of interprofessional collaboration and its educational and practical implications for social work. They point out that interprofessional collaboration is nothing new as far as social work is concerned. Social work is, of its very nature, on the boundaries of a number of disciplines and the success or failure of social workers has much to do with their ability to manage complex collaborative arrangements. They go on to delineate four key dimensions which may be operating in the course of interprofessional and interagency work, showing how they may serve to cause difficulties, misunderstandings and conflicts in both theory and practice.

When considering interprofessional collaboration in practice, it is suggested that the concept of multidisciplinary 'teams' may be of limited use. Care, the authors maintain, is often provided by a multidisciplinary 'network' not a multidisciplinary 'team'. The distinction is an important one since the former is made up of a group of people who work regularly together on a set of tasks. The latter, by contrast, may come together for one or more tasks or work on one case only and can have a broad and changing membership. 'Networks are infinite in their possible connections. Different staff join in or drop out of the networks surrounding any particular case as and when their services become necessary or can be dispensed with' (Hey et al, p. 204). A team, therefore, has different implications for interprofessional education from a network. In the light of this analysis, Hey et al go on to look at the implications for training and education in social work suggesting that Kane's tripartite scheme of necessary attributes—knowledge, skills and actions—is applicable in this case (Kane 1976). The authors conclude that the goal of better patient care will only be achieved if imaginative and relevant programmes of interprofessional education are initiated.

The precise role that the separate education and training of health and social care workers plays in the development of successful or unsuccessful interprofessional collaboration is far from clear, however. Dr Pietroni (Stereotypes or archetypes? A study of perceptions amongst healthcare students, p. 218) investigates this relationship and demonstrates empirically not only that students from the varying disciplines of health and social care (medicine, nursing and social work) develop strong perceptions of one another at an early stage in their training, but also that these perceptions are largely negative. Dr Pietroni suggests that this is possible because the students in the different disciplines have no educational contact with each other before meeting as professionals. Once trained these perceptions may be readily reinforced through professional contacts and hence the negative imagery is never challenged. Dr Pietroni goes on to develop a Jungian interpretation of these perceptions, · which he suggests are archetypal, and explores their implications for interprofessional collaboration. He postulates the need for intermediaries to act

as message-bearers for the various health and social care professionals (like Mercury, the archetypal 'trickster') and, more fundamentally, the development of a new notion of the professional, archetypally associated with the shaman. This he equates with Schön's 'reflective practitioner' and argues that without such an archetypal shift interprofessional collaboration, and indeed education, will always be hampered by discord.

In an earlier paper (Training or treatment?–A new approach, p. 226) Dr Pietroni looks at the implications for training and education of GPs arising out of the growing need for them to be able to make psychological diagnoses of their patients. He describes an essentially reflective programme undertaken by the Department of Family Medicine at the University of Cincinatti, Ohio which attempted to develop a model for this kind of education. This work is closely linked to that of Michael Balint, the difference being that Dr Pietroni accepts that most GPs will not have or wish to seek out personal counselling or psychotherapy which would provide them with space for reflection on how their work is affecting them personally and which of their personal needs or problems they are taking into their work. Pietroni therefore develops an alternative model that enables self-reflection to take place as a normal part of the educational process.

The programme took the form of a group of 10 GPs who met weekly for 2 hours to discuss problems that arose from their work. They were encouraged to explore and share their experiences of the relationship between professional difficulties and anxieties and their private lives. In this way the traditional boundaries between public and private lives were broken down and the inherent links between the two in practice could surface. Although the primary aim of this programme was to enable GPs to make better psychological diagnoses by being aware of the important part that their own personalities played in their relations with their patients, as Pietroni makes clear, the line between training and treatment was broken down. Indeed it was demonstrated that this is in fact a false distinction and that the dictum 'physician heal thyself' has a real and practical applicability. Reflection is not an abstract concept with abstract benefits; it is a necessary skill which can be taught and learnt and which can be used in a concrete way in practice.

Such an undertaking is not, however, without its difficulties. The reality of some of the areas of difficulty in interprofessional collaboration and reflection in a clinical setting are explored in Reason et al (Towards a clinical framework for collaboration between general practitioners and complementary practitioners: discussion paper, p. 230) and Reason (Power and conflict in multidisciplinary collaboration, p. 237). These papers uncover some of the practical difficulties that the Marylebone Health Centre experienced in its endeavour to provide an holistic approach to health care. The different practitioners held varying assumptions about everything from the nature of clinical knowledge to the models of health care being followed to the types of language used to the meanings of that language, and these issues all presented themselves as areas of potential conflict. The experience of the Health Centre suggested that an effective multidisciplinary practice must attempt to develop a model of diagnosis and treatment which recognises the importance of all disciplines while giving supremacy to none. In order to achieve this it will be necessary for clinicians to have knowledge about disciplines in which they are not specialists. It will also, and equally importantly, be necessary for practitioners to negotiate openly around and reflect upon the issues of power and conflict which arise from mulitidisciplinary collaborative efforts. Communication has to be worked at; it will not appear without effort.

The theme of the crucial importance of communication in interprofessional work is taken up by Meek & Pietroni (Communication in cancer care—a reflective learning model using group relations methods, p. 247) The series of seminars which form the basis of this paper were established in an attempt to explore the communication that takes place, or more particularly the communication that needs to take place, in the care of people who have cancer. Participants in

the seminars included patients and relatives as well as doctors, nurses, social workers and complementary health practitioners. The seminars identified issues and difficulties for both the carers and those being cared for and the authors analyse these in terms of the anxiety they induced. They point out that certain areas of potential conflict seemed to become less emotionally charged as communication and understanding between the members of the groups developed. Other issues—both conscious and unconscious—could not be so easily negotiated and areas of real and sometimes strongly held differences emerged. These differences arose from different perceptions of the most appropriate way to deal with a number of dilemmas common in the care of people with cancer. The paper demonstrates clearly that interprofessional collaboration, and indeed interprofessional education, cannot be solely concerned with systems which aim to limit and manage conflict by developing compromise. On the contrary, those who work interprofessionally must recognise that there may be areas of significant disagreement which are not amenable to compromise. These need to be confronted, respected and managed in their own right, not written off as professional intransigence.

It was in the light of all this work, and in an attempt to develop some guidelines for interprofessional education, that Spratley & Pietroni undertook their research (Creative collaboration: interprofessional learning priorities in primary health and community care, p. 257). The two workshops described in this report were asked to highlight and discuss issues for interprofessional learning. The learning priorities which were identified arose from a series of interprofessional projects presented by the participants. The participants included representatives from Social Services and the Health Service, carer organisations, the voluntary sector and educational institutions. A clear theme that emerged from the presentations, as well as from the experience of individual members of the workshops, was that commitment from all parties was necessary if collaboration was to be effective. Facilitation of this, it was argued, would be aided by the development of working environments in which the differences between professionals could be openly addressed. Such an environment would not allow for successful interprofessional collaboration, however, unless supported by interprofessional learning opportunities. These must enable misunderstandings between professionals, and their often prejudiced perceptions of one another, to be identified and challenged. This kind of learning would help to develop interprofessional understanding of cultures, languages and behaviour, which is at the root of creative collaboration. The importance of developing leadership skills suited to complex multiagency networks and teams is identified by the authors as one key priority for interprofessional education and training.

The research methods adopted by Spratley & Pietroni drew on a cycle of action, reflection and feedback; this project is an example of reflective practice in action. It is fitting that this chapter ends, as it began, with a recognition of the importance in theory and in practice of the concept of reflection. It is a concept that encourages individuals to think of themselves as a whole and also as a part of living and changing systems rather than as discrete units. It is a concept that is at its very roots holistic. It is a concept that, in its simplicity and its complexity, sums up both the inspiration for the work here collected and its significance.

REFERENCES

Department of Health and Social Security 1988 Report of the Inquiry into child abuse in Cleveland. HMSO Cmd 412
Kane R 1976 Paper to CSWE conference. Philadelphia
Mattinson J 1992 The reflective process in casework supervision. Headley Brothers, London
Schön D 1983 The reflective practitioner. Temple Smith, London
The Children Act 1989 HMSO, London
The NHS and Community Care Act 1990 HMSO, London

THE HISTORY OF THE PRIMARY HEALTH CARE TEAM

Anne Kilcoyne
Patrick Pietroni

INTRODUCTION

Part of the history with which every primary health care team struggles is embedded in the fact that the family practitioner service began with the single-handed general practitioner. The landscape of primary health care legislation is littered with piecemeal reaction to problems rather than truly pro-active planning. In the 1950s and 1960s Department of Health recognition of the need for a more strongly based community health service gave rise to economic incentives which encouraged general practitioners to form groups and to involve the nursing and social work professions in primary health care practice. This was to give rise to a particular pattern of leadership where the prima inter pares position of the doctor, determined partly by his prior occupancy of the building, but also by virtue of his longer training and history of professional supremacy, gave rise to an assumed leadership of the team.

The potential role, range of skills, background training and conceptual framework of each of the professions was foreign to and frequently misunderstood by the others, the complete absence of any pre-qualifying training in available models and working practices of interprofessional teamwork having much to answer for in this respect. The a priori assumption of leadership within the team by doctors, untrained and unprepared for collaborative teamwork, caused further heartfelt difficulties. Interprofessional disparities in perceived social status, income and legislated responsibility further

undermined the potential for fruitful and easy professional communication.

Salmon (1966) and Seebohm (1968) were to attempt to address these problems by identifying responsibilities through the organisational separating out and restructuring of nursing and social work respectively. This separation has continued and is further underlined by Griffiths (1988) despite the fact that the Royal Commission on the National Health Service (1979) advised one coherent management structure which would knit together the primary health care professions rather than dividing them.

The re-organisation that this organisational division has involved has led to a further deterioration in interprofessional respect and esteem (Richard 1980): for in fact the reorganisation effectively split the health care of the whole person between three camps.

The problem of interprofessional collaboration over a single patient is now compounded by the complexity of the different hierarchical structures within each of the team's professions. There are different contractual obligations, responsibility and accountability to different management systems. Thus the general practitioner is both manager and employer, yet many of his interdisciplinary staff are not employed by him and are accountable to the area health nursing officer or the social services department.

These administrative and organisational separations lead to very particular difficulties for those members of the primary health care team who work between two separate organisations which embody two separate occupational cultures. Quite simple but intractable problems arise, such as physical accessibility. The attached nurse or social worker may not often be in the same building at the same time as the general practitioner, and it may be very difficult to arrange team meetings when this is the case. The records of one profession may be kept in a different location from the records of another; thus vital information which needs to pass from one profession to another may simply not be available at the crucial moment.

Reprinted from the Royal College of General Practitioners Members' Reference Book: 1990, pp. 307–311 with the permission of Sabecrown Publishing.

Huntington (1987) points out other problems. A nurse, for example, working within a general practice is accountable to her immediate area health manager, the nursing officer, who is in turn accountable within her organisation for the deployment of staff. The general practitioner may experience the nursing officer as intrusive and interfering when she asks for the nurse to account for what she does in the practice. It is easy to see how the nurse may be placed in a difficult and conflict-ridden position. She may identify very closely with her role within the general practice and come bitterly to resent the nursing officer's management of her, although this management is inevitable. On the other hand, she may identify more closely with her 'home' organisation, in which case conflict arises with the practice. Her role within it may have to be constantly negotiated, a situation that may appear unwarranted, restrictive and uncooperative; and particularly irksome to other members of the practice.

These difficulties, which apply as much to the social worker as to the district nurse or health visitor, arise not from personality difficulties (which is how they are experienced) (Jones 1986) but from the separations of structure and administration of the professional organisations concerned. Research shows that individuals working on and between the boundaries of organisations experience conflict, crises of identity and stress (Huntington 1987).

DIFFERENT OCCUPATIONS: DIFFERENT WORLD VIEWS

As Fromm (1972) notes: 'Man . . . has a vital interest in retaining his frame of orientation. His capacity to act depends upon it and in the last analysis, his sense of identity. If others threaten him with ideas that question his own frame of orientation, he will react to those ideas as if to a vital threat.'

The contributing professions to primary health care each have a distinct occupational culture. Not only are their contributing roles different, as are their pecuniary rewards and their social status, but so are their styles of learning different. Bligh

(1979) concludes that, as a result, there is a stark contrast in their constructions of reality.

Each profession acts in a sense like a tribe. Members are nurtured in distinctive ways, they develop their concepts in exclusive gatherings (called professional training, or college membership), they have their own leaders and pecking orders. Like all tribal societies they impose sanctions on non-conforming members. If a member takes on the reality constructs of another tribe then he or she may even be threatened with exclusion.

In her 1987 paper Huntington suggests that the occupational culture is made up of:

- its sense of mission, aim and task
- the focus and orientation of the profession
- its ideological knowledge base and its technology
- its status and prestige
- its orientation to clients and patients
- its orientation to other professions.

If one compares these indicators between nurses and doctors, social workers and nurses, or doctors and social workers there are distinct and potentially irreconcilable differences in their occupational identity constructs.

Pietroni's research (1990) with undergraduate students in all three professions indicates that there are already clear and distinct occupational identities at a relatively early stage of professional development. More seriously, however, there are strongly negative stereotyped perceptions of the other professions at this early stage. The sense of inclusion (we belong) and exclusion (they do not); the gathering sense of 'us' and 'them' is basic to the formation of a clear sense of group identity. What is worrying about this research is the negative future of the perceived differences. This augurs badly for the future when such students (with attitudes further hardened through exposure to their occupational culture and having been in receipt of the negative perceptions of other professions), are required to work together in a collaborative setting where issues of life and death are at stake.

Such stereotypic perceptions can be ameliorated only by exposure to and collaboration with the reality of the perceived 'out group'. Pietroni's research indicates that this should take place early in the training of health care professionals. It should also continue throughout post-qualifying education and be framed in such a way that the unconscious tendency to stereotype can be made conscious, and thus be tested consciously against reality.

Although not all members of a single professional occupational group behave in the same way, it is quite clear that each occupation encourages and trains for different modes of professionalism in approach, knowledge, ways of relating to clients and to one another. Nursing training often encourages what Schön (1983) has called the 'practical professional'. This is characterised by a commonsense-based, practical approach to problems arising on the ground. Competence is seen as arising from experience. If a procedure is seen to work well then it will be utilised again. This pragmatic, trial-and-error based approach is likely to predetermine the attitude to interprofessional communication. If the other members of the team value regular team meetings then these will have the support of the 'practical professional'. If the only time when a nurse and doctor have time to talk is in the car park then that is where it will happen. If other members of the team are resistant to face-to-face interprofessional communication then the practical professional will limit himself to noting the relevant facts about the patient in the case notes.

Schön (1983) also describes the 'expert professional': a person who claims expert knowledge. When faced with uncertainty the 'expert' will deal with it by reference to his or her expertise. Distance is maintained from patients and also from other colleagues who do not have the same professional background. Signs and signals of deference to the expert's authority and status are the bread and butter of the interprofessional communication patterns which the 'expert' seeks and encourages. Doctors are traditionally trained for this approach.

The 'manager' professional, also identified by Schön, is familiar from the field of social work. This is based on a two-tier notion. Here an experienced practitioner will become a manager responsible for personnel, planning strategies and the management of resources. He or she provides a supervisory back-up to less experienced practitioners who are engaged in on-the-ground enactment of their policies. Social workers are trained within this culture. The Griffiths Report (1988) further strengthens this style of social work.

Each individual within any of the professions may draw on each of these professional models at different times. But it is clear that each of the professional trainings of the contributing primary health care professions favours one of these approaches above the others.

Schön proposed a fourth model which he calls the 'reflective practitioner'. The person recognises the skills and relevant knowledge of colleagues and seeks for a connection in communication with them, recognising the value of both thoughts and feelings. Respect for their expertise is not predetermined by established status considerations but is allowed to arise from the way the current situation calls forth their skills.

As Hey et al (1990) point out, the reflective practitioner model has profound implications for the training of the multidisciplinary team. The reflective practitioner monitors his or her own response to the situation as well as that of colleagues in the light of the dialogue that is established with the client. The unfolding context and the meaning ascribed to it by all the people involved in it is under continuous review. Action is continually modified by the process; uncertainty calls for communication rather than recourse to previously rehearsed proscription.

The 'network' is a pool from which professionals are drawn for particular patients or groups of patients. The membership is changeable and the frequency of meetings determined by the exigencies of the case. In primary health care the convening part of the network may be a product of crisis management. The defining characteristics of the 'team' are that it works on a multitude of cases, all its members are involved in working together over time, each member has direct patient contact, the team has regular ongoing meetings for case allocation, discussion, management of resources and training.

GRIFFITHS AND THE IMPLICATIONS FOR TRAINING

In Griffiths' opening letter to the Secretary of State there is a stated awareness of the gaps that exist between the professions and the need for training in this area: 'An overriding impression of training is the insularity of training for each professional group.'

Unfortunately, Griffiths' letter goes on to state: 'It may be over-ambitious to talk about common training in skills for everyone working in the community, but an understanding by each profession about the role of the other professions in the community could easily be achieved.'

When the issue of training resurfaces in the report it comes in the final chapter, which is entitled 'Other issues'.

The thrust of the directives for training is threefold:

1. Training during the period of implementation.
2. A re-orientation of social work training to take account of the more 'managerial' character of the job.
3. Particular training for the 'community carers'.

Although Griffiths (1988) again comments on the insularity of the professions leading to failures of communication, the need to understand the roles of other professions, and the necessity for effective collaboration in training matters (para 8.8) he does call for central government to make a full assessment of the training implications for all groups of professionals involved (para 8.5). However, he remains general in most of his own assessments. Specificity is reserved for the changes in social work training. Recruitment and in-service training systems need to change, as does the qualifying training for social workers. They all need to give greater emphasis to management skills to reflect the change in emphasis and role. Social workers will need to be trained in the new skills needed for the buying in of services, the design of successful management accounting systems, and effective use of the information emanating from these systems. General practitioners will need a more 'systematic approach':

... identifying ... all of his patients whose health status means they can be expected to have community care needs. The responsibility for arranging such systematic considerations will be the general practitioners' using the resources available to the practice in the most effective way. (Griffiths 1988, para 8.2)

The systematic approach is likely in the current climate to be a quantitative approach. The responsibility to make a predetermined number of visits each year to the elderly is one example. The system which is not much spoken of is the indeterminate system of communication between patient and practitioner, between disciplines and agencies. The reason why this is overlooked and not properly 'accounted for' has been identified by Schön (1983). The development of professional practice has been driven by a dominant positivist philosophy which privileges a scientific approach. Professional practice is thus conceived of as primarily technical. Deciding gets separated from doing, means are separated from ends, research from practice. Small problems which can be researched are given precedence over the huge, messy problems of a practice which cannot easily be held still and named. Primary health care and the need for a multidisciplinary approach lie in this 'messy' ground. Intuition counts here as much as technology. Theory here is generated by the situation, not by prescription. Uncertainty and confusion are accepted and contained within the multidisciplinary team. The knowledge which is useful is not technological or quantifiable, it is a 'knowing in action'.

Schön calls for an investigation of the notations and conventions that artists and practitioners from non-scientific backgrounds use to create and communicate in worlds with which they work—unlikely in a world where the accountant is pre-eminent.

REFERENCES

Bligh D 1979 Some principles for interprofessional learning and teaching. In: Education for cooperation in health and social work. Occasional Paper 14. London, Journal of the Royal College of General Practitioners

Fromm E 1972 The anatomy of human destructiveness. London, Jonathan Cape

Griffiths R 1988 Community care: agenda for action. A report to the Secretary of State for Social Services. London, HMSO

Hey A, Minty B, Trowell J 1990 Interprofessional and interagency work: theory, practice and training for the nineties. Chapter 11, CETSW Report

Huntington J 1987 Factors affecting interprofessional collaboration in primary health care settings. Delivered to the Royal Society of Medicine Forum on Medical Communications

Jones R V H 1986 Working together—learning together. Occasional Paper 33. London, Royal College of General Practitioners

Pietroni P C 1990 Unpublished research conducted within a multidisciplinary seminar in the undergraduate training of the Department of General Practice. St Mary's Medical School, London

Richard 1980 The NHS and Social Services, Project Paper RC 11. London, Kings Fund

Royal Commission on the National Health Service 1979 Report. London, HMSO

Salmon Report 1966 Report of the Committee on Senior Nursing Staff Structure. London, HMSO

Schön D A 1983 The crisis of professional knowledge and the pursuit of an epistemology of practice. Delivered at the Harvard Business School, 75th Anniversary Colloquium on Teaching by the Case Method

Seebohm 1968 Report of the Committee on Local Authority and Allied Personal Social Services. London, HMSO

INTERPROFESSIONAL AND INTER-AGENCY WORK: THEORY, PRACTICE AND TRAINING FOR THE NINETIES

Anthea Hey
Brian Minty
Judith Trowell
With contributions by:
Helen Martyn
Brian Minty
Alan Rushton
Alan Shuttleworth

'The thrust now must be to ensure that professionals in individual agencies work together on a multidisciplinary basis. To achieve this end agencies need to establish the individual training needs of their professionals and to ensure that they receive necessary training on a single discipline and multidiscipline basis.' (Department of Health 1988).

In this chapter two different viewpoints are interwoven: one is primarily conceptual, drawing on current research findings (AH); while the other (BM/JT) is deeply rooted in practice experience and practice teaching. Four tutors— Helen Martyn, Alan Rushton, Brian Minty and Alan Shuttleworth—then provide experience from their own courses.

INTRODUCTION

AH: Social work, as we know it in the public sector, developed on the boundaries of other institutional services—hospitals, courts and public assistance offices. Interprofessional and interagency practice is for social workers, then, part of their history. The degree to which social workers have, or can be, moved from the margin of these settings to their core, or be pulled away from them altogether, is limited if these other services are going to meet their objectives. This lesson has been regularly ignored and then relearnt over the past 20 years.

The fashion of the 1960s and early 1970s for joining agencies together in the search for unity

Reprinted from Right or privilege? Post-qualifying training with special reference to child care. Pietroni M (ed). pp. 104–129 May 1991 with the permission of CCETSW.

and comprehensiveness, has given way to the establishment of smaller decentralised units of service delivery. In the 1980s, it was realised once again that people have numerous problems which interact and that few social problems can be laid at the door of only one agency. Language has changed in recognition of this fact. The call now is for multiagency responses, for more multi-disciplinary activity and closer working together.

In relation to children, it is 40 years since a Joint Ministries circular first advised local authorities to establish committees to coordinate responses to children neglected in their own homes. Exhortations about the need to collabo-rate in the field of child protection have contin-ued, not least because the list of failures to achieve successful collaboration between different pro-fessions and agencies stretches from Colwell to Cleveland and Carlisle. Furthermore, future ser-vice delivery is likely to be even more complicated culturally and structurally as more voluntary and private agencies and workers become involved in regular mainstream provision.

More analysis of the nature of interprofessional and interagency work is needed and more preparation for it is required if significantly bet-ter collaboration is to be achieved.

THE NEED FOR INTERAGENCY AND INTERPROFESSIONAL COLLABORATION

BM/JT: If children's development becomes dis-torted or seriously delayed, they and their fami-ly situation may need to be assessed and helped by a variety of professional experts. These may well include as well as social workers, general practitioners, health visitors, clinical or educa-tional psychologists, teachers, audiologists, speech therapists and optometrists. Some of these professions may also be involved in trying to assess whether children have been abused. If this is the case, in trying to protect them from further abuse they may need also to involve lawyers and the police. Social workers' dealings with these other professions may be as impor-tant as their dealings with the child or young person and his or her family, because of the part they play in assessment and helping systems.

In those cases where more than one profession has a significant part to play, it is likely that *interagency* cooperation will be necessary, because services for children are shared by many organisations, most obviously health, education, and social services departments, together with voluntary agencies. The police and lawyers within local authorities and private practice also have important parts to play in child protection work. The sharing of information between the professions and a willingness to work together are especially essential in cases of child abuse, if children are to be protected and the possible ill-effects of intervention are to be minimised. Essential information is often scattered through many agencies, and parents and other carers and even the children and young people themselves may attempt to conceal abuse and neglect. Medical, social and criminological information is often essential in order to establish that a child is not safe in his or her own home.

However, interdisciplinary and interagency collaboration on their own are not sufficient to protect children, if the quality of the work undertaken by each agency and professional is not, in itself, good enough. On the other hand, lack of collaboration may negate excellent practice by individual professionals or agencies. There are, of course, important legal and professional reasons why, at times, certain professions or agencies must take independent action when the contrary views of other professionals are recorded at case conferences. Individual practitioners and agencies are professionally and legally accountable in a way that case conferences are not. Social work departments sometimes take unilateral action in relation to children in their care, since they have parental responsibilities and rights. Other considerations apply to other professions.

Working within a multidisciplinary and multiagency context is further complicated by a number of different approaches and viewpoints. These might include the different backgrounds of the professionals involved, the different types and standards of training received, the different

rewards, in terms of both salary and institutional power. Professionals from different fields are used to working within their own particular culture and organisational structure.

A CONCEPTUAL APPROACH: FOUR DIMENSIONS OF INTER-PROFESSIONAL COLLABORATION

Interdisciplinary and interagency work is an essential process in the professional task of attempting to protect children from abuse . . . The experience gained by professionals in working and training together, has succeeded in bringing about a greater mutual understanding of the role of the various professions and agencies and a greater ability to combine their skills in the interest of abused children and their families . . . (DHSS 1988).

AH: A good deal of research has been undertaken into the different dimensions which may be operating when members of different professional groups come together, as they do increasingly in, for example, those committees established to further joint planning between health and local authorities and more recently established area child protection committees. These dimensions are now examined more closely.

Socialisation

Understanding another professional's stance and working comfortably with it is no simple matter. As Robinson (1978) pointed out: 'If socialisation has been at all effective, the professional will simply experience his own view as subjectively, massively real—so real that he cannot help seeing it as obvious, as of critical importance; indeed, as simply the way things really are.' Further, admitting another view of the world is not an easy matter to arrange, for as Fromm (1972) warns us, people have a vital interest in retaining their frame of orientation: 'Capacity to act depends on it, and in the last analysis one's sense of identity. If others provide ideas that question one's own frame, one will react to those ideas as to a vital threat.' Kahn (1977) suggests three prerequisites for interdisciplinary collaboration: 'insight into one's own occupational system, effort to gain insight into systems with which we would collaborate as well as clear definition of and agreement about the reasons, bases and goals of collaboration'.

The challenge then is both to socialise appropriately to a particular profession because this is functional, and at the same time to develop the intellectual scepticism and rigour which provides a degree of objectivity about one's own base and an openness to others.

Structure and culture

From the moment a new member enters the ranks of any profession he or she begins to absorb that profession's own particular organisational practices and attitudes. Some aspects of this process are obvious even to the outsider; others are more subtle and even the initiated may be unaware of their impact. A number of research studies are relevant in the context of multiagency working. Huntington (1981), for example, provides a useful framework for analysing the structural and cultural dimensions of occupational groups. Although derived from her research work on general medical practice and social work, it can be generalised to analysis of other professions. For instance, Taylor (1986) and Holdaway (1986) take some of these elements in considering relations between social workers and the police, which have been recognised as increasingly important in child protection work.

Elements of structures and cultures which Huntington suggests are pertinent to a consideration of interprofessional collaboration are given in Box 6.1.

As Huntington in a later work (1986) points out, concentration of workers in any setting contributes to the development of a specific occupational consciousness arising out of 'the common experiences and sentiments which derive from a shared work situation' (Mungham 1975).

Clearly these features of any occupational group change over time. Currently planned joint training and joint investigative work in the field of child sexual abuse are achieving closer relationships between social workers and police officers. This is happening at the post-qualifying stage. At the basic

---

> **Box 6.1** Structures and cultures pertinent to interprofessional collaboration (Huntington 1981)
>
> **Structure**
> Age of occupation
> Age of membership
> Size
> Location and distribution
> Marital status
> Class of origin
> Educational attainment
> Work setting
> Income size and type
> Clientele
>
> **Culture**
> Mission, aims and tasks
> Focus and orientation
> Knowledge
> Technology and technique
> Ideology
> Identity
> Status and prestige
> Relational orientation to patients and clients
> Relational orientations to other occupations

professional stage an American professor of social work, Marian Kahn (1977) described attempts to enhance the mutual understanding of social workers and various 'allied health professionals'. Discussions were framed around a set of 10 questions pertinent also to more experienced practitioners:

1. What do you want us to learn about you? (what you do? know? believe?)
2. What do you want to learn about social work? (what we do? know? believe?)
3. Your unique role? Unique contribution to human service field? Ours?
4. Your contribution to the knowledge base of other health professionals? Ours?
5. Common denominators? Core knowledge? Skills? Common issues? Values? Meeting ground? Overlap?
6. Differences? Incompatabilities? Sources of conflict?
7. Are there aspects of your field to which you think social work can make a contribution? Vice versa?
8. Is there anything in your training that prepares you to work effectively in collaboration with members of other professions? Any emphasis on interpersonal communication? Group process?

9. Incongruities between how you define your professional role and how you are perceived by others?
10. Actual or hypothetical case examples or practice situations which we can address together?

Professionalism

Applying the cultural components listed earlier by Huntington shows that different occupational groups espouse quite different modes of approach, knowledge, ways of relating to clients and to each other. This is not to say that all members of one particular group always approach their work in the same way. Research has identified four different professional models which may be summarised briefly as follows:

The *practical professional* has a commonsense approach and a belief that competence is best acquired by long experience of coping with actual situations where working solutions must be found by trial and error.

The *expert professional* is presumed to know and claims to do so regardless of uncertainty, maintains a distance from the client and looks for deference and acknowledgement of his or her expertise and status. This model is familiar and has been much criticised, notably by Illich (1976) summarised by Schön (1983).

The *managerialist* model involves a two-tier motion. In the higher tier are professional leaders who apply their decision-making expertise to planning, resourcing and training for primary operational tasks defined by reference to their views of what constitutes effective intervention. The lower tier of practitioners then perform these tasks (Jones 1985).

Schön and his collaborator Argyris have, however, proposed a fourth and arguably more requisite model: the *reflective practitioner* (Argyris & Schön 1978, Schön 1983). The world view of reflective practitioners offers a stark contrast to the professional expert. The professional who is presumed to know, now:

recognises that others have important and relevant knowledge to contribute and that allowing this to emerge is a source of learning for everyone. Reflective

practitioners look for a sense of freedom and real connection with, rather than distance from clients, they actively seek out connections with clients' thoughts and feelings and allow any respect for their own expertise to emerge from discovering it in the situation (Schön 1983).

These four models are, of course, expressed as ideal types. In practice they may become much more blurred. Each may be appropriate to differing sorts of work, agencies or specific social or professional contexts. Each has some propensity for inappropriate use, or, indeed, abuse.

Important from the education and training perspective is Schön's suggestion that reflective practitioners should monitor all situations and their own conduct in them in the light of dialogue with the client. They are expected to select their responses having reflected about the situation as it unfolds, so no single set of rules for action is prescribed. It follows that education and training should emphasise the principles involved and encourage the use of reflection in order to understand how action is dependent upon, and continually modified by, context and the meaning ascribed by other participants in the situation. Both the process itself and education for it are tough and demanding as Schön in his latest work on the subject (1987) makes plain.

Social work is not the only profession which has striven to address its own foundations and modes of relationship with clientele or users. In medical practice the relevance of the models established in basic medical training which are essentially of the expert kind have been significantly questioned. Metcalf (1979), now a Professor of General Practice, developed an alternative model. Pietroni (1989) has developed multidisciplinary training models designed first to make unconscious stereotypes explicit and then to work on altering them. In a recent development, Joss & Jones (1985), of Brunel University Centre for the Study of Community and Race Relations, adapted Metcalf's training model to the context of police training.

The reflective model makes good sense for social work practice and education. It represents not so much a new model of professional practice as a restatement of some earlier principles which have perhaps been submerged by other competing demands and the uncertainties and exigencies of present day practice.

This model offers the hope of a much fuller and active role for clients. However, pursuing this model either diagnostically or therapeutically requires time and well-developed skills as for example with conciliation work. It, therefore, carries direct and indirect cost consequences for service and for education and training. Yet it may be effective because it seeks, through negotiations, acceptable rather than imposed solutions whenever those are achievable. It may be essential in child and family care and child protection, the primary concern of this report, where there are so many competing interests in both the client and professional systems and their interface. The Children Act 1989 strongly encourages such an approach. However, echoing other parts of this report, too, such an approach requires that managers, supervisors and trainers are themselves educated and trained to use the approach.

Older and longer established professions, such as medicine, have tended to conform to the 'expert' model. Professions surrounding medicine, including social work in clinical settings, have tended to follow suit. In other sectors of social work, even to some extent in clinical settings, a more reflective model (perhaps less defined than the one advanced by Schön) has had greater influence. As a result, social work has had to contend with criticism from traditional professions of a lack of expertise. In response, social work has tended to deny the importance of expertise rather than engaging in a debate on how best it should be used. Social work's divergence from traditional models has been further reinforced by new models of intervention introduced by social services departments since Seebohm reflected in different terminology. 'Patients'/'clients' become 'users'/'consumers'; 'professionals' become 'workers' or 'carers'.

Organisation

When professionals from different groups come together in a working environment, the way in which the multidisciplinary and multiagency workers are organised has a direct bearing on how the work is done. When the need for interprofessional and agency work is recognised, 'teams' are often called for. In health authorities, for example, the interdisciplinary working group has been the preferred organisational model, at least in clinical settings. Social workers have been involved in such groups since the turn of the century (Kane 1975). However, it is questionable whether all such groups should properly be called teams. Nor are the conditions which call for team approaches clearly distinguished from other conditions in which the necessary contact can be achieved by less structured and permanent means from a larger network of staff.

BM/JT: This confusion calls for a distinction to be drawn between multidisciplinary teamwork and multidisciplinary networks. *Multidisciplinary teams* work over time on a range of cases, and are involved not only in working with clients, but in regular on-going meetings for case allocation, discussion and management of resources, and training. A *network of different disciplines*, usually from more than one agency, may be involved in a particular case or in several cases, and there may be joint work and case discussion, one form of which is case conferences. The network has as its *raison d'être* a particular case or groups of clients or patients, but the group of professionals do not continue to work together over a range of activities other than work with that individual client, group or community. Often in child abuse work a group of specialists at managerial level meet regularly in case conferences and at policy-making meetings. They do not usually work face-to-face with clients; nor are they usually in daily contact with each other. They may refer to themselves as, and in some senses are, a team. But they are not a multidisciplinary team in the usual sense, rather a coordinating group representing a range of agencies and professions.

AH: Kane (1975) in her study of interprofessional team work quotes Friedson (1970) as suggesting that the idea of team work is a myth in the health field . . . 'since the medical profession holds a dominant position and because of the doctor's clinical autonomy, both other professions' and clients' interests cannot be safeguarded.' This argument implies that 'genuine teams' are composed of groups of equals. However, equality may not be a defining characteristic. Indeed, this conception of teams as collaborative and flexible forms of role and authority interaction is an essentially twentieth century idea. An older tradition sees teams as competitive concerned with winning and losing, within a framework of rules of interaction, under strong leadership and direction (Emery & Trist 1973).

Before discussing different forms of collaboration and the educational consequences which may flow from them, it is worth rehearsing differing degrees of collaboration which may be needed. In Davidson's typology (1983) there are five degrees:

1. communication/consultation
2. cooperation
3. coordination
4. federation/teamwork
5. merger.

Tibbit's matrix (1983) combines these five degrees along one axis with three levels of work on the other axis (see Table 6.1)

These levels of work can be related to the different work strata identified (Jacques 1976, 1986, Rowbottom & Billis 1978). It seems as though three different organisational forms can be distinguished at the service delivery level (conceivably at the higher levels too). First, there are genuine teams composed of small groups of people from different originating disciplines who are now sharing common tasks and involved, therefore, in continuous face-to-face interactions. However, it has been noted that in some settings, particularly in mental health and child guidance, these teams often turn out to be 'unidisciplinary' in practice, members having all espoused the same approach to practice. Others remain wholly or largely multidisciplinary with members' different knowledge and skills constituting their primary contribution (Rowbottom & Hey 1978).

Secondly, larger working groups may have clients in common, but not shared tasks, with collaboration between workers less tightly ordered. Work may be conducted sequentially or in parallel. In these groups, here called networks, 1–3 of Davidson's typology may be embraced according to need. The more interactions that are required the more sensible it is for members of networks to be located close together. Networks are infinite in their possible connections (see for example the *ecomap* on p. 85 of DHSS 1988). Different staff join in or drop out of the networks surrounding any particular case as and when their services become necessary or can be dispensed with.

A third model—the case-related team—in some ways combines the first two. Pairs or very small groups from a larger group which may include members of teams or networks who at other times pursue a wider range of tasks, work together to pursue joint or co-work with a particular case. This model has been used frequently for investigative and assessment work, for example

Table 6.1 Matrix of degrees of collaboration (Tibbit 1988)

	Communication	Cooperation	Coordination	Federation	Merger
Strategic planning (WS 4/5)					
Operational management (WS 3)					
Service delivery (WS 1/2/3)					

in crisis interventions in mental health and more recently in the investigation of child sexual abuse. The Cleveland Report (DHSS 1988) specifically advised that this model be used in this field because such work tends to be very distressing and is, therefore, potentially unbearable as a permanent field of endeavour. For the purpose of designing education and training the considerations applying to teams will clearly apply to some degree to these more transient groupings.

Establishing ideal model teams tends to be costly in terms of staff resources as by definition two or more staff are being deployed on each task or case. Effective teams also require a specific institutional base, good leadership and lines of accountability, all of which can cause problems (Rowbottom & Hey 1978). Case-related teams which make less taxing demands may, however, be just as effective in a wider range of situations than currently applied. Indeed, in high anxiety work or for the specific purpose of development and learning such models may be highly beneficial. Co-working may be not only more effective but more efficient. By holding and supporting workers to task, cases may be open for shorter periods. It could not only improve the supply of therapeutic skills, but restore confidence in them.

Roles and relationships within teams may, and should, vary in line with employment and work assumptions and be carefully specified. With an agency the leader may have a full managerial role. Between agencies and/or when the current work is truly multidisciplinary, the team leader should be strong on coordination, with managerial relationships continuing to be held within originating disciplines. These more complex forms of organisation and accountability require the exercise of very fine discretion and well-developed negotiating and communicating skills. Social workers operating in these groups need to be especially competent and confident if they are to hold boundaries, negotiate priorities and avoid 'buck passing'.

THE SOCIAL WORKER'S CONTRIBUTION TO INTER-PROFESSIONAL COLLABORATION: A PRACTICE PERSPECTIVE

BM/JT: In many aspects of work with children, the social worker's role overlaps with that of other professions, but certain tasks and responsibilities are specific to social work. These are related to the use of social workers' statutory powers to protect children, or to act in a parental role to children in care. Social workers are expected to have particular skills in assessing family and other social situations and to have special knowledge of a range of national and local services for children and their carers.

In some tasks undertaken by social workers, such as communicating with young children, members of other professions are often more skilled. Also in areas such as child development and the law, essential for social workers who deal with children to know something about, members of other professions are the acknowledged experts. A range of information needs to be collected from various professions if the serious and persistent problematic behaviour or symptoms in a child are to be fully understood. It will often be necessary to provide:

1. A social history (including an appreciation of the cultural and material environment in which a child is growing up).
2. A family history of the current family and of the parents' previous families.
3. A medical assessment of the child and a full medical history.
4. A psychiatric assessment of the child and a history of any previous disturbed behaviour.
5. A psychological assessment, involving the use of appropriate psychometric and other tests and scales such as self-esteem inventories.
6. An assessment of the child's current functioning, including his or her intellectual and cognitive functioning and any learning difficulties, his or her peer group relationships, and behaviour and achievements at school and elsewhere.
7. An assessment of parenting capacities, parental physical and mental health, any

learning disabilities of the parents, and an assessment of other members of the household and of the family interactions.

A complete assessment will not be required in *all* cases, but there are cases where little or no progress will be made without one. An inadequate appreciation of the problems of a child and his or her family will almost inevitably lead to an inadequate intervention. Social workers, who will often be the key worker in child abuse cases, must, as part of what Barclay called their 'social care planning' role, ensure that the necessary information and reports are assembled. They must then be involved in decisions about intervention strategies as well as carrying responsibility for the social work aspects of intervention.

DIFFICULTIES FOR THE SOCIAL WORKER IN INTERAGENCY COOPERATION

Although cooperating with other professions can pose difficulties for any of the recognised social work tasks, the main difficulties seem to arise when information is shared and cases are referred for additional help or resources. Part of the problem is that many pay lip service to the notion of interdisciplinary cooperation without always appreciating the implications. Cooperation is assumed to be easy, when, in fact, as the analysis on page 201 has clarified, it is a complex and often difficult process. Its advantages are in general valued, so long as it is on one's own terms. Some of the problems are now examined in more detail.

Conflicts about values and procedures

Real cooperation between professionals requires common goals, shared values and agreed ways of proceeding. The struggle for a common view and agreed means of proceeding is most keenly felt when negotiating new ventures, because the ground rules for sharing the work have to be worked out from scratch. Value conflicts may

arise which can be difficult to resolve. For example, most area review committees have established agreed rules of procedure for dealing with suspected physical and sexual abuse, but until recently agreement on procedures for physically examining children suspected of being sexually abused was not always achieved. The Butler Sloss report (DHSS 1988) describes how the paediatricians, social services and the police in Cleveland were unable to cooperate for a period, due to disagreement over procedures and the validity of the anal dilation test in diagnosing child sexual abuse.

The goals and values implicit in protecting children, and in working with their families are still not universally agreed. Sexual abuse exposes the considerable disagreements, both within society and among the professions involved, as to how best to deal with the perpetrator, and sometimes where to place the abused child. Some wish to see many more sexual abusers being given treatment, albeit in secure conditions, to try and prevent them re-offending, while for others the only proper response to such a terrible abuse of power is to prosecute and punish. The value conflicts can become polarised between the professions, since society appoints policemen to apprehend and punish those who break the law, and trained doctors and probation officers to treat offenders who have psychological problems. The conflicts are heightened by practical difficulties: for example, lack of treatment facilities and difficulties in obtaining convictions because children often have to say things in court which cut across the most basic attachments and loyalties, although the practice of questioning children by means of video links will remove some of the stress on child witnesses.

Deciding on the best balance between listening to the wishes of the child as to where he or she should live and doing what is considered best in spite of his/her wishes can generate unresolved tension because the perpetrator of intra-familial abuse will often wish to return home. Where wishes and needs conflict, there is a danger that agencies will take the decision which is easiest to defend in public. An obvious implication of these difficulties is that values in relation to child care and child protection work, and their basis in emotions and experience, have to be discussed in any post-qualifying training relating to children. They should also be discussed with regard to the unequal power and status of the professions involved.

Resource and agency control problems

Difficulties can arise when one service requires a particular facility provided by another service as monopoly supplier. For example, a clinical psychologist or child psychiatrist employed by a health authority may be the first professional person to suggest a child has special education needs, when the supplier, an education authority, may be reluctant to accept the suggestion. Even more contentious might be a request by a social worker to an education authority for a boarding school place for a child who is unhappy at home and disruptive at school. In this case, the LEA might regard it as the responsibility of social services to find the child another home. They may be unaware that the social worker already knows that the parents are unwilling to place the child voluntarily into care and believes they lack evidence to apply for care proceedings. Moreover, the social worker may feel admission to care would not be in the best interest of the child or of his or her family. While there may be strengths in the parent/child relationship, in the social worker's view, the child needs to be distanced from mismanagement, constant criticism or gross over-protection.

Current tight financial constraints on all services involved with children are not conducive to generosity between them. Social workers undertaking interprofessional and interagency work, therefore, need to understand the structure of power, decision-making, and responsibilities in the different agencies if they are to intervene effectively.

Social defences

When working closely with other professionals, social workers need to recognise the tendency of organisations and professions to foster distorted views of one another. It is a means of coping with their own members' anxieties, and protecting their sense of worth and status in the face of emotionally threatening situations. The notion of 'social defences' was put forward over 30 years ago by Jacques (1955) and was applied to the management of anxiety in the nursing profession (see Menzies 1960). Social workers will require the ability to see through organisational and professional projections of this kind if they are to cooperate effectively across disciplinary and agency boundaries. Otherwise, those who build bridges between agencies and disciplines may be accused of distancing themselves from their true colleagues and values, and identifying with others, and so lose access to much-needed support from within their own professional group.

Fears of loss of control

Almost all cooperation, whether at policy level or the level of the individual client, must involve each of the cooperators in some loss of control and influence which may have legal and ethical implications. The social worker who refers a case to a psychiatrist may fear that the psychiatrist is planning to ask him or her to drop out of treatment, or to prescribe drugs without psychotherapy. The psychiatrist who shares the case with an independent-minded social worker, may wonder in what direction the case is going, and who (if anybody) is in control. Professions working together on the same case may not always cooperate, since they may on occasion be pulling in opposite directions. While the social worker may have decided that the child needs to be at home, the GP or educational psychologist may be working with the parents to prevent this outcome.

Unresolved leadership issues in multidisciplinary teams and networks

Over the years considerable conceptual effort has gone into trying to resolve the problems of managing multidisciplinary teams working with children and families. Teams may operate best where the need for 'primacy' and 'leadership' is acknowledged, and where it is possible to make a distinction between these two concepts. Primacy occurs when one person is primus inter pares among the senior members in each profession. It is often determined by the setting, i.e. who owns the building and provides the administration. In health settings this person is usually the senior doctor and in educational settings the senior educational psychologist, whereas in residential units, family centres, or specialist child protection units, it will usually be a senior social worker. He or she is responsible for accepting or rejecting referrals, and so forming the boundary of the team. This person is also usually held responsible for the overall quality of the work of the team, which implies an ultimate right to control the allocation of cases to workers with what he or she considers are the appropriate skills, and the right to intervene if things go drastically wrong.

Some heads of teams see themselves as consultants or advisors. In some teams leadership may be more shared and cooperative, taken by various members, depending on the extent to which they command the respect and acceptance of their colleagues. When members of different professions work together on a case, the leadership issue is more complex. Even though a social worker from an area team may be nominated as key worker for a given case, his or her accountability for coordinating the work and his or her network leader status for the particular case may not be fully accepted by more senior members of the network from other agencies or professions. Even in multidisciplinary teams in clinical settings, the leadership issue is complex since some members such as teachers or social workers may be accountable to both the clinic team leader and a team leader in the professional hierarchy of the education department or social services department which employs them. The resulting confusion as to who leads the team or network can reflect on the quality of the work.

Differences between the professions

The different models of professionalism and Huntington's framework (1981) for analysing differences have already been referred to under 'Structure and culture', page 206. Some of the specific differences she observed between social work and general practice which made it difficult for social workers to feel at home as members of primary health care teams, included differences in theoretical outlook (psychological versus social or emotional explanations of problems); status (high versus low); their view of respective responsibilities towards the client or patient; their means of remuneration (independent practitioner versus salaried employee) and the level of remuneration (high versus low). Many of these points would apply to the relationships between social work and a large part of medicine. Closely observing a traditional ward round in an adult psychiatry setting, Fisher et al (1984) found that the psychiatrist dominated the discussion, even though much of the content related to psycho-social issues rather than to narrow medical or psychiatric matters.

With goodwill and patience the differences can be overcome, but there has to be genuine respect for each other's contribution, and openness to each other's theoretical position. Many social workers say they relate poorly to doctors because the latter rely supposedly on the medical background. In fact, a number of models are used by doctors, including several forms of the medical model. Equally, many doctors find it hard to use social workers except in routine ways. Relations between social workers and members of other professions may be similarly fraught.

However, the fact that doctors and social workers do not share the same explanatory models need not be a barrier to cooperation, so long as each values the expertise of the other. The setting in which a social worker is based will influence the range of professions he or she must work with. For guardians ad litem and long-term child protection workers, for example, good working relationships with solicitors will be especially important. At its best, interprofessional work may lead to creative dialogue in which several theoretical positions jointly appreciated generate new insights.

Mirroring conflicts

It should not be supposed that relationships and understanding between the various disciplines and agencies will necessarily be built up in an atmosphere of calm rationality. Powerful emotions can be stirred up by work with people in severe distress, particularly abused and neglected children, who frequently feel lost and desperate. The issue of removing children from their parents frequently arouses enormously strong feelings not only in the parents and children concerned, but also in the professional people involved, especially when distressed people appeal implicitly or explicitly to the common humanity of the worker. Some professionals will identify strongly with or against the parent, and others with, or even against, the child. Indeed, as suggested by Reder & Kramer (1980), the different professions and agencies may come to mirror among themselves the conflicts that exist within the family. Or they may project on to one another their frustration when the parents and the children cannot be helped effectively. The work clearly requires empathy but also objectivity to counterbalance the strong conflicting emotional pulls when families and individuals are in conflict with themselves.

EDUCATION AND TRAINING FOR MULTIDISCIPLINARY AND INTER-AGENCY PRACTICE

BM/JT: Training for all professions involves a process of socialisation into the norms of the particular professional group. This tends to produce a professional identity, and a sense of loyalty to the rest of the group which, at least by implication, excludes non-members. In fact, that certain aspects of professional training serve the same functions as tribal initiation ceremonies is hard to deny. So, at all levels of training, any tribalist tendencies should be balanced by inculcating an appreciation that professions are interdependent, a process assisted when social workers are taught by members of other professions—psychologists, doctors, teachers, lawyers, and police officers. Team teaching, for example between a

lawyer and a social worker, or a psychiatrist and a social worker, can help to model collaboration and emphasise that all knowledge is interconnected.

Teaching by members of other professions will be of greater benefit at post-qualifying level because social workers will, by then, have gained a strong social work identity as a result of employment. Members of post-qualifying courses will also need to experience systematically through joint working as well as observation visits multidisciplinary networks or multidisciplinary teams as part of their assessed practice. A Sioux Indian proverb says that we have no right to judge somebody else until we have worn his moccasins for a long time. Shared cases is the professional equivalent of shared shoes. A necessary condition for effective collaboration with social workers is for the other professions to have some appreciation of the social dimension and the legal obligations of social services both to protect children and to act as parents to those in care. Learning how to work collaboratively comes from working with other professions, either as a member of a multidisciplinary team, or through carefully worked out arrangements for collaborative work as part of a multiprofessional network providing a range of services to a particular child or family. It is, therefore, valuable for course members on post-qualifying courses to have experience of both interdisciplinary networks and multidisciplinary teams. The former offer opportunities to listen to the points of view of and to work alongside a wide range of professionals. The latter enable members to develop a shared area of competence, while retaining their own expertise. The relationships of shared skills and knowledge can be envisaged as overlapping circles.

Indicators for education and training: a policy perspective

AH: The Association of Directors of Social Services briefly addressed the requirements of multiagency collaboration in its policy statement Competence in Caring (1985). It suggested that such collaboration required:

Table 6.2 Organisational and educational parameters of multiagency collaboration

Networks	Teams
Involve procedural contacts (embracing sequential involvement and work in parallel)	Involve shared common tasks and reciprocal interaction
Low to moderate degree of collaboration in order to achieve formal coordination of work	Suggest the highest degrees of collaboration
Imply interagency approaches	Imply multiagency approaches
Predominantly involve enhanced networking	Predominantly involve enhanced teamwork skills
Training needed is for basic working knowledge of a wide range of agencies	Training is for in-depth understanding of the few other professions in membership of the team

- shared vision and values
- delineation of responsibilities to avoid overlapping and duplication and ensure best use of resources
- development of collaborative working relationships at all levels within respective organisations
- awareness of the changing role and tasks of other agency professionals . . . which suggest the need for joint training programmes.

Finer discrimination is needed to transform these generalised objectives into appropriate organisational and educational responses. Some of the parameters are summarised in Table 6.2 extracted from Joss & Hey (1986).

Having established the parameters, it is thus necessary to specify more clearly what breadth and depth of knowledge and skills might be expected at different developmental stages. *The Statement of Requirements for Qualification in Social Work in CCETSW Paper 30* touches, but does not much elaborate on, aspects of issues analysed in this chapter. For example, part of the relevant knowledge base is identified as 'organisational content' and incorporates some of what previous generations of social workers were taught by way of understanding of agency function. Practice competence includes ability to:

- 'contribute to the formulation of programmes of care in collaboration with users, carers and other professions' (para 2.4.2)
- 'clarify the mutual responsibilities of all involved in the implementation of such programmes' (para 2.4.2)

- 'understand and where necessary take part in procedures for interprofessional collaboration' (para 2.4.4.).

In today's climate it would be necessary to plan and arrange, for example, the formal learning and skill development possible in short courses needed for improved networking. Some of the training could be done jointly with the other professionals involved and could include agency exchange placements. Models are offered from recent developments in ASW and child protection training. However, for improved teamwork more substantial and sustained experience may be necessary. For staff appointed to teams who have not previously acquired the range and depth of required competences, mentoring and skilled supervision must be provided. The higher order competences which such supervisors and trainers will require are therefore urgently needed.

Rosalie Kane (previously quoted on p. 203 for her research in interprofessional teamwork) has developed a comprehensive analysis of the knowledge, skills and attitudes required of members of interprofessional teams in a paper delivered to the CSWE Conference in Philadelphia in 1976 (see Box 6.2).

Box 6.2 provides an elaborate schema of how much development is generally necessary if the standard of competence in social work is to match that of the other disciplines commonly involved in teams, who benefit from much longer, deeper and more structured education and training. However, some of the items on Kane's schedule, for example teaching about

---

Box 6.2 Knowledge, skills and attitudes required by members of interprofessional teams (Kane 1976)

Knowledge

Participants should understand:

1 *Group process:* the dynamics of small face-to-face groups, including individual behaviour in groups, group norms, leadership, communication, decision-making, and harmony in relationship to productivity; normal phases of group development.

2 *Professions:* the nature of professions and evolving professions; the relevance of concepts such as status, autonomy, role clarity, role gratification, and professional ethics to teamwork; methods to find out specific information related to a particular profession with whom one collaborates.

3 *Organisations:* various administrative arrangements and their effects on teamwork; concepts such as line and staff authority and delegation of responsibility; levels of practice within different agencies and community groups.

4 *Teamwork:* growing body of literature on interprofessional teamwork per se; theoretical models for interprofessional teamwork.

5 *Evaluation methods:* validity and reliability of data; biases in evaluation designs; ways of documenting the effectiveness of the contribution of one's own profession.

Skills

Participants should be capable of:

1 *Group process skills:* utilise group process to achieve team goals and participant's goals; facilitate participation; exercise leadership directed towards both group process and task achievement; move towards conflict resolution and, when possible, consensus.

2 *Communication skills:* communicate clearly, accurately and without jargon; present information, clarify own professional role, express feelings, give and receive feedback; communicate clearly and succinctly in writing.

3 *Resource management:* mediate effectively between resources so as to manage group and own tasks smoothly and in keeping with clients' needs.

4 *Team analysis:* apply concepts about interprofessional teamwork to analyse a given team's functioning and suggest changes when appropriate.

5 *Problem-solving skills:* formulate a problem, set goals and priorities, implement tasks, and evaluate results.

Attitudes

1 Confidence in one's own ability as a professional and a person.

2 Respect for the abilities and motivations of persons with a different professional training.

3 Acceptance of the need of all team members for recognition and self-esteem.

4 Willingness to share a task with others.

5 Tolerance of disagreement and conflict.

6 Tolerance of ambiguity.

7 Flexibility—willingness to allow modification of one's role to evolve within the framework of one's professional values.

8 Research-mindedness—recognition of the importance of testing the effectiveness of different interprofessional arrangements and commitment to participating in such work.

9 Favourable attitudes towards recognition of, and the importance and complexities of each other's work.

---

organisation, occupational sociology, group process, are more commonly included in the social worker's basic training than in that of doctors and nurses. Others, for example knowledge of evaluation methods and the inculcation of research-mindedness, are less well developed in social work than in psychology or medicine.

Supervisory, leadership and resource management skills and the basic knowledge requirements underpinning them are not, however, exclusive to interprofessional teamwork. Their presence in the schema serves rather to highlight the general paucity of formal and substantial educational and training opportunities available to the able

and motivated staff member who prefers preparing for managerial level work to being pitched in at the deep end. Lack of preparation may not only incur the individuals concerned in higher cost, but also their colleagues and the more junior staff whose work they are now expected to frame and develop.

In short, skills in leadership and supervision relevant to team settings have the same components as those required by other managers and consultants in other spheres of practice. These competences must, of course, be built on the in-depth knowledge and skills in direct work and the special understanding Kane suggests are necessary to interprofessional practice. Areas of practice requiring such skills may now be found not just in health and clinical settings but in special child protection units and day and residential resource centres as well as more traditionally residential therapeutic establishments. The newer working patterns and demands of these settings point to the need for staff who can sustain a variety of different roles and relationships and move in and out of teams and networks effectively. They need to do so with confidence, feeling neither threatened nor the need to dominate. In essence, these requirements match those of society at large as Pietroni (1989) has pointed out in a private communication: 'More lateral relations, expert-'ease' without patronage, the management of constant transitions in organisations, different relationships between men and women and more pluralist models of society, within and between nations, based on exchange rather than colonisation and dominance'. In organisational theory these forms are usually referred to as matrix (see e.g. Knight 1977). It follows that, as the range and complexity of work and context grows, so do the numbers of staff requiring further and higher post-qualifying training opportunities.

THE EXPERIENCE OF THE FOUR POST-QUALIFYING COURSES

The four tutors were provided with a draft of this chapter and asked in particular to compare the Kane chart (Box 6.2) with the content of their own courses. A summary of their replies is given below. In addition to these subjective views, it should be pointed out that two of the tutors (Rushton & Martyn) recently conducted empirical research among course members and their employers (1990). This research indicates that 59% of former students now report improved or increased collaboration with other disciplines.

Diploma in advanced social work (children and families), University of London, Goldsmiths' College

Helen Martyn

Teaching of interagency and interprofessional work suffuses the whole course, both taught sequences, seminar work and tutorials and, most certainly, in the practice component. I do not want to claim a false specificity for I cannot give amounts of time devoted to these particular subject areas but what I can do is to indicate the parts of the course where these issues are particularly live.

Regardless of the type of agency from which they come, all our course members contribute experience of interagency and interprofessional work. Guidelines for the course assessment require that such work be given attention: *Is the course member able to think about and conceptualise her or his work coherently to colleagues in social work and other professions?*

Next, I would single out practice skills which are the main sequence of the course, comprising some 9 days out of a total of 52 days' teaching. A range of methods are used from some formal didactic teaching, through workshops and task-centred groups, to such experiential methods as sculpts and role plays. Much of the teaching in this sequence focuses on interagency and interprofessional work, for example, assessing borderline parenting. In addition, a taught sequence on organisations focuses mainly on how large politically-controlled organisations discharge their task. Current concerns about child abuse and child sexual abuse, not to mention the enquiry reports which focus ever more sharply on the need for interagency and interprofessional collaboration are certainly addressed in these sessions.

Lastly, a substantial proportion of the course is taught externally, often by lecturers from different disciplines, e.g. doctors and lawyers, so providing a different professional perspective from social work. As an example, I would cite the Working with Families sequence, 3 days of which are taught by a psychiatrist. In trying to apply Kane's analysis *very roughly* to the learning and teaching on our course, under Attitudes, I have ticked the whole list with a query about research-mindedness. Under Skills, we can include Group Process, Communication skills and Problem-solving skills, and under Knowledge, Organisations, but our students would leave the course also with knowledge of group process and of professions.

MSc in psychiatric social work, University of Manchester, Department of Psychiatry

Brian Minty

Our course is situated within a Department of Psychiatry, which is itself multidisciplinary, since it contains clinical psychology and psychiatric social work as well as psychiatry. Teaching and practice are fairly regularly multidisciplinary for all the professions concerned. In addition, the MSc functions in the schema of University regulations as the second year of a 2-year course of which the Diploma in Psychiatric Social Work (CQSW) is the first. In order to meet CCETSW regulations, students from the Diploma who wish to do the MSc have to take a break of at least 2 years. Students who have qualified elsewhere have to be deemed to have achieved a level of knowledge and skill in social work in relation to mentally disordered people, including emotionally and behaviourally disturbed children, roughly equivalent to students leaving the Diploma course.

The MSc course in itself is mainly concerned with learning research methods and undertaking a piece of empirical research, with a practice element, comprising half-a-day a week for 1 year, or its equivalent, always in a multidisciplinary setting. There is also a short series of seminars relating to practice, in which issues such as role confusion, overlap, teamwork and collaboration are discussed.

An applicant's knowledge of child and general psychiatry, and experience of working with children and disturbed adults is assessed through the application, correspondence and interview. Applicants whose training and experience lack knowledge of either child or adult psychia-

try and experience related to these subjects have to attend the lecture and demonstration seminar series in these subjects, which extend over two terms, and which are assessed by examination at the end. $3\frac{1}{2}$ hours a week for 20 weeks is a sizable amount of teaching which is done by psychiatrists, psychologists and social workers.

No specific teaching on group process is provided on the MSc course, although there is a sequence on the basic course, including an experiential element, of $2\frac{1}{2}$ days. There is no specific sequence devoted to teamwork on the MSc except for the series of seminars relating to practice.

Evaluation methods are specifically taught on the MSc both by lecture and by seminars on the critical analysis of social work-related research.

The skills and attitudes referred to by Kane would be to some extent developed by MSc students in practice placements that are supervised and assessed. 'Problem-solving skills' and 'research-mindedness' would be highly developed through teaching around research method, and the actual practice of research. The MSc students will already have made considerable progress in developing most of the other skills referred to by Kane through their basic training and experience before joining the course.

Diploma in post-qualifying studies in social work in mental health settings, the Maudsley Hospital/Institute of Psychiatry

Alan Rushton

The Maudsley course shifted from a full- to a part-time course in 1987 leaving us now only two-fifths of the time to cover the mental health field, including multidisciplinary work. Members of the full-time course were exposed to such multidisciplinary work in both more traditional consultant-led hospital psychiatric teams and less hierarchical, often local authority established, community mental health agencies in supervised practice placements in the Maudsley/Bethlem hospital and community agencies. Many opportunities were afforded to compare the course members' experience of different modes of operation, e.g. rigidity v. overlap of roles; quality of service relative to different professional structures; different ways of handling conflict.

Some settings provided poor or uncertain models of the social work role and status while others showed social workers in leadership roles, possessing much expertise and confidence. This learning method had problems because the uneven experiences of members sometimes led to rivalry, resentment and disappointment.

We also organised role-play exploring relationships between the five main professional groups in mental health, using mostly the child guidance setting as an example . . . although it was also helpful to explore issues such as the 'statutory/therapeutic' question: incompatibility or purposeful integration?

On the part-time course we continue to emphasise the importance of multidisciplinary work on the grounds that no one discipline possesses all the necessary knowledge and skill. We encourage a positive attitude towards relating to the professional network, collaborative therapeutic work and respect for the empirical knowledge base of the other disciplines. On the other hand, we encourage the members to identify strongly with their own professional group (rather than the all-purpose mental health worker idea); to maintain a critical stance towards the claims and aspirations of other groups and to argue the necessity of strong social work involvement in mental health care.

Perhaps the strongest element in multidisciplinary work that the Maudsley has to offer, and which the members appreciate, is the teaching by practitioners who have good awareness of the process by which cases are referred to a team (why here? why now? whose needs? etc) and the process by which aspects of the case become allocated to various team members. These sorts of consideration, often cast in a systems framework, play a large part in discussion of case material.

Discussion of professional roles, power and influence also finds a place in the sociology seminars and in the social policy sequence.

Child care practice, policy and research (with MPhil option), Tavistock Clinic/Polytechnic of East London

Alan Shuttleworth

The central aim of the CCETSW-recognised part of the course is to enable students to practise better by thinking about the connections between their practice and its organisational and policy environment. This environment continuously shapes what happens to individual cases. Social workers need to be able to grasp those processes if they are to work on cases effectively. Conversely, what happens to individual cases continuously affects social workers' relationships to their organisational and policy environment and that needs to be grasped too. It is clear that those environments need to be understood as multi-agency/multiprofessional environments. The concept of task and of difference of task is essential for useful work in such situations.

Current teaching as it bears on collaborative work

There are currently no lectures. Teaching is entirely learning-from-experience based. In seminars and differing forms of tutorial-supervisions, students bring their own experience for discussion. Areas of the course where collaboration issues are explored are:

1. *Work discussion seminars:* students take turns to bring for discussion the current situation on a case they are needing help with. Multiagency and multiprofessional issues naturally arise in the course of these seminars.
2. *Fortnightly tutorial/supervision plus periodic agency-liaison meetings:* the collaborative enterprise of course/students/employing agency is regularly reviewed in these meetings. The modelling of collaboration across major boundaries, undergoing varying vicissitudes— the pains or pleasure of learning/conflicts of various kinds/being on the receiving end of assessments/holding the power to review the course—is a central feature of the course.

3. *Group relations event:* during the second year of the course all students are required to take part in a 4-day group relations event in order to deepen their understanding of group, intra-group and institutional processes.

4. *Issues in child care seminar:* an agenda of current policy and organisational issues in child care social work is established with students. These values are then explored in a reading seminar, a group discussion or presentation of prepared work by the individual students. Multiagency and multiprofessional issues are frequently explored on these occasions.

5. *Research project:* students are required to carry out a research project into some specific area of child care social work practice. In doing so, the organisational (including multiagency/professional) context of that area of practice requires their attention. In my experience, students seem to be naturally able to get a grip on it at this stage and are certainly encouraged to do so.

Possible future developments

Bearing in mind what has been said about the need to balance the formulation of *what should be* with the exploration of *what is*, we are currently exploring ways of formulating more clearly views of what should be. This is likely to take two forms:

1. *A lecture series* which sets out to explore the developing argument about the form child care social work practice should take. This will, of course, entail giving systematic attention to the developing argument about the nature of the problems such practice addresses, its appropriate goals and what policies and organisational frameworks are appropriate to their accomplishments. Multiagency/professional issues will necessarily play a significant role in this.

2. A clearer *statement of the target-skills* we are aiming to help students acquire. This will entail a clear process of assessment as to whether they have been acquired by the end of the course. Capacity for multiagency/professional work will be among these skills.

CONCLUSIONS

AH: The issues addressed in the earlier part of this chapter are given a more focused and central place in the four courses than their outline curricula might suggest. In general the emphasis in all four is tilted towards influencing attitudes and improving skills. They are less concerned to pass on or make available the type of knowledge highlighted in the first part of this chapter at least in specific content and structured form.

Three of the four courses operate within multidisciplinary clinical settings which are also part of teaching hospitals associated with universities. Post-qualifying social workers in training work alongside, and may share, some teaching with students from other disciplines. In assessment of preparation for interdisciplinary/interagency practice using Kane's framework, teaching of social workers is likely to score quite well compared with basic and post-qualifying training of doctors.

Formulating proposals for educational and training development from the four courses' experience, however, runs into a number of conceptual and practice-related issues. In 1978, Thomas Briggs, of the Syracuse School of Social Work's Continuing Education and Manpower Development Division, suggested to a London seminar on teamwork, that neither concepts nor practice of teamwork within social services agencies were well developed (Briggs 1978). Although his own views may have reflected a largely American experience, he also drew heavily on research by Gundy (1975) in area teams in Scotland in the early 1970s. One of the threads of Briggs' analysis was that social workers were too individualistic to be good team members, because they were likely 'to view the central purpose of social work as counselling' and usually referred to themselves as 'caseworkers or group workers'. He went on to suggest that 'this identity has led to a 'process' rather than a 'goal' orientation, the former seeing clients as having psychological problems with social consequences and the latter emphasising social problems with psychological consequences.'

Since then DHSS-sponsored research studies (1985) suggest that the pendulum has swung too far the other way, that goal orientation has pushed out process. Middle and senior managers with responsibilities in the field of child abuse who attended a workshop run by Brunel Social Services Consortium in 1989 were agreed that abilities and methods required for identifying, investigating and securing first interventions in cases had improved significantly but had out-stripped capacities to undertake sustained therapeutic work. However, recent major disasters have given new focus to process because of the impact of trauma, not only on victims and the people they are close to, but on the staff involved.

An interest in process (not necessarily at the expense of goal) is a shared concern of all four courses and indeed is a major interest of the con-tributors to this chapter. Most authors are associated with multidisciplinary clinical settings, and have been keen to keep alive and develop 'process' skills. Alan Shuttleworth of the Tavistock speaks strongly on their behalf below.

AS: Our experience is that students come to post-qualifying courses in profoundly tangled states of mind about interagency/interprofes-sional matters, reflecting both the tangles of the environment within which they are continuing to work and their own individual tangles. They are, more often than not, struggling with varying degrees of despair and cynicism about the gap between the fine words they know and the but-terless parsnips that fill their plates. This despair and cynicism usually adds to the muddles they are in. Our philosophy and experience is that by paying close and sustained attention to the tan-gles that actually arise in their own work prac-tice students' capacity to untie these tangles for themselves grows. Only after considerable progress in this direction do students begin to think with reasonable comfort and sense about the link between what is and what should be. Before reaching this stage, students characteristically feel a disabling degree of persecution at having to look closely at the very distressing situations they are coming to think they have been, to dif-ferent extents, mishandling badly for some time.

I would not want to quarrel with any of Kane's *shoulds* but have, as yet, not met anyone who straightforwardly deploys the complete set of knowledge, skills and attitudes. The problem is partly one of specifying what *should be* but is equally one of specifying what the state of affairs is that we are addressing. What are the resources in staff and students and students' agencies for dealing with it? Who are these post-qualifying students who are coming on courses? What are their pre-occupations? What is problematic to them? Who are these teachers who are offering them some-thing? What do they have available to teach them with? What time-scale is involved in that? What methods of teaching help in practice? A teaching method that focuses on articulating what *should be* may be weak on struggling with what *is*. Conversely, a method that is good at the lat-ter may be weak on the former.

AH, BM and JT: Perhaps the most that can be hoped for is a better balance between the poten-tially competing approaches. The various features which affect interagency/disciplinary practice were articulated on pages 210–211. This was not prescriptive about how, when or over what time-scale the relevant knowledge, skills and attitudes can or should be acquired. Nonetheless, the gen-eral thrust of the analysis was that planned devel-opment opportunities should be provided which are relevant to the nature and context of the work being undertaken.

The Kane framework, at least, provides a com-prehensive overview out of which staged devel-opment can be built. Some opportunities will be provided by unidisciplinary training events, others by events shared with members of other disci-plines. Given the difficulty in managing intera-gency and interprofessional work, it follows that training events will need to have skilled design-ers and facilitators who can co-lead and model collaboration and hold, interrupt and illuminate relevant theories and concepts. In short, the general training continuum recommended in this report needs to incorporate training relevant to enhanced interprofessional and agency practice. Training policies should also seek to enhance the opportunities for interdisciplinary training through proactive extension of mutual accreditation systems. The ultimate goal is improved client service but this is only possible if members of different professions can, as Kahn (1977) puts it, 'delight in another's work and in connecting their own to it.'

REFERENCES

Argyris C, Schon D 1978 Theory in practice: increasing professional effectiveness. Jossey Bass, London

Briggs T 1978 Obstacles to implementing the team approach in social service agencies. Personal Social Services Council, London

Davidson S 1983 Planning and coordination of social services in multiorganisational contexts. Social Services Review 50 (1) pp 117–137

Department of Health and Social Services 1985 Social work decisions in child care. HMSO, London

Department of Health and Social Security 1988 Protecting children: a guide for social workers undertaking a comprehensive assessment. HMSO, London

Emery F, Trist E 1973 Towards a social ecology. Plenum, London

Fisher M, Newton C, Sainsbury E 1984 Mental health and social work observed. George Allen and Unwin, London

Friedson E 1970 Professional dominance. Atherton Press, New York

Fromm E 1972 To have or to be. Sphere, London

Gundy J 1975 Social service delivery in Scotland: a study of four area social work teams. University of Toronto

Holdaway S 1986 Police and social work relations—problems and possibilities. British Journal of Social Work 16 (2) pp 137–160

Huntington J 1981 Social work and general medical practice: collaboration or conflict? George Allen and Unwin, London

Huntington J 1986 The proper contribution of social workers to health care practice. Sociology and Medicine, Spring

Illich I 1976 Disabling professions. Marion Boyars, London

Jacques E 1955 & 1971 Social systems—a defence against persecutory and depressive anxiety. In: Klein M et al (eds) New directions in psychoanalysis. Tavistock, London

Jacques E 1976 A general theory of bureaucracy. Heinemann, London

Jones S 1985 Professionalism. Brunel University (unpublished)

Joss S, Jones R 1985 Do police officers survive their training? Policing 1 (4)

Joss R, Hey A 1986 Clarifying the purpose of multiagency exchange systems. Brunel University (unpublished)

Kahn M 1977 Towards collaborative health practice: 9th annual meeting of the American Society of Allied Health Professionals. Journal of Allied Health Workers, winter

Kane R 1975 Interprofessional teamwork. Syracuse University School of Social Work, New York

Kane R 1976 Paper to CSWE Conference. Philadelphia

Knight K 1977 Matrix management. Gower, Farnborough

Menzies I 1960 A case study in the functioning of social systems as a defence against anxiety: a report on a study of the nursing service in a general hospital. Tavistock Institute of Human Relations, London

Metcalf D 1979 The long term view. Journal of the Royal College of General Practitioners. Occasional Paper No. 9

Mungham G 1975 Social workers and political action in Jones H (ed) Towards a new social work. RKP, London

Pietroni P 1989 Flow-chart of general practitioner training. Personal communication

Reder R, Kramer S 1980 Dynamic aspects of professional collaboration in child guidance referral. Journal of Adolescence 3 (2) pp 165–173

Robinson T 1978 In worlds apart. Bedford Square Press, London

Rowbottom R, Billis D 1978 The stratification of work and organisational design. In: Jacques E (ed) Health services. Heinemann, London

Rowbottom R, Hey A 1978 Organisation of services for the mentally ill: a working paper. BIOSS, Brunel University

Rushton A, Martyn H 1990 Two post-qualifying courses in social work: the views of course members and their employees. British Journal of Social Work 20 (5) pp 445–468

Schön D 1983 The reflective practitioner. Temple Smith, London

Schön D 1987 Educating the reflective practitioner. Jossey Bass, London

Taylor T 1986 The police and social workers. Gower, Aldershot

Tibbit R 1983 Health and personal social services in the United Kingdom: interorganisational behaviour and service development. In: Williamson A, Room G (eds) Health and welfare state in Britain. Heinemann, London

STEREOTYPES OR ARCHETYPES? A STUDY OF PERCEPTIONS AMONGST HEALTH CARE STUDENTS

Patrick Pietroni

BACKGROUND

A review of the literature on interprofessional work reveals a degree of frustration and failure that leaves the reader with little room for hope (Batchelor & Mcfarlane 1980, Kilcoyne 1990). Numerous reports on the disasters that enter public debate from Cleveland to Rochdale identify the lack of effective communication between the professionals involved as well as the absence of interagency cooperation.

The implementation of the Griffiths report on community care has been partly interrupted by the Government's failure to provide or identify appropriate funding. This has also led to the curtailment of several educational and training initiatives that were started in anticipation of Griffiths' report. His report focused primarily on the need for change in managerial and organisational structures and very briefly mentioned the need for a rethink of our health care training practices (Griffiths 1988).

Most of the surveys on collaborative work highlight the need for training and recent developments amongst professional groups suggest that this focus is at least on the educators' agenda.

A survey of interprofessional training in the UK revealed an encouragingly high level of interprofessional courses although the majority of these were for district nurses and health visitors only (CAIPE 1989). In addition, very few of these courses occurred at the undergraduate level and the literature suggests that 'tribal allegiance' has been well and truly formed by the

Reprinted with permission from the Journal of Social Work Practice: 5 (1) pp. 61–69 Spring 1991, published by Carfax Publishing Company, PO Box 25, Abingdon, Oxfordshire, OX14 3UE.

time a health care practitioner has qualified whether in social work, medicine or nursing (Bligh 1979).

The different professions contributing to primary health and community care each have a distinct occupational culture. The differences in social status, pecuniary rewards and basic assumptions all lead to distinct tribal groups. Each group will develop its own characteristic style of communication and language leading to stereotypical judgements and the consequent problems that this degree of fixity encourages. Many of these stereotypical judgements are negative and give weight to the view that unless they are addressed early on in the training of all health care workers the future of teamwork is indeed poor. This paper describes an attempt to uncover these stereotypes at an undergraduate level and goes on to discuss how such stereotypes may be a manifestation of much more powerful archetypal forces which require a level of understanding so far absent in much of the literature.

METHOD

The Department of General Practice at St. Mary's Hospital Medical School organises a 4-week attachment to General Practice for medical students. Within those 4 weeks a half-day seminar on multidisciplinary teamwork is held with nursing and social work students. The objective of the seminar is to highlight the unexpressed views amongst the students regarding their perception of each other. Once these views are consciously available a discussion is encouraged to explore how far these views reflect actual transactions and how much they reflect prejudice and stereotypical behaviour.

Students are initally kept in single discipline groups and asked to create a list of adjectives to describe the three disciplines i.e. 'write down what comes into your head when you think of a medical student/nurse/social worker'. Students are discouraged from discussing amongst themselves and encouraged not to censor their spontaneous associations. Occasional prompt questions are suggested by the tutors (a mixture of doctors, social workers and nurses) such as 'what sort of car do medical students/nurses/social workers drive?', 'what sort of clothes do they wear?', and so on.

Following this exercise the sheets of adjectives are pinned on the wall of the room and the large multidisciplinary group then discuss the implications of the views expressed. Students are then invited to discuss their own personal experience of each other's disciplines. Finally, students are divided into multidisciplinary groups and given the desert survival game to complete, a group task used to explore issues of leadership and group process.

FINDINGS

During a 2-year period over 372 students completed the seminar: 196 medical students, 104 nursing students and 72 social work students. Table 6.3 includes the most commonly mentioned adjectives used by each group to describe each other and in Table 6.4 the adjectives and attributes have been separated according to categories reflected by the participants' choices. An analysis of group discussion and the desert survival game did not form part of this study although

reference to these sections of the seminar will be made in the discussion below.

DISCUSSION

It is clear from the findings that a large degree of uniformity existed among students' views of each other and that the negative attributes identified with each discipline were consistent with the students' perceptions of their own disciplines. The uniformity and consistency of the listed attributes, together with the largely negative perceptions, augur badly for practice when such students are required to work together in a collaborative setting where issues of life and death are at stake. On several occasions students protested that the findings were 'only stereotypes' and did not reflect their true beliefs. In the subsequent discussions, however, several instances were described which occurred between medical and nursing students who had most contact on hospital wards where the negativity of the perceptions was reinforced by actual exchanges. For the majority, however, the seminar was the first occasion where they had actually met a member of another discipline.

The raising to consciousness of these issues

Table 6.3 Adjectives used by health care students to describe students of social work, medicine and nursing

	Social worker students	Medical students	Nursing students
Social worker students	overworked caring scapegoats Guardian readers health foods	beer drinking immature intelligent rugby players arrogant	hardworking unimaginative gentle caring female
Medical students	2 CVs left wing self-opinionated intellectual lesbians caring	arrogant underpaid lazy heavy drinking rugby players naive	chip on shoulder overworked hard working underpaid smokers
Nursing students	overworked Guardian readers 2 CVs caring vegetarians	arrogant snobby overworked rugby players	caring underpaid hardworking overworked apathetic bicycles

Table 6.4 Categorised adjectives used by health care students to describe students of social work, medicine and nursing

LIFESTYLE	APPEARANCE	POLITICS	MONEY/CLASS	PROFESSIONAL	EMOTIONAL	
health foods jogging drinkers	jeans sandals long hair	Guardian Labour CND	2 CVs middle class working class	jack of all trades blamed hardworking	gullible diplomatic honest	**SW/SW**
drink a lot rugby	tweed jackets cord trousers attractive	Conservative Times	middle class public school social class 1	intelligent caring patients as objects	arrogant nervous frightened	**SW/MS**
fun loving chain smokers	black stockings strong physically uniforms	Mirror Telegraph Mail	underpaid Minis Fiats	hardworking dedicated exploited	nervous insecure bossy	**SW/N**
vegetarian lentils health foods	tweed suits sexy bohemian	left wing feminist racist	middle class Morris Minor Mirror	find problems much maligned analytical	officious sensitive chip on shoulder	**MS/SW**
drunken sporty live in squalor out of choice	square poorly dressed	Telegraph Times Sun	underpaid bicycles Morris Minor	hardworking naive intelligent	nervous arrogant lazy extrovert	**MS/MS**
smokers promiscuous eat chips	dirty sexy uniformed	Sun Liberal non political	do not drive poor live in homes	hard working over protective of patients dedicated	angelic brusque stroppy	**MS/N**
muesli / brown rice brigade do not smoke dope	weird clothes leather jackets long haired	left wing Guardian CND	middle class bicycles average pay	hardworking meddlers disorganised	egotistical wishy-washy well meaning	**N/SW**
rugby high standard of living	self conscious God's gift untidy	Tory right wing Conservative	poor middle class rich upper class	competent overworked not patient oriented	big headed snobby arrogant	**N/MS**
eat chips and tomato sauce sleep with anyone	sexy dirty shoes uniformed	politically apathetic apolitical Daily Mail	poor bicycles mixed class	caring hardworking failed Drs	cynical kind submissive	**N/N**

allowed for a testing against reality in the group of the basis on which these judgements were made. It also addressed, albeit temporarily, the unconscious tendency to stereotype present amongst all the students. Not dissimilar studies have been undertaken by other researchers.

Patterson & Hayes (1977) studied discussions of single discipline and multidiscipline groups of students from occupational therapy, social work, speech therapy and dietetics. Students were given 10 minutes in which to write down all the words which came to mind in connection with the word 'illness'. These word lists were then analysed and allocated to one of several categories. What the study identified was that not only was the difference in the words used amongst each discipline significant but also the context (i.e. whether the group was multi or single discipline) resulted in different word lists. The importance of the context in which communication occurs has been emphasised by many researchers. For example, whether a case conference takes place within a health centre, social services department or ward room will affect the choice of words used and decisions made.

A second study was conducted amongst nursing and medical students looking after the same patient (Lewis & Resnik 1966). They were asked to complete a questionnaire after having conducted an interview with a patient. This questionnaire asked for:

1. adjectives to describe the patient, e.g. fat, anxious, dirty, pleasant
2. objectives of care in decreasing importance
3. the student's own feelings concerning the important factors likely to influence the outcome of the patient's illness.

Altogether, 29 pairs of students evaluated 163 patients.

Student nurses were significantly more positively orientated towards their patients than medical students, and there was an almost complete reversal of the relative orientation between the students—the medical students were disease-centred in their objectives whilst the nurses were patient-centred.

The authors went on to examine whether any shift occurred between individual pairs during the course of this experiment (8 weeks), i.e. would pairs of students working together increasingly share the use of common adjectives, identify common objectives and factors related to medical care. They found no evidence that this occurred and concluded that 'the orientation and attitudes of students are primarily shaped during the first few months of their professional careers'. Indeed there is evidence to suggest that the attitudes of new medical students when compared to students in the arts and social sciences are significantly different with regards to the ability to tolerate change, uncertainty and lack of structure (Parlow & Robertson 1974).

I will now go on to explore what these studies suggest using Jung's concept of archetypes and archetypal images.

For Jung, his theory of archetypes represented his most important theoretical contribution and hastened his break with Freud. For many analysts, even those well predisposed to Jungian ideas, archetypal formulations can have the feel of 'high-faluting portentous language' that obfuscates rather than enhances discussion (Rycroft 1982). Even within the Jungian field there is much debate as to the usefulness of archetypal formulations within clinical work. For example, Fordham, one of Jung's principal followers in London, is cautious regarding an analyst's tendency to relate personal imagery to myth, folklore or legend. Such a focus in Fordham's view can lead to the patient losing contact with the personal context of his unconscious material (Fordham 1957).

Where archetypal formulations can help to enhance debate, however, is where they are linked to ethological concepts of human behaviour, especially when they draw on universal themes that transcend individual as well as cultural norms. Thus archetypes can be described as 'biological norms of psychic activity' that exert an influence on experience tending to organise it according to pre-existing patterns.

Whether archetypal behaviour should be viewed as instinctive or not is one of the major debates within Jungian circles and cannot be fully explored within the constraints of this paper. Jung's theory of archetypes in some ways resembled Plato's notion of 'Original Ideas', Bastian's concepts of 'Elementary Ideas' and Schopenhaur's 'Prototypes'. Similar concepts can be identified in some Kleinian writers— Isaac's 'unconscious fantasy' and Bion's 'preconceptions' being the closest.

The common thread which I wish to develop in relation to this particular study is that certain behaviour patterns seem to exist within the human species which are sufficiently common, occur sufficiently regularly, are environmentally stable and exert such a force on human growth that they act as a template for subsequent experiences. Within clinical work Jungians recognise a 'hierarchy of archetypes'—the persona, the shadow, animus/anima and the self. Other archetypal motifs are to be found in a variety of literary and artistic forms. In relation to the material identified in this study I would like to explore the motif of the medical student/doctor as hero-warrior-god, the nurse as great mother and the social worker as scapegoat.

THE DOCTOR AS HERO-WARRIOR-GOD

Notwithstanding the presence of white witches and midwives, medicine has always been a masculine-dominated preserve. Although there were goddesses of healing such as Isis, the Gods of Medicine, i.e. Apollo, Aesculapius, Chiron, were all male and, equally important, were warrior-gods. Perhaps not surprisingly therefore, the language of medicine emphasises a kind of aggressive invasion or penetration: 'fighting the disease', 'the war against cancer', 'the magic bullet' and 'stamping out infection'. The 'heroic nature' of medical advances, transplant surgery, in vitro fertilisation, genetic engineering, all challenge the boundary between god and man—the task of the hero in myth and legend.

From Adam to Prometheus and Icarus the task of the hero has been to transcend proper human limits. 'Hubris' is the consequence of this unfettered heroic activity. For the Greeks, hubris occurred when man appropriated to himself what rightly belonged to the gods. It manifests itself as human arrogance. So that when medical students are described as 'arrogant', 'beer-drinking', 'rugby playing' (battlefield) and 'God's gift' they can be seen as fulfilling the role not only they, but thousands before them, have had ascribed to them by human beings in cultures as diverse as Greece, India and Egypt. It is interesting to note that the additional set of attributes identified in this study—'naive, immature'—fit the 'as if' personality or *puer aeturnus* often linked with the hero. The *puer aeturnus* 'denotes an attitude that is innocent of responsibility towards the circumstantial facts of reality as though these facts are provided for either by the parents or the state or at least by Providence (it is) a state of childish irresponsibility and dependence' (Baynes 1950).

'We can identify a state of inflation whenever we see someone (including ourselves) living out an attribute of deity, i.e. whenever one is transcending proper human limits' (Edinger 1973). It is interesting to note that for the Ancient Greeks, it was unethical for a doctor to treat a patient who was in the grip of a deadly disease; for to do so the doctor pitted himself against Nature and ran the risk of that fateful hubris that waited for those mortals who challenged the gods. Thus I would argue that the doctors' use of high-tech medicine continually challenges the limits of the natural phenomena of life and death and the archetype of the hero still maintains a great hold on medical behaviour and the culture and philosophy of the medical profession.

THE NURSE AS GREAT MOTHER

The nursing profession has a long and well established link with the medical profession. It is still predominantly a female profession and, in spite of rigorous efforts to produce social and professional change in the doctor/nurse relationship, the role of the nurse as the mother/wife/servant to the father/husband/master (doctor) still forms the basis of working relationships observable in most clinical settings.

The word 'nurse' itself, with the connotation of mothering and suckling, reflects the link between the role of nursing babies and nursing the sick. The word nurse is derived from the Latin word *nutrire*—to nourish or to suck—and links in with the eighteenth century role of the housemaid, situated as it was in a specific class position, whose responsibilities included the suckling and wet-nursing of the children of the great house. Florence Nightingale's influence on nursing roles further reinforced the twentieth century approach to nursing, that of the organised housewife, caring mother *and* obedient servant, exemplifying at one and the same time the virtues of Victorian upper-class women and their upwardly mobile working sisters. Thorner (1955) suggests:

the nurse like the mother in relation to the infant caters to the patient's needs and therefore presents the most convenient object of cathexis on whom he may discharge his craving for response as well as aggressive impulses. This situation predisposes the patient to the transference phenomenon (falling in love) with the nurse (Thorner 1955).

For Jungians, the great mother serves as the most powerful archetype of feminine. The image and idea of woman as body-vessel is the natural expression of the human experience of woman bearing the child within her and of man entering into her in the sexual act.

The identity of the female personality with the encompassing body-vessel in which the child is sheltered belongs to the foundation of feminine existence— 'woman is not only the vessel that like everybody contains something within itself but both for herself and the male is the life such in which life forms' (Neumann 1955).

The equation woman=body=vessel=world therefore generates the most powerful hopes and fears for which the word 'nurse' often serves as a kind of catch-all carrier. The 'gentle, caring, overworked, underpaid' association of students to the word 'nurse' lacks, however, the power usually implicit in the image of the Great Mother but links well with the 'Angel of Mercy/Madonna/ Lady with the Lamp' image associated with Florence Nightingale.

Like all archetypes, the Great Mother possesses elemental negative as well as positive attributes. We see the emergence of these negative attributes in the association 'brusque, sloppy, cynical' and together with the 'black- stocking, sexy, promiscuous' cluster we have the picture of *Kali*—the devouring Indian goddess representative of the dark and terrible mother. That nurses act as containers for both individual and institutional terror within hospital settings has been well recognised and written about (Menzies 1960).

THE SOCIAL WORKER AS SCAPEGOAT

The notion that we can transfer our guilt and suffering to some other being who will bear it for us is familiar to the savage mind (Fraser 1923). The scapegoat is the powerful archetype whereby the existence of the shadow can be projected and discharged. Within myth and folklore the scapegoat is often dressed in odd clothes, is linked with a disability or bodily defect or plays the part of the gaudy fool or jester. In addition, Bronowski suggests that: 'In the fight against natural chaos the guilt of society is that it is a society. The guilt is order and the guilty are those whose authority imposes order'. (Bronowski 1955).

Barbara Wooton (1980) in her popular critique of social work linked the emergent profession with the 'Daddy knows best' image and accused social work of imposing its own attitudes, values and order on the client. In fact, social work and state authority have to co-exist in a complex, intimate and sometimes fraught dynamic within this general debate.

Thus two powerful ingredients ensure that the social worker is destined to serve as a vehicle for the powerful scapegoat archetype. The first, an identification with the 'outsider' and the second, this link with state authority.

The students' associations include the word 'scapegoat' as well as the 'health food/ vegetarian/2 CVs/long haired/sandals' image. The link with the state/authority is reflected in the attributes 'nosey, self-opinionated, officious'. Is it any wonder that we celebrate like our ancient forefathers the ritual sacrifice/slaughter of the social worker/scapegoat in the repeated child abuse enquiries that have become so familiar to us all. I am sure many social workers will recognise the descriptions of ceremonial sacrifice derived from anthropological literature:

Finally, the scapegoat hotly pursued by men and women beating gongs and tom-toms is driven with great haste out of the town or village (Fraser 1923).

On the eve of Ascension Day a man disguised as a devil was chased through the streets which were narrow and dirty in contrast to the broad and well kept thorough-fare lined with imposing buildings which now distinguish the capital of Bavaria. His pursuers were dressed as witches and wizards and provided with the indispensable crutches, brooms and pitchforks which make up the outfit of these uncanny beings (Fraser 1923).

So, if social workers did not exist we would indeed need to invent them. Since as a profession social work is new, if my thesis is correct, social workers must have taken on the role of scapegoat from a previous group of unfortunate health care workers. It appears historically that there are some grounds for thinking that this may well be the case. The first recorded execution of a witch occurred around 430AD and over the next 12 centuries thousands were persecuted and killed. *The Malleus Maleficarum* (The Hammer of

Witches) is the treatise which laid down how such poor creatures could be identified. It was not until 1736 that the laws against witchcraft were repealed. The midwife then took on the role of the 'scapegoat' and during the nineteenth century the 'itinerant healer' became the butt of all that was wrong with medicine. As medicine reconstructed itself on the high ground of 'hard science', social work seems to have been developed to occupy the vacancy thus created.

IMPLICATIONS FOR PRACTICE

If the students' associations with the words social worker, medical student and nurse reflect, as I am suggesting, archetypal images that form part of our collective unconscious, we will need to review our approach to the concept of inter-professional work. Certainly we should at least cease to be surprised that teamwork is so difficult—because the warrior/god, the great mother stripped of the animal aspects of her power, and the scapegoat do not make for easy bedfellows.

Pursuing the archetypal motif, I would suggest that we shall not arrive at a functioning team until two further archetypal images surface within the team. I perceive that both are emerging and I do not personally share the 'hopelessness' that pervades the relevant literature. In this area, the fourth archetypal image closely linked with healing is that of the trickster—in ancient mythology symbolised by Hermes or Mercury, the carrier of messages between god and man and identified with the Caduceus, the staff with two snakes, not just the one snake associated with the medical profession.

The trickster can be seen as connected though opposite to the scapegoat—slippery, cunning and linked, I suspect, with the emergent discipline of psychotherapy. It is, I believe, no coincidence that many social workers seem to 'escape' into psychotherapy. The description of Odin, the Norse/trickster/god suggests a mode of operating not unfamiliar to psychotherapeutic work: 'Odin constantly interfered in the affairs of men treating them like puppets to bring about the effects he desired. Generous with gifts at the outset

he withdraws them without compunction when they have done their work' (Williams 1979).

Loki, another Scandinavian trickster/god was noted for his ability to see what was hidden and for his gift of verbal dexterity which enabled him to speak in riddles.

It is interesting to note that when the students were asked to suggest the attributes they would wish a team leader to have, the following cluster of adjectives were most often used : 'good communicator' 'listens', 'calm' 'cunning', 'knows a little about everything', and when asked which of the disciplines were most likely to possess these attributes social workers were invariably identified, clearly in the trickster aspect of their role rather than the scapegoat aspect.

I do believe however that the emergence of the trickster in the team (whether or not in the profession of social work) may not be alone sufficient to enable the warrior-god, the great mother and the scapegoat to work together. The fifth archetype image which is also the earliest associated with healing is that of the shaman or wounded-healer.

The shaman is found in almost all cultures and is closely linked to the trickster, acting as a mediator between mortal man and the supernatural. The role of the shaman was not taken lightly for often it involved a descent into the underworld. The shaman's place amongst the tribal group was of great importance, sometimes being female and on occasion an ex-patient, although equally likely to be the son of the previous shaman. The shaman's 'art' was acquired through an apprenticeship which at times was exceedingly hazardous.

Two special features distinguish the shaman from the previous archetypal images described. First, the shaman's relationship to healing was *to the group* and was not always individualised. The orchestration of a 'collective healing ceremony' formed part of the shaman's skills—and it may be that we could learn much about teamwork if we were to study the meanings and format of these collective healing ceremonies. Secondly, the role of the shaman involved a 'descent into the underworld' and enabled him to confront his wounds. The shaman was and is also the representation of the wounded-healer archetype. The essential fact is not merely that the healer has endured affliction but has gone on to assimilate the experience of it either to be cured or to learn to live with the wound as a creative part of the healer's being' (Bennet 1988).

It is this 'living with the wound' that typifies the shaman and allows for a level of integration and change that is not present in the other archetypical images so far depicted. Its modern equivalent is perhaps also depicted by Schön's notion of the 'reflective practitioner':

He/she recognises that others have important and relevant knowledge to contribute and that allowing this to emerge is a source of learning for everyone. Reflective practitioners look for a sense of freedom and real connection with, rather than distance from, the client. They actively seek out connection with the client's thoughts and feelings and allow any respect for their own expertise to emerge from discovering it in the situation (Schön 1983).

'Living with the wound' implies a recognition of the limitation of each of our disciplines; the willingness to descend into our own underworlds and the recognition that if we are to come together to form a group, we need, as Kane (1975) so eloquently phrased it, to develop the ability to 'delight in another's work and in connecting our own to it'.

REFERENCES

Batchelor I, McFarlane J 1980 Multidisciplinary teams. King's Fund Project Paper No. RC12

Baynes H G 1950 The provisional life. In: Analytical psychology and the English mind. Methuen, London

Bennet G 1988 The wound and the doctor. Routledge & Kegan Paul, London

Bligh D 1979 Some principles for interprofessional learning and teaching. University of Nottingham, CCETSW

Bronowski J 1955 The face of violence. George Brazillier

CAIPE 1989 A report—national survey on interprofessional education in primary care. (Available from King's Fund, 126 Albert Street, London. NW1)

Edinger E 1973 Ego and archetype. Penguin, Baltimore

Fordham M 1957 New developments in analytical psychology. Routledge & Kegan Paul, London

Fraser J 1923 The golden bough. Macmillan, New York

Griffiths R 1988 Community care—agenda for action. HMSO, London

Kane R 1975 Interprofessional teamwork. Syracuse University of Social Work, New York

Kilcoyne A 1990 Post Griffiths : the art of communication and collaboration in the primary health care team. Marylebone Monograph I, Marylebone Centre Trust, London

Lewis C E, Resnik B A 1966 Relative orientation of students of medicine and nursing to ambulatory patient care. Journal of Medical Education 41 pp 162–166

Menzies I E P 1960 A case study in the functioning of social systems as a defence against anxiety. Human Relations 13 pp 95–121

Neumann E 1955 The great mother—an analysis of the archetype. Routledge & Kegan Paul, London

Parlow J, Robertson A 1974 Personality traits of first year medical students. British Journal of Medical Education 8 pp 8–12

Patterson M, Hayes S 1977 Verbal communication between students in multidisciplinary health teams. Medical Education 41 pp. 205–209

Rycroft C 1982 Review of archetype: a natural history of self by Steven A (q.v.) New Society 20th May, London

Schön D A 1983 The reflective practitioner. Temple Smith, London

Thorner I 1955 'Nursing' the functional significance of institutional patterns. The American Sociological Review 20 pp 531–538

Williams P 1979 The fool and the trickster. Brewer, Rownan & Littlefield, London

Wooton B 1980 Social science and social pathology. Allen & Unwin, London

TRAINING OR TREATMENT?—A NEW APPROACH

Patrick Pietroni

INTRODUCTION

In the last two decades great emphasis has been placed on the education of general practitioners in the area of psychological diagnosis and management. At the same time, an increase in the teaching responsibilities of general practitioners has involved their undergoing further training in educational methods and leading small groups. Many different approaches to conducting such courses have been described and discussed (Bacal 1971, Marinker 1972, Watson 1973, Fabb et al 1976, Freeling 1976, Cox et al 1982).

The best known approach for teaching psychological diagnosis has been the Balint group (Balint 1957). Other methods have involved the use of role-play, simulated patient interviews and video-tape playback. Heron (1973) has described his approach to developing a 'peer learning group' using some of the 'growth exercises' that arose out of the Human Potential Movement.

Initially, seminars on teaching skills relied heavily on the methodology developed by educationalists. Many general practitioners learnt about 'defining educational objectives', 'giving feed-back' and preparing 'assessment questionnaires'; Marinker (1972) described the outcome of the London Teacher's Workshop in which an attempt was made to look at the problems of trainer/trainee relationship in some depth.

Subsequent courses included Freeling's (1976) *Nuffield Course for Trainers* and Byrne's work at Manchester (Byrne & Long 1973). The tasks of these courses can be summarised by one of the following categories:

1. To increase the doctor's sensitivity to the overall needs of the patient/trainee.

Reprinted with permission from the British Journal of Holistic Medicine: 1 (2) pp. 109–112 1984.

2. To increase the doctor's sensitivity to the important part his personality plays in managing the problems of the patient/trainee.
3. To increase the doctor's skill in being a member of and leading a small group.

Whatever the organisers' or members' expectations may be, during the course of such groups both soon recognise that the boundary between professional matters and personal issues is difficult to maintain. As doctors reveal information concerning their approach to their patients or trainees, they inevitably reveal and face their own values, personal prejudices and belief systems. This may lead to an uncomfortable realisation that the defence systems they choose to adopt in their professional lives are similar to those in their personal lives. For some this is a new and public discovery that is nevertheless welcomed. For others it is a shock.

Balint (1957) was aware of this problem from the outset but was determinedly against his groups developing into therapy sessions. He attempted to select and screen out those doctors who were seeking therapy and discouraged personal revelations in the group work. Bacal (1972) challenged the accepted wisdom of keeping separate these two tasks of professional development and personal growth, but did not suggest an alternative model.

The purpose of this paper is to describe the structure of a group of general practitioners who met weekly over a period of 3 years, in the hope that it will provide such a model. In addition to the three tasks outlined above, the group agreed to examine and explore the doctor's personal and professional life as it impinged on the first three tasks.

OUTLINE AND BRIEF DESCRIPTION

The Department of Family Medicine at the University of Cincinnati, Ohio, was formed in 1976. By June of 1977 there were six full-time and six part-time faculty. Apart from the Chairman and the author, none had held previous academic posts, although all had been involved with teaching students. A Faculty

Training Group was started by the author and from then on a group of 10 general practitioners met weekly for 2 hours to discuss problems that arose out of their work.

A timetable was developed in which each month a different theme would govern the task of the group for that month:

1. *Theme I—Patient care:* Each doctor would have the opportunity to present and discuss individual patients that he had treated over a period of time. Much of the work done in this phase resembled a traditional Balint group. In addition, the group had access to video-tape consultation by each doctor.
2. *Theme II—Teaching:* Each doctor would have the opportunity to discuss teaching problems occurring in individual supervision or small group seminars. The emphasis in these sessions was on the comparison between the doctor/patient and trainer/trainee relationship.
3. *Theme III—Small group experience:* In these sessions each of the doctors in turn took over the leadership of the group and either presented a topic or led a discussion. The author became member and recorder. In the following week the author spent 15 minutes discussing his observations on the leadership style and group process of the previous week.
4. *Theme IV—Personal growth:* These sessions began with a series of structured exercises with the aim of building trust and facilitating group cohesion. Later, interpersonal issues relating to members of the group and the leader were discussed. Eventually as the group developed, more intimate and personal issues were revealed by members, reflecting their day-to-day concerns relating to their families, partners and staff.
5. *Application meeting:* At the end of each 4-month cycle, a further meeting was held to review the previous 4 months' work. At this meeting, each doctor described how he/she had applied any information gained during the weekly meetings to his/her daily activities.

DISCUSSION

The three innovations introduced to this group were:

1. Time given for members' own personal issues to be expressed and explored.
2. Structure provided which guided the task of the group and changed each month.
3. An application meeting held after every 4-month phase of the group's work.

The acceptance of the structured exercises used at the beginning of the group's life was high and the participation very active. A total of three doctors left after attending a few sessions. Their comments indicated that they found the methods used unacceptable and, as one stated, 'mickey-mouse'. The attendance of the remaining members averaged over 75%.

There is an understandable and natural reluctance to removing the boundaries between training and treatment. The group could find itself dealing solely with one individual's problems. Many doctors would not agree to participate and would almost certainly withdraw if the group's work revolved around personal issues. And yet there is an unwritten and unexpressed belief that if change is to occur it is very difficult not to stray into the personal life of the members. All too often groups operate with a hidden agenda—at times even hidden from the group leaders.

A very necessary first step in this group's life was the development of trust between members and myself. This was encouraged through the risk-taking necessary in some of the initial exercises. The mixture of structure provided by the timetable and looseness inherent in the process of some sessions led to the development of a 'potential space for play' (Winnicott 1971). This allowed sufficient loosening of the boundary between professional and personal areas for creative exploration to occur. At a later stage the members were given the opportunity to engage in disclosures. This enhanced their feelings of being part of an active growing group and allowed them to explore issues of concern to them.

On several occasions it proved possible to relate the work done in one particular month to situations described during another month. Some brief examples are given.

1. A trainer who found himself angry with a trainee who on occasions failed to attend and was consistently late for supervision was asked to consider how he would respond to a patient who behaved in a similar way. His insight into the patient's likely problem for non-attending helped him to manage the same situation with a trainee.

2. A father described his frustration over an incident in which his alarm had been set to wake him up in the middle of the night by his young son. This particular doctor/parent had been unable to show his anger in other than 'impotent rage'—to both his family and patients. One of the younger doctors role-played the son and re-enacted the scene which had caused him turmoil. He was helped through this approach to develop a more assertive rather than aggressive stance and subsequently reported a beneficial outcome in a number of doctor/patient encounters.

3. One doctor described how a trainee had labelled him as a 'puffed up old windbag' and seemed to be asking for reassurance from the group that this was not so. One of the members of the group helped him become aware of some of his sadness and feelings of insecurity that lay beneath this label. This particular doctor then described his feelings of professional inadequacy and his attempts at combating them.

These brief examples illustrate how problems encountered by doctors in one area of their life can surface in a totally separate area.

Was this aspect of the group's work training or treatment? It would be very difficult, if not impossible, to be clear of the boundary between these two tasks. By including as legitimate the task of 'personal growth', the door was open for any member to explore if he so chose. That so many of the group did choose to 'open the door' suggests that it certainly became an

acceptable task. By providing the external structure of the monthly themes, the anxiety created by an open 'growth group' with an open-ended commitment was allayed. There are seminars for general practitioners where each of the different themes form the focus of the group's work: patient care (Bacal 1971); teaching (Marinker 1972, Cox et al 1982); small group dynamics (Freeling 1976); personal growth (Heron 1972). In this group the four different themes formed part of a rotating structure and thus provided a method of looking in depth and yet at the same time at different aspects of the members' work and life—thus helping to draw them together.

The application groups allowed a link to be made between the work in the group and life outside. The use of application groups has been a major element in the work of group relations workshops organised by the A. K. Rice Institute (Coleman & Bexton 1975). It is important to give members attending intensive long-standing groups an opportunity to detach themselves and comment on the process. This allows for the development of objectivity toward their own learning and growth and counteracts any tendency for the group to become, as Freeling (1976) describes, 'a place for intellectual masturbation'.

Underlying the need for this approach in working with doctors is my belief that it is only insofar as we are able to accept and heal our own problems that we can begin to accept and heal those of our patients. This is by no means a new concept and has been widely recognised and referred to in most cultures.

In the East, both training and treatment are embodied in the concept of the guru. In the West, one of the highest accolades that can be given to a doctor is that 'he was a great teacher'. We have, it seems, at least at that level, recognised the link between training and treatment. The literature on the need to humanise medical education is vast and by no means recent. If the impetus to produce doctors who respond to their patient as-a-whole is to be maintained, it is necessary for us to devise methods which allow us to respond to doctors and medical students as-a-whole. This necessitates the exploration of the boundary between professional issues (training) and personal issues (treatment) to further facilitate the changes to which Balint (1957) addressed himself.

It is hoped that the model described will stimulate discussion for, as Oliver Cope so succinctly stated: 'The practice of medicine today reflects the education of yesterday'.

ACKNOWLEDGEMENTS

I am particularly grateful to my colleagues in the seminar group who encouraged and made possible this study. Their own honesty and contributions were the hallmark to the outcome of this venture. I am also grateful to Professor Robert Smith who provided the opportunity and created the environment that was necessary for the group to function.

REFERENCES

Bacal H A 1971 Training in psychological medicine. Psychology in Medicine, 2, 13–22

Bacal H A 1972 Balint groups: training or treatment. Psychology in Medicine 3, 373–377

Balint M 1957 The doctor, his patient and the illness. London: Pitman

Byrne P S, Long B E 1973 Learning to care. London: Churchill Livingstone

Colman A D, Bexton W H 1975 Group relations reader. California: Grex

Cox R, Kontianen S, Rea N, Robinson S 1982 Learning teaching. Institute of Education; University of London

Fabb W E, Heffernan M W, Phillips W A, Stone P 1976 Focus on learning in family practice. Royal Australian College of Practitioners: Melbourne

Freeling P 1976 Language and communication in general practice. London: Hodder and Stoughton

Heron J 1973 Course for new teachers in general practice. University of Surrey

Marinker M 1972 A teacher's workshop. Journal of the Royal College of General Practitioners, 22, 551–559

Watson H J 1973 Small group methods in medical teaching. Association for the Study of Medical Education

Winnicott D W 1971 Playing and reality. London: Tavistock Publications

TOWARDS A CLINICAL FRAMEWORK FOR COLLABORATION BETWEEN GENERAL PRACTICE AND COMPLEMENTARY PRACTITIONERS: DISCUSSION PAPER

Peter Reason
Derek Chase
Arnold Desser
Chrissie Melhuish
Sue Morrison
David Peters
Dorothy Wallstein
Vivien Webber
Patrick Pietroni

Keywords: Complementary practitioners, general practice, collaboration, cooperative inquiry.

INTRODUCTION

The Marylebone Health Centre (MHC) was established in 1987 as a general practice within the NHS aiming to develop and assess innovative approaches to primary health care. Among the principles developed as part of the 'Marylebone Model' is the commitment to offer patients a wide range of approaches to health care, including both educative strategies and treatment by disciplines which may be described as 'complementary' to general practice. At MHC these include homoeopathy, traditional Chinese medicine (TCM), osteopathy, counselling, and therapeutic massage.

Over the years multidisciplinary practice at MHC has taken several different forms. Complementary practitioners have held sessions there, seeing patients referred by general

practitioners and taking part in the development of the Marylebone practice, and the centre has established a multidisciplinary clinic. The Marylebone practitioners have a degree of familiarity with each others' disciplines through working together over several years, and also usually have some experience and competence in a range of complementary and orthodox healing practices; thus, for example, the osteopath is also a general practitioner, and the TCM practitioner a family therapist. In the autumn of 1989 a new multidisciplinary clinic, the MHC Research Clinic, the subject of this paper, was established.

THE PROBLEM

A central question in all of these collaborative endeavours concerns the nature of multidisciplinary practice. What is involved when practitioners with very different assumptions and practices try to work together? In particular, what kind of clinical models should inform such practice? Another concern was to explore the balance between expert knowledge and patient empowerment, and the extent to which patients might choose between different approaches to treatment.

The MHC Research Clinic was established to explore these issues of multidisciplinary practice. At this clinic patients, referred by their GP, were seen for individual assessment by each complementary practitioner. Following the assessment each patient met with the clinical team, with his/her GP in the role of advocate, to hear feedback from the practitioners and jointly to agree a management plan.

It was decided that this clinic should also be explored by the clinicians involved using co-operative inquiry, in order to identify and learn from the opportunities and problems of clinical practice facing such a venture. It was also to be the subject of a clinical trial in order to determine its impact on practice issues such as attendance at the centre and prescription rates, as well as on patient well-being.

Reprinted with permission from Journal of the Royal Society of Medicine: 85 pp. 161–164, March 1992.

COOPERATIVE INQUIRY

In traditional research, the roles of researcher and subject are mutually exclusive. The researcher contributes all the thinking that goes into the project, while the subject contributes the action being studied. In cooperative inquiry [1, 2] these mutually exclusive roles give way to a cooperative relationship with bilateral initiative and control, so that all those involved work together as co-researchers and as co-subjects. As co-researchers they participate in the thinking that goes into the research—framing the questions to be explored, agreeing on the methods to be employed, and together making sense of their experiences. As co-subjects they participate in the action being studied. The co-researchers engage in cycles of action and reflection: in the action phases they experiment with new forms of practice; in the reflection stages they reflect on and explore their experience critically, learn from their successes and failures, and develop theoretical perspectives which guide and inform their work.

Ideally in cooperative inquiry there is full reciprocity, with each person's agency—their potential to act as self-directing persons—fundamentally honoured both in the exchange of ideas and in the action. This strongly contrasts with traditional approaches in which all agency is held by the researcher, and the subjects of the inquiry are treated as objects.

The inquiry team for this research consisted of the three practice GPs and the four complementary practitioners, with the Director of Clinical Research as facilitator. The inquiry engaged in five cycles of action and reflection between November 1989 and June 1990. Each action phase consisted of two or three clinics attended by up to four patients; each reflection stage consisted of a 3-hour meeting at which the experience of the previous clinics, and the experience of the whole venture to date was discussed in detail. The meeting with the patients in the clinic itself and the reflection meetings were all tape-recorded and the transcripts circulated to the clinical staff involved in the clinic, who were thereby able to reflect more thoroughly on their experience.

It is important to note that the patients who attended the clinic were involved only minimally in the inquiry, although without them the inquiry could not have taken place. They were involved with their GP in agreeing their expectations for the clinic and in making a joint assessment of their health both before and after the clinic.

Among the guiding assumptions of cooperative inquiry is that valid knowledge is formed in action and for action [2–4]. It follows that the outcomes of the inquiry importantly include the group members':

1. experiential or tacit understanding of the process of multidisciplinary practice
2. individual and collective practical knowledge, including the skills of collaborative practice developed together
3. conceptual or propositional knowledge of the issues involved in this multidisciplinary process.

All these forms of knowledge are valuable and important outcomes of the cooperative inquiry process. A written article can only address the last of these three forms of knowing.

An overview of the whole inquiry has been provided in a working paper [5], and an exploration of issues of power and conflict in the clinic in a separate article [6]. The present article describes a clinical model for the kind of multidisciplinary work which was developed in the course of the inquiry. The ideas in the paper evolved during the inquiry process: the first draft was written at the end of the inquiry proper, and was refined in several later meetings. Thus the clinical model presented here is based on the experience of the group, but has not been critically tested in action as thoroughly as a fully rigorous application of the cooperative inquiry method would demand. For a fuller discussion of issues of validity in cooperative inquiry the reader is referred to the working paper.

VARIETY OF CLINICAL MODELS

At the start it seemed, on the surface, that there was a relatively clear and shared idea of what the clinical team were setting out to do and how this was to be accomplished. It soon became evident, however, that there were many different models for the clinic in team members' minds, some quite explicit, some tacit; some widely shared, and others more idiosyncratic.

For example, in one view the clinic was based on a multidisciplinary model of practice, and its purpose was to extend the treatment available to patients to include appropriate complementary therapies. Another view was that while the complementary viewpoints were important, the key process of the clinic was the empowerment of the patient to take charge of his/her own health.

Thus there was a degree of initial confusion, with different team members, unwittingly, operating with different objectives and from different assumptions. Through the research process the inquiry group clarified the different models which were being used, and with a developing sophistication explored their interrelationships.

Thus a first, and maybe most important, finding of the inquiry is that any multidisciplinary team involving general and complementary practitioners needs to work very hard in the initial stages to agree what it is setting out to accomplish and to find ways to explore and understand the different models and assumptions its members bring to any joint exercise. In our experience this is more problematic and requires more attention than may at first appear.

A MODEL FOR MULTIDISCIPLINARY PRACTICE

There appear to be three arenas of concern and attention in the consultation between a practitioner and a patient in which some kind of assessment may be made. It is necessary for the purposes of discussion to consider these separately, which is, of course, artificial since they must be integrated in practice.

First there is a specialist diagnosis from the perspective of the practitioner's chosen discipline, made with the authority of his/her expertise: the bio-medic may diagnose in terms of disease entity, the osteopath in terms of body structure, the acupuncturist in terms of energy, and so on. Each practice has a unique perspective on the problem, elicits a different set of signs and symptoms, and has its own particular way of investigating and understanding them.

The second arena for attention is the psychosocial context in which the symptoms occur—the patient's current predicament and response to it, mediated as it will be by his/her individual and cultural history. Thus there may be a current problem of housing, of poor relationships, of unemployment; and these may be exacerbated by a history of physical abuse or psychological neglect which may make the patient particularly vulnerable in these circumstances.

While in this arena there is more likely to be general agreement concerning the issues which need attention, practitioners with different personal experiences or political perspectives are likely to identify or emphasise different issues: a woman might be seen as clinically depressed by a male GP but as suffering from oppressive male domination from a feminist perspective; an unemployed black youth might be seen as malingering and delinquent from a right wing viewpoint, but as severely underprivileged from a liberal perspective. The issue here is what meaning is placed on the patient's life, and by whom [7].

The third arena for concern is the relationship between practitioner and client, which is critical in influencing the extent to which any clinical intervention is likely to be successful. This relationship is also important in its own right, since practitioners may wish to influence it in particular directions. Several issues may need consideration, for example:

1. the extent to which the practitioner is willing and able to develop a close and empathic relationship
2. the patient's belief systems concerning health and illness
3. the practitioner's intention and skills in relinquishing control and empowering the patient; and the patient's intent and capacity to take power
4. the patient's physical and mental condition— there are occasions when a patient may be

quite appropriately dependent on the practitioner for life-sustaining intervention or containment of distress

5. the manner in which the relationship is influenced by earlier and childhood experiences (although an in-depth treatment of these issues would most likely fall within the expert realm of a psychotherapist).

In conventional one-to-one practice, be it orthodox medical or complementary, all these factors may be taken into account by the practitioner and to some extent by the patient. The diagnosis, or 'knowing through', is (or should be) the synthesis of the three perspectives. In multidisciplinary practice the same diagnostic concerns are present but with a greater variety and richness of alternatives. Some of these issues are addressed in the remainder of this paper.

PERSPECTIVES FROM DIFFERENT DISCIPLINES

A multidisciplinary practitioner group will have available a much wider range of resources than a single practitioner, and is thus faced with the challenge of how to use them. There is a wide variety of possibilities, some of which are identified as follows:

1. It may be possible to make a 'match' between patient condition and therapy; to say, for example, that conditions of menopausal imbalance are best treated with homoeopathy. Some such matches are beginning to emerge in practice, although much more research is needed before such statements can be made with confidence.
2. Treatment by one discipline may be supplemented and supported by treatment by a second. On occasion in the MHC Clinic homoeopathy was twinned with osteopathy, the homoeopathy (for example Rhus tox and Bryonia, low potency) aiming to help with fibromyalgia and myofascial pain; similarly homoeopathy was used to support counselling, with Natrum muriaticum being used to help a patient in counselling let down his defences. In addition, all the complementary

disciplines were used at times in conjunction with more orthodox general practice approaches.

3. The involvement of several experienced clinicians working from quite different perspectives may enable all the practitioners, and thus potentially the patient, to deepen their understanding of the patient's condition. This may result in more effective long-term treatment of a patient with a chronic condition:

A patient was seen in the clinic with a variety of physical symptoms and a fear that she had MS. A history of debilitating childhood illnesses including meningitis and rheumatic fever, of physical and psychological abuse, and physical injury combined with very poor housing conditions resulted in an experience of physical pain, exhaustion, and deep-seated anxiety. Some of the physical pain was diagnosed osteopathically, and treatment relieved one layer of the pain symptoms.

However, further reflection in later inquiry sessions suggested that long-term treatment was required and that, while held and supported by her general practitioner, this patient would ideally receive care and attention over several years, with treatment probably including psychotherapy, maybe family therapy, acupuncture, and further osteopathy. All this would need to be carefully orchestrated to meet her life situation and ability to respond and change.

It was not possible to design such a programme within the limitations of the Research Clinic, although the patient continues to see her general practitioner, whose understanding of her condition has been deepened, and who has access to the wide range of resources of the Marylebone Health Centre (for a fuller description see ref. 5).

4. The clinicians are able to use their colleagues' differing clinical expertise in order to support, inform and develop their own expert judgement.

On the other hand there are possible negative consequences of the multidisciplinary model, the most likely one being that instead of developing a creative synergy between the different disciplines, difficulties of communication and understanding cause the team to dilute the skills of its practitioners to conform to some lowest common denominator and the particular differences of the different disciplines get lost. In the

Marylebone experience it proved very difficult fully to appreciate and integrate the clinical skills and experience of the different practitioners: we simply did not have the concepts or the language. In consequence all the practitioners felt that they were educating their colleagues at the same time as trying to understand the patient, and that they had greatly to simplify their technical explanations in order to be understood.

Because of these difficulties of communication across professional disciplines, there was also a tendency to discuss the patients in terms of their psychosocial predicament (because that was the arena of most shared understanding) to the detriment of careful diagnosis from the perspective of the different disciplines. Also, there was at times a feeling that the general practitioners in particular did not appreciate the distinctive expertise and clinical contributions of the complementary practitioners, especially of the homoeopath and the TCM practitioner. As one of these practitioners reflected toward the end of the inquiry, the implication was that their approach could not have any *medical* validity, but what it could have was psychosocial validity.

PSYCHOSOCIAL ISSUES

There is likely to be a greater uniformity of understanding and perspective in this arena, and less likely to be differential expertise to contribute to the diagnosis (although a systemic family therapist might well have a professionally informed opinion). However, the collaboration of practitioners as individuals with different life perspectives may make possible a much deeper understanding of the patient's predicament. As pointed out above the danger appears to be that, just because this is an area of common understanding, it will come to dominate discussion.

RELATIONSHIP ISSUES

Relationship issues are greatly complicated by multidisciplinary practice, certainly in the form of the Marylebone Research Clinic, involving as it did the meeting between the patient and a group of practitioners. In addition to issues in the relationship between individual clinician and patient, there is the broader question of the management of the relationship between the patient and the team as a whole, and also between the clinicians themselves.

First, patient/clinician relationships now take place in the context of the multidisciplinary clinic. Thus the traditional personal relationship between GP and patient may be disturbed. While the positive side is that the patient may be supported by more people, one danger is that they may get 'lost', with no one clinician taking responsibility for overall care; another is that the patient may (consciously or unconsciously) play one clinician off against another.

Secondly, it is important to manage the meeting between patient and team with the utmost care, because it is clearly much more complex to establish a healing relationship between one patient and a group of practitioners than it is one to one. The patient is confronted by a possibly overwhelming array of clinicians, each with their different clinical perspective, and the danger is that they will in some way compete to 'sort out' the patient.

The initial view of the meeting with the patient which followed the assessment interviews was that the patient, having heard from the clinicians, would make his or her own choice of treatment. This was an attempt to guard against the danger that the clinicians would in some sense 'take over'. However, this rather simplistic notion confused patients and sent the clinicians into turmoil. A new more business-like and problem-solving structure for the meeting was then adopted: each clinician in turn would report from his/her perspective, and then the GP orchestrated a decision, with the team making great efforts to include the patient as an equal partner in the decision process. This format was acceptable for a while, but its limitations became apparent: it was a compromise, and more seriously a defence against the anxiety of uncertainty, of working together in a new way.

It is evident that a completely new language is needed if the clinicians are to be able to meet the patient as a group and work together with her or him in the room. While the inquiry team was not able to explore this with any degree of rigour, it does appeal as a possible focus for future inquiry. Such a new language might look to ceremonial and ritual processes for inspiration, creating what might be termed a transitional space or an alchemical vessel [8]. It might mean drawing on the thread of clinical work which comes from models of brief psychotherapy, family therapy and systems thinking [9–12]. It would mean much more careful strategic planning of the meeting as an intervention by the practitioners.

The third relationship question concerns the clinicians themselves and their capacity for creative collaboration. Certainly in the early days of this clinic the team really did not know how to work together: there was the inevitable awkwardness of people working together in a new and challenging situation and this was compounded by the absence of a clear and shared model of practice, and compounded again by the failure to realise the extent of this absence. The establishment of the Clinic within a framework of cooperative inquiry, with its phases of systematic reflection, enabled the team to identify these problems and work toward their resolution. One outcome of the inquiry is the clinical model described in this paper.

HEALING RELATIONSHIPS: WHO HAS THE 'JUICE'?

The multidisciplinary model as described so far is a useful logical and analytical tool. However, careful diagnosis and analysis need to be linked to subjective considerations which the team encapsulated in the question 'Who has the juice for this patient?' This notion of *juice* is not just about having the most appropriate treatment, or about empathic relationships and a good bedside manner. It is about a personal integration of the specialised skills of a discipline with an understanding of the patient's predicament and containing these within a healing relationship, so that empathy and personal expression are channelled through the healing discipline.

CONCLUSION

A creative and effective multidisciplinary practice would work together to integrate these arenas in its work. It would develop an expertise in collaboration over and above the separate expertise of the individual clinicians. It would take time to educate itself in some depth into the perspectives of each of its specialised disciplines, and in discussion of each patient would allow adequate time for each clinician's viewpoint to be fully developed. This would lead to a joint 'expert' choice of appropriate treatment (or combination of treatments). This judgement would be integrated with a psychosocial diagnosis and with an assessment of which clinician is best suited to develop a healing relationship with the patient.

The cooperative inquiry described in this paper has laid a firm foundation for further work to develop the understanding and skills required for this kind of multidisciplinary practice. The following questions in particular merit further consideration:

1. What steps can a multidisciplinary team take to deepen members' understanding of the diverse clinical practices of its members, and of the manner in which these are expressed by each practitioner? Clearly, some of this can be accomplished in a straightforward manner through reading and discussion; however, we suspect that the more subjective aspects of these healing skills are more difficult to communicate and can only be learned through extended and sympathetic collaboration.
2. How can a multidisciplinary team as a whole best relate to a patient? Are there therapeutic practices outside primary health care—in systemic family therapy or group psychotherapy, for example—on which a team could draw?

ACKNOWLEDGEMENTS

The authors are grateful to Dr Peter Davies, John Heron, Dr John Horder, and Dr Judi Marshall, who read various drafts of this paper and made helpful comments.

REFERENCES

1. Reason P, Rowan J. Human inquiry: a sourcebook of new paradigm research. Chichester: John Wiley, 1981.
2. Reason P. Human inquiry in action. London: Sage Publications, 1989.
3. Macmurray J. The self as agent. London: Faber & Faber, 1957.
4. Heron J. Philosophical basis for a new paradigm. In: Reason P, Rowan J, eds. Human inquiry: a sourcebook of new paradigm research. Chichester: John Wiley, 1981.
5. Reason P, et al. Marylebone Health Centre Research Clinic 1989-90: the cooperative inquiry. London: Marylebone Centre Trust, 1991.
6. Reason P. Power and conflict in multidisciplinary collaboration. Complementary Medical Research 1991; 5 (3).
7. Aldridge D. Making and taking health care decisions: discussion paper. J R Soc Med 1990; 83: 720–732.
8. Samuels A. Jung and the post-Jungians. London: RKP, 1985.
9. Burnham J B. Family therapy: first steps toward a systemic approach. London: Tavistock, 1986.
10. Palazzoli M S, Cecchin G, Prata G, Boscolo L. Paradox and counterparadox. New York: Jason Aronson, 1978.
11. Watzlawick P. The situation is hopeless but not serious: the pursuit of unhappiness. New York: Norton, 1983.
12. Watzlawick P, Weakland J, Fisch R. Change: principles of problem formulation and problem resolution. New York: Norton, 1974.

POWER AND CONFLICT IN MULTI-DISCIPLINARY COLLABORATION

Peter Reason

A multidisciplinary clinic was established in an inner city general practice. Using the approach of cooperative inquiry, the clinicians involved explored their joint practice to understand better the nature of multidisciplinary practice. This paper focuses on issues of power and conflict which arose in the course of this work, and makes suggestions for future practice.

INTRODUCTION

In this paper I want to explore some of the group and interpersonal issues which arise when general medical and complementary practitioners work together. Particularly I want to look at this in terms of power and power conflicts, and to attempt to understand some of the deep-seated causes of misunderstanding which may arise between practitioners who are good working colleagues and who hold each other in considerable respect.

However, before exploring these issues of power and conflict I shall first describe the setting and briefly discuss cooperative inquiry, which was the method used for this inquiry.

MARYLEBONE HEALTH CENTRE

Marylebone Health Centre (MHC) is a general practice established in 1987 working within the NHS in central London. As part of the Marylebone Centre Trust (MCT), MHC aims to develop and assess innovative approaches to primary health care. Thus, for example, the work of MHC is the subject of continuous audit: comprehensive patient computer records are maintained which provide accurate information on clinical,

Reprinted with permission from the Complementary Medical Research: 5 (3) pp. 144–150, published by the Research Council for Complementary Medicine.

social and economic aspects of the practice. Similarly, practitioners meet regularly to discuss issues in the practice and patient groups of various kinds have been established.

One outcome of these discussions and reflections has been the articulation of a statement of practice called the Marylebone Model. This model sets out a number of working principles which underpin the work of MHC, and includes two statements of interest to our present concern: offering a multidisciplinary approach and empowering people to take control of their own health and well-being.

Thus a multidisciplinary approach is an important part of the Marylebone Model of primary health care and over the years multidisciplinary practice at MCT has taken several different forms. At the time of writing five complementary practitioners—a homoeopath, an osteopath, a practitioner of traditional Chinese medicine (TCM), a psychotherapist and a masseuse—hold sessions at Marylebone Health Centre, seeing patients referred by general practitioners and taking part in the development of the practice. A series of multidisciplinary clinics were held which are described and evaluated by Wallstein et al [1].

In the autumn of 1989 a new MHC Research Clinic, based on this earlier work, was established to explore issues of multidisciplinary practice. At this clinic patients, referred by their GP, are seen for assessment by the complementary practitioners. Following the assessment the patients meet with the clinical team, with their GP in the role of advocate, to hear feedback from the practitioners and together agree a management plan. The idea behind this joint meeting, which was a bold step in its own right, was to see if it was possible to empower patients by involving them in decisions about their health care.

The MHC Research Clinic was planned to be the subject of a clinical trial to determine its impact on practice issues such as attendance at the Centre and prescription rates, as well as on patient well-being [2]. In addition, it was decided that the clinic should also be explored by the clinicians involved using cooperative inquiry, in order to identify and learn from the opportunities and problems facing such a venture.

COOPERATIVE INQUIRY

In traditional research, the roles of researcher and subject are mutually exclusive. The researcher contributes all the thinking that goes into the project, while the subject contributes the action being studied. In cooperative inquiry these mutually exclusive roles give way to a relationship based on bilateral initiative and control, so that all those involved work together as co-researchers and as co-subjects [3, 4]. As co-researchers they participate in the thinking that goes into the research—framing the questions to be explored, agreeing on the methods to be employed, and together making sense of their experiences. As co-subjects they participate in the action being studied. The co-researchers engage in cycles of action and reflection: in the action phases they experiment with new forms of clinical practice; in the reflection stage they reflect on their experience critically, learn from their successes and failures, and develop theoretical perspectives which inform their work in the next action phase.

Ideally in cooperative inquiry there is full reciprocity, with each person's agency, his or her potential to act as self-directing persons, fundamentally honoured both in the exchange of ideas and in the action. This strongly contrasts with traditional approaches in which all agency is held by the researcher and the subjects of the inquiry are treated as objects. Cooperative inquiry is one method of several which is informed by a radical participatory worldview (see, for example refs 5–7).

While there is not the space within this article to explore these issues fully, it should be noted that because of the emphasis on self-reflective agency, this is a method particularly suitable for practitioner research and for the development of innovative approaches to practice.

The inquiry team for this research consisted of the practice GPs and the five complementary practitioners, with the Director of Clinical Research (the author of this article) as facilitator.

The inquiry engaged in five cycles of action and reflection between November 1989 and June 1990. Each action phase consisted of two or three clinics attended by up to four patients; each reflection stage consisted of a 3-hour meeting at which the experience of the previous clinics, and the experience of the whole venture to date, were discussed in detail. Both the meeting with the patients in the clinic and the reflection meetings were tape-recorded, and the transcripts circulated to the clinicians, who were thereby able to reflect more thoroughly on their experience.

Among the guiding assumptions of cooperative inquiry is that valid knowledge is formed in action and for action [3–9]. It follows that the outcomes of the inquiry importantly include the group members' experiential or tacit understanding of the process of multidisciplinary practice; their individual and collective practical knowledge, which includes the skills of collaborative practice they developed together; and the conceptual knowledge of the issues involved in this multidisciplinary process. All these forms of knowledge are valuable and important outcomes of the cooperative inquiry process. A written article can only address the last of these three forms of knowing. While this paper addresses specifically issues of power, as full an account as possible of the inquiry has been provided in a working paper [10].

A further issue in reporting cooperative inquiry concerns ownership of any reports which are made. While an inquiry group may be able to prepare a report to which every member subscribes, individual members may also wish to make individual reports in papers such as this one. In addition, it will be clear that each member of the inquiry group will speak from their unique personal perspective. I believe it is important that any report purporting to come from a cooperative inquiry group includes a statement of how it was written and to what extent it represents the shared views of the group. Thus this paper was written by myself as single author; it was based firmly on the work of the inquiry group, and has been discussed in detail at a meeting with most of the inquiry group members. While many of their comments have been incorporated and they agree broadly with the content of this paper, the theoretical reflections on the work are entirely my own responsibility.

POWER, EMPOWERMENT AND POWER CONFLICTS

The inquiry group, in its reflection meetings, agreed that issues in the management of power were central to the conduct of the clinic. Of particular interest was the question of whether the attempt to empower patients was leading to disempowerment of complementary practitioners.

The empowerment of patients

The clinic was established with the clear intent of empowering patients to make their own health choices. The GP who initiated the clinic felt that the arrangements in the earlier multidisciplinary clinics, in which the practitioners discussed the patient's case in private before suggesting a treatment package, was fundamentally disempowering and that it was wrong for the patients to be told what was good for them on a 'Doctor knows best' basis. It was also argued that it is fundamental to the treatment of patients with chronic conditions that they experience the capacity to do something about it themselves.

On the other hand, it was argued that patient choice is meaningless unless based on knowledge and understanding of the options, which was clearly often not the case with patients at this clinic. But since it was often impossible for anyone, even the most knowledgeable practitioner, to make a fully informed choice about the appropriateness of different therapies to a particular patient, it may make much more sense for the patient rather than for the practitioner to make the choice on the basis of his or her own subjective wisdom.

In the event we agreed that, even with the (for some) dramatic intervention of inviting the patients to discuss and agree their treatment with the group of practitioners, we did not actually make much impact on their sense of empowerment.

Power and disempowerment of practitioners

One of the questions which arose very early was whether, in attempting to empower the patient, the process of the clinic was disempowering the complementary practitioners (CP). The meeting with patients was a rich and complex event, which required considerable skill and understanding to work well. On a few occasions the intent was met, and the patient appeared to leave with a fuller understanding of his or her predicament, a sense of empowerment, and a sensible management plan. On some occasions the meeting was simply flat and embarrassing. Other occasions were confused and unsuccessful, with the clinicians left feeling upset and sometimes angry.

One source of difficulty was that the complementary therapists felt unsure of their ground, unsure of the extent to which they could use their clinical expertise and unsure of when this would be seen to be disempowering the patient. They were uncertain how to describe the possible benefits of their therapy to the patient, and about the extent to which it was acceptable for them to disagree with their colleagues in front of the patient. In addition, there was always the possibility that, in offering an alternative form of treatment, they would be experienced as criticising the GPs' treatment strategy over several years. There was at times a sense of considerable anxiety, with all the practitioners feeling unsafe, awkward and de-skilled.

Whether this was an intentional strategy of the general practitioners (conscious or unconscious) or simply an unintended consequence of the clinic structure was fiercely debated:

CP1: . . . on a fundamental level (it's) about safety . . . (to GP) Do you have an agenda about making us feel unsafe . . . ?

CP2: (amid laughter) You like to make us squirm!

CP1: . . . If that is part of the experimental model, let's get it on the table! You want to empower the patients and disempower the practitioners. I think you can empower the patients without disempowering the practitioners. I think there has to be a balance struck, or else the dynamic of this meeting will always be difficult.

It was also argued by the complementary practitioners that their power was legitimate and not to be discounted lightly:

CP3: I know knowledge is power, but knowledge is being somehow used pejoratively here . . . I've studied, for Christ sake, there is stuff that I know, and how is it going to be put into practice here . . . ?

A vignette

It may help to offer an example of conflict as it occurred in the clinic, and how different layers of conflict reverberate with each other. The clinic session in question took place at a particularly busy time, when all practitioners were feeling more or less harried. The clinic was full, with four patients attending that afternoon, which always added to the pressures to timetables and keeping in touch with a lot of diverse information. There was further awkwardness because the first patient had been referred by a GP with whom relationships were uneasy, and who had not been referring to the clinic very regularly.

The second patient appeared on the surface to bring structural problems to the clinic which needed osteopathic treatment; release of tension in the lower spine would improve circulation and diminish back pain, as well as possibly helping with pain in the knees. However, from the perspective of the TCM practitioner, supported by the homoeopath, there was stagnation of energy in the whole body, due to both initial weakness and also the incidence several years earlier of typhoid and malaria. From this perspective the question was not simply structural, it was energetic, emotional and spiritual as well. The conflict was between a view of someone simply needing some adjustment, and of a deeper constitutional deficiency requiring energetic work. There was considerable confusion in the debate about which form of treatment to adopt, because there seemed to be no framework, conceptual or intuitive, which encompassed all the different possibilities. This confusion added to the prickly feeling between the clinicians that day.

The third woman had been experienced by all practitioners as difficult to work with; also, she had arrived late, and then harshly criticised one of the practitioners for giving her very little time. She had complained to her GP about this, rather than directly to the person concerned. Dealing with this added to the awkward atmosphere.

Finally, the fourth patient who attended appeared very passive and unclear about what she wanted, so that it was difficult to reach a decision about appropriate treatment. The GP concluded that, because of this indecisiveness, she should not be offered treatment at this stage. The complementary practitioners reacted strongly against this, seeing his attitude as unprofessional and almost sadistic, in that he had not responded to her need for help. He in turn felt that the CPs were inappropriately 'rescuing' the patient and not confronting her with the possibility of taking charge of her predicament.

There had been hints of this difference during the meeting with the patient; they emerged more explicitly (and quite explosively) immediately afterwards and were explored in depth in the subsequent reflection meeting. At that time it was realised that, in addition to the various group and interpersonal issues that were influencing the situation, there was a difference in clinical understanding of the patient's condition:

GP: I think the thing I remember most about that clinic was that after she'd gone I commented on the fact that I felt we should have left her untreated and you said that you thought that was a bit sadistic. And I thought about that afterwards and . . . I assume it was because you felt that you had something very clear to offer and that you could treat her indecision as well as her physical symptoms. I was feeling that here was a woman who wasn't putting out anything at all. It was very clear that she didn't want to take a position on anything as I saw it and I would therefore have waited until she moved in some direction. That, it seemed to me, was a reflection of two very different models.

Homoeopath: Yes, that indecision would be seen as a homoeopathic rubric; in other words, a basis for a prescription, and was in a hierarchy of symptoms—in her case, a very highly marked symptom, and therefore from a homoeopathic management point of view would have to be covered in any prescription. But it wasn't just the indecision. It was mirrored right through her case, if I remember . . . there were a lot of ill-defined symptoms . . . and very changeable. It was a very changeable picture and had a very yielding manner. But from a homoeopathic point of view it was quite a clear picture . . .

Similarly, the disagreement over the second patient became clearer much later as we prepared this paper:

TCM practitioner: I remember having a disagreement with you (the osteopath) over patient X who came in with the sore knees . . . You talked about the structure of her back in relation to her neck, and I talked about other things, seeing it much more as an emotional and depression illness (with) stuck liver and heart . . . I felt that structure followed on from what was going on inside (which is not always the case). And I criticised you because of how absolutely structural, how unbendingly structural, you were with her, and didn't see any of the other stuff.

(I need, in passing, to make two important qualifications to these examples. First, while in the main example I have given the clash was between the homoeopath and the GP, there were equally heated debates between the other clinicians, particularly the homoeopath and the TCM practitioner. Secondly, the members of the group were adamant that they could not be defined simply as osteopath or psychotherapist; each called on a wider range of skills than is simply encompassed by the label of their discipline.)

EXPERIENCES OF THE CLINIC IN THE LIGHT OF MODELS OF POWER

I want now to reflect on these experiences in the light of some of the commonly used models of power that a group facilitator might use to understand what was happening. In making these reflections, and in focusing to some extent on the conflicts which arose in the group, I want to emphasise again that this group of practitioners were intimate colleagues who by and large liked and respected each other. Despite this, conflicts emerged which were not easy to manage.

French & Raven

French & Raven's model of the bases of social power [11] is a basic but still useful starting point. From their analysis, we can identify *reward*

power, as in the ability to provide material or non-material benefits (wages, gifts, approval, love); *legitimate* power, as in the ability to validate or approve behaviour based on acceptance of cultural values and social structure; *referent* power through association or access to a high prestige group; *expert* power in giving advice or help based on particular skills or knowledge; and finally *coercion*, power based on physical force.

We can use this framework to look at the processes involved in the clinic and see that the senior general practitioners (who are responsible for the management of the Health Centre and the policy of the Trust), are in a powerful position in relation to the complementary practitioners. They hold reward power in that they control the work contracts, and thus whether the CPs continue to work at the Health Centre. In addition all GPs hold reward power as gatekeepers for the clinic in that they control access to patients. All GPs hold legitimate power, since they are generally recognised in society as the senior and most prestigious of the healing professions. However, this legitimation is ambiguous: for some CPs there is considerable prestige and kudos to be gained in working for a well known 'holistic' general practice; others are attacked and criticised by their complementary colleagues for joining the 'establishment'. Finally GPs also have expert power based on their professional training and experience in family medicine; they might be described as 'expert generalists'.

In contrast, the complementary practitioners hold primarily expert power, in that they offer skills and competence in their specialised fields of practice. When they experience this expert power as misunderstood and as challenged by the attempt to empower patients at their expense, they naturally respond with vigorous resistance.

This relatively simple analysis based on French & Raven's categories shows that there may be a fundamental power imbalance in a multidisciplinary team. This should lead us to look for ways in which this imbalance may exacerbate differences of opinion or perspective within the team, making them more intransigent. The creative management of differences is of course of particular importance in multidisciplinary teamwork, and so ways must be found to explore these issues and to share power in appropriate ways, and care must be taken not to attack the power bases of any of the practitioner groups. If it is not possible to remove the power imbalances, the group must develop a sophistication such that it is able to attend to and manage them effectively.

Power and group process

A second way of looking at power and power conflicts in a situation such as this is to turn to theories of group process and group development. Generally speaking, it is agreed that groups develop through a series of phases in which certain issues of relationship are dominant and need resolution, often through a crisis in the life of the group. Srivastva et al [12] see group life as primarily concerned with issues of identity and influence. They describe how in the initial phase of group life each member is essentially alone, wondering with considerable anxiety which other members are similar and dissimilar to themselves. This phase gives way to a phase of pairing, in which people reach out to the most similar other, moving away from those they experience as dissimilar. The primary issues here are in *inclusion* and *exclusion*.

If these phases are successfully negotiated, these pairings join together in offensive and defensive cliques, and the group may enter a phase of considerable conflict as these cliques vie for control. This struggle may be very important for the effective life of the group, as fundamental issues of principle and practice are thrashed out. The primary issue here is *influence.*

Again, if these phases are successfully negotiated the hard differences between the cliques will begin to dissolve, and the group will have an opportunity to move into a situation in which all members have an acceptable position and effective voice within the group. The structure of the group can now be seen as a complex network of inter-relationships based on a deep understanding of members' needs and their offerings, and tasks are shared on the basis of skill. The primary issue now is the development of *intimacy.*

Srivastva and his colleagues are at pains to point out that, even though the development of a group can be seen as proceeding through phases in which certain issues become salient, nevertheless all these issues are present to a greater or lesser extent in the life of the group at any particular time. And it is certainly so for the multidisciplinary group at MHC. Issues of inclusion were evident in concerns about being liked or disliked by colleagues, and in concerns about whether one's clinical skills and the practice one represented were being honoured and properly used. To some extent the group could always be characterised as a group of separate practitioners, each with their own skill looking for membership. Issues of influence were expressed in the conflicts about the nature and purpose of the clinic; to some extent the cliques developed as complementary practitioners against the GPs, and this masked some of the conflict between the complementary practitioners themselves. Also, issues of intimacy were expressed in the very genuine regard members of the group had for each other both as individuals and as clinicians, although this was hindered by lack of in-depth understanding of each other's practice.

So from a perspective of group process and development a multidisciplinary team is a very complex animal. Our stance as a cooperative inquiry group helped us to attend to these issues of process, although it is very clear that we could have profitably spent even more time on them than we did. We would recommend that any group of diverse practitioners intending to work together attend very closely to these questions of group process.

Organisational conflicts

A third way to look at questions of power is in terms of the wider organisational processes and the place of the inquiry group within these. There was continual debate at MCT about the role and value of complementary disciplines within general medical practice, about the appropriate allocation of resources and about competing demands on funding. At times these debates were experienced as battles for survival.

The struggle for definitions of reality

However, these perspectives on the power issues within the group do not go far enough or deep enough; there are other more subtle issues to attend to. Listening one day to the tape of a reflection meeting as I prepared it for feedback to the group, I thought to myself, 'I can see the different power bases, I can see the interpersonal, group and organisational conflicts, but something else is going on as well!' I was struck that there was some underlying and unexpressed conflict. My notes at the time read:

My feeling on going through these tapes is that there is a power struggle for defining what this clinic is all about. Yet this power struggle is kept under the table. If it is about empowering the patient, does this imply that the GPs . . . want to disempower the CPs . . . ? Again, if it is about a psychodynamic rather than a clinical intervention, this again disconfirms the GPs' clinical skills. But if it is a clinical setting, does this mean that the GP risks being overshadowed by the CP practice . . . ? What happens, I think, is that the discussion flip-flops between the different definitions of what the clinic is all about . . . because this is the fundamental ground of conflict. The conflict is about practice, about skill, and ultimately about self worth. I think the very design of the clinic has pointed to this fundamental subscript . . . I think therefore that any future clinic, or any model we would offer to the medical and complementary community, would have to take this essentially covert conflict very seriously indeed.

In order to understand this kind of covert power struggle we may turn to Lukes [13] who discusses three dimensions of power. At a very simple level, power can be seen in terms of who gets their way when a disagreement arises: who can make decisions when there is an overt conflict of interests? But this is an over-simplified view, since power is frequently exercised through 'non-decisions'; for example, by preventing issues coming to a public forum for debate and thus 'fixing things' beforehand. In this second dimension, power can be defined in terms of who can control the agendas for public debate, as for example the orthodox medical establishment has attempted to control the debate on complementary practice [14].

However, both these are inadequate views of power for three reasons:

1. Power arises not only in decision-making or non-decision making, but in the overall bias of a social and political system toward consideration of certain issues and the exclusion of others.
2. Power is not only associated with observable conflict, but may also be used to shape desires and opinions and so stop conflict from arising.
3. Power is not only present when there are grievances and differences, since it may be used to shape the way people see their world so that they may accept things as they are because they see no alternative, or because they accept that the way things are is natural and unchangeable.

It seems to me that Lukes' third view of power may help us get a perspective on the power conflicts in the multidisciplinary group. I think it is arguable that there is an underlying power struggle going on for who was to define reality for that group. And by that time I mean not just an argument about role and purpose of the clinic, not just a struggle for self-esteem and recognition by others, although these are both important. I mean a struggle about the ground on which any discussion in the clinic is conducted: whose worldview, whose ontology and epistemology, as well as clinical method, would dominate; and whose would be relegated to a subordinate position. This kind of struggle clearly falls within Lukes' third dimension. The possibility of its resolution lies in the ability of the group to develop a framework of ideas shared among the participants, but this is not at all easy.

The point about struggle is that it is inchoate, confusing, and almost inexpressible. We do not have the language (yet) to explore these issues clearly, and in another paper [15] we have argued that further cooperative inquiry into clinical models in this kind of setting is needed in order to develop such a language. But the struggle surfaces now and again, as in the examples above: the whole group gets into a difficult argument because there is no framework for agreement; or clinicians from different disciplines clash because, while they may agree about what the patient needs, they interpret those needs through quite different frameworks, and bring to the situation fundamentally different assumptions about what an intervention may do.

The symptoms of such a power struggle are the feelings identified above that beyond the interpersonal disagreements and the structural differences something else is around (although these more superficial conflicts will multiply the effects of the deeper ones). People will suddenly find themselves in conflict which they did not expect. They will not be able to express themselves in words clearly. They will feel their world is taken over. I think this might well be called a *paradigmatic* power struggle.

Bateson's theory of learning

We may gain some further illumination on this notion of paradigmatic power by borrowing from Bateson's discussion of logical categories of learning and communication [16]. Bateson bases his work on the theory of logical types, the notion that no class may be a member of itself, and thus that a 'chair' and the 'class of all chairs' are at different levels of logical typing. He argues that many errors of understanding and of communication are caused by failure to see that phenomena are at different logical levels. Using this perspective to discuss the nature of learning, Bateson uses the curious term *Zero Learning* to describe a specific response, as when I 'learn' from the clock striking that it is 6 o'clock. *Learning I* involves changes in *Zero Learning*, as in habituation and rote learning. *Learning II* is a change in the process of *Learning I*, a change in the set of alternatives from which the choice is made, and is therefore about learning how to learn:

the phenomena of *Learning II* can all be included under the rubric of changes in the manner of which the stream of action and experience is segmented or punctuated into contexts together with changes in the use of context markers [16].

For example in acupuncture, *Learning I* might be exemplified by knowing where to insert needles to 'cure' particular symptoms: *Learning II* would involve a wider and deeper understanding of

the theory of Chinese medicine and an ability to apply it creatively to a particular patient.

Beyond *Learning II*, *Learning III* involves a corrective change in the system of sets of alternatives from which the choice is made. So if *Learning I* is habituation, *Learning II* is learning to punctuate and conceptualise experience so that a system of practice can be formulated, then *Learning III* is about moving beyond a system of practice, learning that alternative systems of practice are available and that it is possible to move between them. This means, following our example, being able to see Chinese medicine as one of a set of alternative healing disciplines, to understand their relationships, and being able, in the end, to choose which perspective to take without diluting any of the individual perspectives.

Learning III is not simply moving from one system of practice to another:

it is necessary to distinguish between mere replacement without *Learning III* and that facilitation of replacement which would be truly *Learning III* [16].

Nor is *Learning III* a compromise between systems, or a reduction to a 'lowest common denominator'. Rather, it is a shift of comprehension and of consciousness that permits a more encompassing view of practice.

Now Bateson points out that *Learning III* is a pretty tall order, because it involves going beyond the bondage—and thus beyond the safety—of a particular paradigm, and importantly also beyond the taken-for-granted-sense of self, because the Self is, after all, a pattern of characteristic ways of understanding and acting in the world:

If I stop at the level of *Learning II*, 'I' am the aggregate of those characteristics I call my 'character'. 'I' am my habits of acting in context and shaping and perceiving the contexts in which I act. Selfhood is a product or aggregate of *Learning II*. To the degree a (person) achieves *Learning III*, and learns to perceive and act in terms of the contexts of contexts, (their) 'self' will take on a sort of irrelevance. The concept of 'self' will no longer function as a nodal argument in the punctuation of experience [16].

Learning III, in the context of multidisciplinary groups, concerns the ability to develop and work with *meta-frameworks* which encompass the different clinical frameworks of the group members, show their relationships and enable clinicians to move with some ease between them. Bateson's analysis suggests that in seeking such a meta-framework we need to look for a quite different quality of conceptualising from the frameworks of individual practices.

DISCUSSION

This issue of the management of paradigmatic conflict has serious consequences for multidisciplinary collaboration, and not just in the field of primary health care. The perspective presented in this paper suggests that multidisciplinary practice is very difficult, that it requires highly evolved practitioners who are in significant ways non-attached to their paradigms of practice and to their Self. More than this, it requires a social setting which supports and encourages such detachment: an evolved multidisciplinary group.

We really do not know much about the design and maintenance of such settings, although studies of some religious institutions might help [17]. However, if we consider again the phases of group development discussed above, it would seem that a group whose members are engaged primarily in the self-oriented anxiety of *inclusion*, or the power struggles of the *influence* stage, is unlikely to support the necessary capacity for detachment. Such detachment is more likely to be nurtured in a mature group well into the *intimacy* stage of group development.

What we can also say is that if there are serious imbalances in the bases of power as in the French & Raven analysis (and currently power imbalances between established and complementary medical practice are clearly present and significant), then the development of the group is likely to be hindered. In particular I would suggest that struggles over legitimacy and formal power, or even simply the presence of formal power differentials as in a bureaucratic style of organisation, tend to freeze the development of groups in all organisational settings. They become cautious committees rather than creative teams, 'intermediate' groups as Randall & Southgate [18] describe them, unlikely to be

destructive, but unlikely to be creative either, and certainly unlikely to evolve a culture which will support *Learning III*.

I would also argue that the presence of conflict at the level of Lukes' third dimension of power, or what I have termed here paradigmatic conflict, is likely to throw the group process repeatedly back to concerns about the earlier issues of inclusion. Group members may from time to time feel they are accepted and appreciated members of the group, able to move freely into the contentious space of a group in the influence stage; then the strange misunderstandings that derive from the lack of a shared framework will result in feelings that 'I don't really belong here . . .' These feelings may have almost the formal characteristic of a double bind [19, 20]; one message from the group tells me I am valued and appreciated, while another demonstrates I am totally misunderstood, and I cannot speak clearly about these confusions.

I suggest that there are two possible strategies for working with the impact of these conflicts on the life of a multidisciplinary team. Let me call them the 'realistic' strategy and the 'idealistic' strategy.

The realistic strategy involves accepting that these conflicts will exist and that they will have a limiting impact on the life and work of the group. In order to mitigate their impact, the group will have to pay considerable attention to its process and to the organisational setting in which it works. It needs to find the language to recognise this kind of conflict, to learn to stand back when it arises, and begin to find words to express what is going on. Otherwise what will happen is that the differences may be put down to personal or professional pathology, and the people involved—often the complementary practitioners—may be seen as too difficult to manage by those who hold formal power.

The idealistic strategy aims to move beyond the conflicts to a higher level of group operation. The group and the managers of its organisational setting would make every effort to ensure that structural power differences were removed, and to create an environment in which the group could develop open relationships. The group itself would devote time to those disciplines which help cultivate non-attachment—meditation and other 'mindfulness' exercises. It would devote time to seeking ways of exploring the paradigmatic differences through imaginal and meditative exercises such as those described by Jean Houston [21]. These might facilitate analogic and 'right brain' thinking which may be less attached to an immutable sense of Self, and enable practitioners to find and share images of their healing process. This would add a second and powerful communication channel to the overstrained verbal channels, and maybe through that facilitate new mutual understandings analogous to Learning III, for as Bateson points out, '. . . no amount of rigorous discourse of a given logical type can 'explain' phenomena of a higher type' [16].

The realistic strategy lies within the competence of any reasonably sophisticated group of practitioners, although competent group facilitation is probably essential if it is to be successful. The more ambitious idealistic strategy can only be sketched out as a possibility at the moment, and clearly requires considerable development work before it could be fully implemented.

ACKNOWLEDGEMENTS

I am most grateful to the members of the inquiry team at Marylebone for the privilege of participating in their explorations: Derek Chase, Arnold Desser, Chrissie Melhuish, Sue Morrison, David Peters, Dorothy Wallstein, Vivien Webber; and to Patrick Pietroni as Chairman of the Marylebone Centre Trust who invited me to contribute to the research programme. John Horder, Peter Davies, Judi Marshall and Margaret Stacey read drafts and made helpful comments. This paper was originally presented at the Conference on *Social Aspects of Complementary Medicine*, Keele University, January 1991.

REFERENCES

1. Wallstein D, Desser A, O'Brian J et al. The collaborative assessment of NHS patients by general practitioners and complementary practitioners. London: Marylebone Centre Trust (in preparation).
2. Chase D et al. Paper on the MHC Research Clinic. London: Marylebone Centre Trust (in preparation).
3. Reason P. Human inquiry in action. London: Sage, 1989.
4. Reason P, Rowan J. Human inquiry: a sourcebook of new paradigm research. Chichester: Wiley, 1981.
5. Lincoln S Y, Guba E G. Naturalistic inquiry. Beverly Hills: Sage, 1985.
6. Skolimowski H. The interactive mind in the participatory universe. The World and I, February, 1986.
7. Skolimowski H. The methodology of participation and its consequences. In: Collaborative inquiry, Vol 3. Bath: Centre for the Study of Organisational Change and Development, University of Bath, 1990.
8. Heron J. Philosophical basis for a new paradigm. In: Human inquiry: a sourcebook of new paradigm research, edited by P Reason and J Rowan. Chichester: Wiley, 1988.
9. Macmurray J. The self as agent. London: Faber, 1957.
10. Reason P, Chase D, Desser A et al. The MHC Research Clinic 1989–90: the cooperative inquiry. London: Marylebone Centre Trust, 1991.
11. French J, Raven B. The bases of social power. In: Studies in social power, edited by D D Cartwright. Ann Arbor: University of Michigan, 1959.
12. Srivastva S, Obert S L, Neilson E. Organisational analysis through group processes: a theoretical perspective. In: Organisational development in the UK and USA, edited by C L Cooper.
13. Lukes S. Power: a radical view. London: Macmillan, 1974.
14. British Medical Association. Board of Science and Education. Alternative Therapy. London: BMA, 1986.
15. Reason P, Chase D, Desser A et al. Clinical models for multidisciplinary practice. London: Marylebone Centre Trust, 1991. Also in J Roy Soc Med (in press).
16. Bateson G. The logical categories of learning and communication. In: Steps to an ecology of mind. San Franciso: Chandler, 1972.
17. Goswell M. Motivational factors in the life of a religious community. PhD dissertation: University of Bath, 1988.
18. Randall R, Southgate J. Cooperative and community group dynamics . . . or your meetings needn't be so appalling. London: Barefoot Books, 1980.
19. Bateson G. Toward a theory of schizophrenia. In: Steps to an ecology of mind. San Franciso: Chandler, 1972.
20. Laing R D. Self and others. London: Tavistock, 1961.
21. Houston J. The possible human. Los Angeles: Tarcher, 1982.

COMMUNICATION IN CANCER CARE—A REFLECTIVE LEARNING MODEL USING GROUP RELATIONS METHODS

Harriet Meek
Marilyn Pietroni

INTRODUCTION

In this paper we discuss a series of working seminars which were organised to explore the communication which takes place or needs to take place in the care of people who have cancer. Special attention is given to the application of a group relations approach in designing the reflective learning model used in the seminars.

The seminars were held at the Commonwork Centre, near Edenbridge, Kent, about an hour from London. The comfort of the accommodation, beauty of the surroundings and removal from the bustle of the world were important in establishing a containing environment for the work of the weekend.

SEMINAR DESIGN

From their experience as doctor and psychotherapist, patient and relative, respectively, the seminar organisers believe that many of the communication difficulties which take place in cancer treatment emerge because of the primitive nature of anxiety produced in both patient and care-giver as a result of their common preoccupation with a death-dealing illness. They felt that if a psychologically similar framework to that of the cancer patient and care-giver could be created within the seminars it might be possible to examine this anxiety and the associated communication difficulties at a more reflective distance than that provided by home, hospital or consulting room.

The reflective learning model of replicating and testing out in a practical way the study situation was developed largely from the field of group relations which forms a temporary institution to study its own functioning as a means of better understanding organisational life (Bion 1975, Miller & Rice 1975, Rice 1975, Bridger 1978). While it is usual to look into rational and irrational processes which take place in organisations during group relations conferences, it is perhaps less usual to apply these techniques to a topic such as the investigation of communication in health care. Perhaps this is especially so if the membership boundary is extended (as in this instance to be described) to include patients, relatives and representatives of self-help groups as well as a variety of staff from in-patient and out-patient professional teams.

MEMBERSHIP

Four residential weekend seminars took place, with 20 participants in each. As Table 6.5 shows, a broad cross-section of participants were invited. During each weekend a balance of professional and lay participants were present. Initially the names of those invited were selected by staff and later were provided by participants themselves. There was no charge for participation although donations were accepted.

In addition to the stated roles in which participants defined themselves and for which

Table 6.5 Seminar membership

Participants	
Patients	7
Relatives	7
Self-help group workers	4
Nurses	13
Medical	17
General practitioners	6
Hospice doctors	1
Hospital doctors	2
Medical students	8
Complementary therapists	10
Social workers	2
Psychology students	1
Researchers	2

they were selected ('patient', 'relative', 'doctor', 'nurse', 'alternative care-giver' etc) it soon emerged that several professionals also were, or had been, patients or relatives of someone who was suffering from or had died from cancer. Thus common assumptions about the professional/personal role boundaries were called into question. Once made explicit within the seminars, this discovery fostered an atmosphere of mutual understanding between participants.

Members were assigned to one of two small groups on the basis of their initially stated roles. In deciding which participants should be invited to a particular weekend, an attempt was made to provide a similar broad mix of background and experience in each small group and within the membership of each weekend.

The basic staff team for each weekend seminar comprised two facilitators and two research recorders. A staff facilitator and researcher were assigned to each group. Additional continuity was provided by the presence of several staff members at all four seminars. For a Saturday evening event only, a creative therapist (once a massage therapist and another time an art therapist) was present.

In the UK this is a novel staff team for work which is derived from a group relations approach, just as it is also fairly unusual to combine a group relations approach with other methods of inquiry and learning within the same event. The staff team and the combination of methods represented both the funders' and organisers' commitment to address body as well as mind in seminars on such themes as this one. So, let us look more closely at the timetable, methods and design of the seminars.

Participants arrived at the Centre on Friday evening. Dinner was followed by simple opening exercises designed to enable people to leave their work behind and emotionally to enter the seminar event and prepare for the task ahead. No other formal activity was planned for the first evening, which allowed participants to meet off duty under relatively relaxed conditions prior to the anticipated intensity of the weekend's work.

The important feature is the small group timetable. As Box 6.3 shows, the timetable of small group meetings which began on Saturday morning followed thematically the progression of a cancer

---

Box 6.3 Timetable and method

Friday evening

7.30–9.00 p.m.	*Supper*
9.00–10.30	Large group I: semi-structured entry group

Saturday

8.15–9.00 a.m.	*Breakfast*
9.00–9.30	Plenary I: beginning
9.30–10.45	Small group I: first knowledge
10.45–11.00	*Break*
11.00–12.45 p.m.	Small group II: bad news
12.45–3.00	*Lunch*
3.00–4.15	Small group III: from out-patient to in-patient (change of room and facilitator)
4.15–4.45	*Break*
4.45–7.00	Large group I: semi-structured activity group (e.g. art therapy; massage)
7.00–9.15	*Supper*
9.15–10.30	Optional evening event (e.g. talk)

Sunday:

9.00–9.30 a.m.	*Breakfast*
9.30–10.45	Small group IV: at home and at work, facing remission, anxiety or death (change of room and facilitator)
10.45–11.00	*Break*
11.00–12.30 p.m.	Small group V: continuation of IV or theme decided by membership
12.30–1.00	Plenary II: ending and review
1.15–2.30	*Lunch*

---

patient from initial diagnosis to in-patient treatment, discharge, then on to recovery or death.

Participants and staff were given the two-fold small group task continually used by Harold Bridger during group relations conferences, namely *investigate a topic and examine the here-and-now processes which take place as you do so*. The facilitators' task was to ensure that each small group worked at both aspects of this task, especially when anxiety was high and communication became more difficult.

The plenaries at 'top and toe' were, in contrast, actively led and more conceptual in approach. This provided a chance for an initial brainstorming of issues and an end-point review.

The small groups were therefore more ortho-dox group relations events—unstructured and freely associative, albeit around specific themes. The facilitators' method in the small groups (in contrast to the plenaries) was reflective, often using here-and-now content and process as a basis for interpreting pre-conscious and uncon-scious material and linking it to the prior and current experiences of participants, both profes-sional and lay.

The small groups focused in sequence on the following themes (see Box 6.3):

1. On Saturday:
    i. First knowledge
    ii. Bad news
    iii. Transfer of care from out-patient to in-patient *(members moved rooms and changed facil-itators at this point; the group membership remained the same)*
2. On Sunday:
    i. At home and at work *(members returned to their original room and facilitator)*
    ii. Facing death or remission with uncertainty.

Each small group focus represented a phase in the experience of cancer care and generated similar anxieties in patients, relatives and professionals alike. Some of the communication difficulties common at each stage of care emerged during the seminars, allowing further exploration. The points at which communication broke down or became difficult undoubtedly highlighted areas in which, in real life, particular care needs to be taken.

Again, in contrast to the small groups, a large group activity session was held late Saturday afternoon on pain relief. One weekend this con-sisted of a 'hands-on' lesson in simple massage; another weekend an art therapy session was included. Both the periods of relaxation and 'free' time, and the 'hands-on' sessions were important in providing a chance to reflect inter-nally on the weightiness of the small group work.

The Sunday morning small group session saw a return to the original room and facilitator, mir-roring the patient's return home to face the uncer-tainties of remission or the further upheavals of recurrence. This session produced particularly clear communication and uncluttered truths, per-haps because it followed a close examination of the turbulence produced by the moves, the inti-macy of the off-duty time and body or image work and a chance to sleep and to dream.

The final plenary provided an opportunity to gather emotional understandings and conceptu-alise issues identified during previous discus-sions. After a relaxed lunch, participants departed, allowing a few hours of weekend time at home. This proved to be a very powerful model but one which was also very containing.

A THEORETICAL BRIDGE

At this point, we would like to change gear slightly and mark out a theoretical framework suggested by the raw material of the seminars, with regard both to their thematic *content* and to the *changing atmosphere* of communication between participants. In the light of this theoretical framework, the thematic content will then be mapped into areas of convergent understanding and areas of divergence between participants. The *changing atmosphere* will be used as a kind of diagnostic tool or barometer which indicates the presence of different levels of anxiety in the membership associated with more or less primi-tive states of mind.

Theoretically the content and changing atmo-sphere of the seminars was reminiscent of the patterns and rhythms of clinical work described by Bion (after Klein) in his formulation of the paranoid-schizoid/depressive anxiety continuum (Ps<->D). This formulation is used by Bion (and after him by Donald Meltzer) to describe changing states of mind that reflect temporary shifts in the nature of internal object relationships.

At one end of the continuum, paranoid-schizoid anxiety prevails and is associated with part-object relationships in which only one small aspect of a relationship can be seen (such as the satisfying or frustrating aspect), at the expense of all others. Paranoid anxiety is thus usually associated with an intense and rigid identifica-tion with a single viewpoint, a loss of the capacity to reflect, and a concomitant loss of concern, empathy or understanding of another. Such primitive anxiety is also associated with particular forms of *mental organisation*, characterised by primitive forms of splitting and projection and, at worst, fragmentation. As a result, as Bion vividly describes in several papers, the atmosphere becomes chaotic and brittle, and thought processes become impoverished and concretised and sometimes disordered.

At the other end of the continuum, so-called depressive anxiety is associated with whole-object relationships in which dependence on others, and even more importantly, *interdependence* can be recognised and mainly tolerated. A less omnipotent atmosphere prevails so identifications are firm without being brittle or rigid. In this state of mind, creative intercourse of all kinds becomes possible since there is a genuine interest in individual differences and the potential for complementarity and new connections arising from them. *Mental organisation* at this end of the continuum is also rather different. The tendency toward splitting, fragmentation, and primitive forms of projection and identification is diminished, so the integrity (or unity) of self and other is more enduring. Thus an atmosphere is created in which it is possible to bear, and even to be interested in, significant differences between people or points of view and to reflect and even to learn from these differences. Bion goes on to propose that the capacity for depressive anxiety and hence for sustaining states of mind in which whole-object relationships predominate can be fostered by the quality of *containment* provided for the bits and pieces of the self cast out under duress. Containment is provided by a kind of free floating attention which Bion calls 'reverie' (Bion 1978).

In the seminars on Communication in Cancer Care it was therefore also a task of the facilitators to sustain their own reverie in order to provide a quality of containment so that even the most difficult differences could be noted, borne, and attended to by the participants.

Taking this theoretical perspective (and also bearing in mind the title of this conference: Community or Chaos), I hope it is now possible to examine some of the content and changing atmosphere in more depth, noting when there

was convergence and participants worked together as a heterogeneous community, and where there was divergence and even a threatened chaos when very high levels of anxiety were present.

CHAOS

Let us begin with the chaos. Perhaps not surprisingly, one of the peak moments of anxiety was when the small groups had to change both rooms and facilitators, mirroring the external real-life shift between out-patient and in-patient treatments. In spite of very simple and clear instructions, several people went to the wrong rooms altogether, some failed to recognise members of their own group with whom they had been working throughout and who had shared the move with them, and one or two became very hostile towards the new facilitator or retrospectively towards the one they had left behind. When the link between the transference and the real-life situation was made by the facilitators, a quite profound exploration of the experience became possible with evident working through on the part of some participants. Retrospectively, hospital staff or hospital care could be 'forgiven' a little for being so different from family and home; consultant physicians and other hospital specialists were recognised and understood as people doing very difficult jobs in very difficult circumstances.

Similarly, on the Sunday morning, when the groups returned to their *original* room and facilitator, instead of feeling simply relieved to be back, several participants expressed a further sense of loss and disorientation similar to that experienced when discharged home from hospital. This experience somewhat surprised the members and gave rise to further exploration of the depth of disorientation they felt and how it interfered with apparently straightforward communications.

There were several other moments when the dynamic relationship between past experience and the seminar experience was dramatically enacted in chaotic communication, but rather than go into these in detail, we will now move on to other areas of convergence and divergence, since these will provide a more complete view of the content and changing atmosphere in the seminars.

CONVERGENT THEMES: A SENSE OF COMMUNITY

Convergent here means that a significant amount of either agreement or mutual understanding across differences was established between participants, regardless of whether they were lay or professional and regardless of status or role. The convergent themes have been divided into conscious and unconscious to differentiate between material brought by participants themselves in a fairly straightforward way and those inferred by the facilitators as a result of the content and the changing atmosphere during the course of the seminars. It will not be possible to go into all of these themes in detail, so one or two will be selected from each figure.

CONVERGENT THEMES: CONSCIOUS

During the first two small group sessions, focused on 'First knowledge' and 'Bad news', participants readily came to recognise a shared pressure regardless of role or status—the pressure of omnipotence. Patients felt their lives were under threat. Relatives felt they were going to lose someone close to them. Professionals felt their expertise—their sense of professional survival—was under fire. Each recognised the tendency to *seek* power and control when what they *felt* was fear, a certain amount of helplessness and confusion. Each participant recognised his/her different but often parallel quest for knowledge, when at best he/she could know only a part of the whole picture and at worst had to live with long periods of uncertainty or ignorance. It was not difficult for professional and lay members to recognise these shared defensive patterns and to see how easily communication in the consulting room could flounder as a result of the level of anxiety with which they were grappling and the brittle, tense atmosphere it generated.

A less expected but nevertheless also consciously convergent theme was the discovery of a mirroring process between the hierarchical structure of the professional team and power relationships in the family. Thus patients present at the seminars complained of the god-like scarcity of hospital consultants in contrast to the greater availability of minor hospital doctors and nursing staff. Patients found it frustrating that their reasonable questions were often evaded by junior hospital doctors and nursing staff, only to be answered briefly and sometimes abruptly or even brutally by senior doctors who then disappeared from sight for days at a time, leaving them with no chance to follow up on the dialogue after further reflection.

On the other hand, hospital staff and family practitioners described how it was sometimes difficult to decide to whom bad news should first be given—to spouse or to patient, for example. What if the patient wanted to know all, but the relative, also present at the consultation, produced vigorous reassurance even when given clear cues by the doctor that all was not well? Consultation time after all was scarce. Should they break the family hierarchy there and then to provide the information the patient was apparently asking for? And was it appropriate to do so? Or should they wait until later when they could catch the patient alone?

That doctors and nurses could discuss these dilemmas with patients and relatives in the room was very moving. It drew the small group together in recognition of their common problems and their desire for communication rather than isolation. It would probably not have been possible however, had they not already discovered that bad news often makes the holder, whether lay or professional, feel extremely lonely, even isolated with it, like carrying some sort of nasty poison around that would do damage if let out of its container.

It was by no means agreed that diagnostic bad news once established, should be given out always, or as a rule. Sharp differences of opinion emerged here. Members reluctantly accepted that all they could agree was that there were no rules in this respect, except that individuals are unique and the art of communication in cancer care lies in recognising this and relating to the individual patient accordingly.

It was perhaps surprising that early on in each seminar a distinction was made between different meanings of the end of life. For some, the end of life was clearly and simply death itself, no more, no less. For others, the end of life was like investigating a subtle question with different layers of meaning in relation to body, mind and spirit. For them death was tolerable if life itself was felt to have meaning right to the end and so on. Although vast, these emotional and philosophical differences seemed to be recognised and accepted as a fact of communal life.

CONVERGENT THEMES: UNCONSCIOUS

The unconscious themes, as previously explained, have been inferred by the facilitators on the basis of the content of the small group discussions. They will therefore only be briefly outlined here since, though they may seem fairly obvious, they were not discussed with participants. It is important to remember that the seminars were brief and their task was investigative rather than psychotherapeutic. We believe this distinction over task is a very important one—as important as it is in all forms of all group relations work. Participants were not psychotherapy patients and staff were facilitators and not clinicians.

Just two of the unconscious themes held largely in common were as follows:

1. Patients, relatives and professionals were clearly engaged in working relationships that were saturated with phantasies of the hero-doctor-god, the saintly nurse, the patient who was damned and beyond salvation and the relative doomed to suffer in purgatory. Phantasies of the father-doctor, mother-nurse and child-patient were also present. These phantasies often structured the power relationships in the room and seemed to restrict communication. It is at times difficult to ask a doctor-god questions when he appears in person, or to hate a saintly nurse who reminds you of someone who has caused you to suffer some unpleasant treatment procedure. Better to regard that treatment as a penance, a form of necessary cleansing than a wilful treatment intervention.

2. Other phantasies concerned the cancer itself. Patients and relatives spoke freely of cancer of all kinds as if it were not only a malignant disease but also a malevolent one, actively malicious, devouring and insatiable, almost human in fact. Professionals spoke of different cancers with more apparent precision but their comments, and indeed the professional language itself, conveyed the sense of being engaged in a struggle with something actually aggressive with which they were at war or by which they were sometimes beaten.

Each party here seemed locked into its own phantastic [sic] script that limited its capacity for reflection, for understanding the other parties and hence for communication.

DIVERGENT THEMES

Splits and reversals will be addressed in more detail under the heading of divergent themes. Needless to say, nearly all participants were caught in polarised thinking at some point during the weekend. Thus hospitals were 'very bad' or 'very good', doctors even more so. The strength of transferences at work in the doctor–patient relationship, whether in hospital or during home-care, was utterly tangible and deserves to be the central topic of another paper. Yet participants varied greatly in the extent to which they sensed the complexities at work here. For many, it must be said, hospitals and doctors were simply by definition 'bad' and the programmed shift of room and of facilitator proved it, rather than illuminating certain aspects of why this was so. For them, the atmosphere surrounding these issues was totally rigid. To question their viewpoint, or to hold another, seemed to threaten both individual and group with chaos through the breakdown of communal understandings and respect for differences.

There was also significant divergence of views over the right of relatives and the management of information, over the value of orthodox treatment and its underlying phantasised meanings and over the efficacy and appropriateness of image work and positive thinking or the dangers of negative thinking. One vivid example here was a young woman who came with her husband. Early in the session they announced that they had transformed her cancer themselves when they christened it Daisy and made it a friend instead of a foe in their minds, such was the power of positive thinking. The small group atmosphere became acutely anxious when these ideas were often repeated by this couple as the only worthwhile view, a panacea for all—'You too can make friends with your cancer and cure it' they seemed to say. Meanwhile the rest of the group was left to carry the scepticism, fear and helplessness and, of course, the anger. The facilitator had to work very hard to help the group restore a more flexible atmosphere in which individual differences of view could be tolerated and clinical realities of different kinds could be recognised and borne.

SUMMARY

In summary, the seminars can be said to have mapped a number of unconscious dilemmas along the paranoid-schizoid/depressive continuum. When the dilemmas were recognised communication deepened. When major differences emerged, the atmosphere changed, and became brittle and defensive, the content was split or fragmented and the participants could easily have gone to war with each other had containment not been provided.

These dilemmas can be summarised as follows:

1. To tolerate differences of all kinds or to split and polarise?
2. To bear mutual understanding and misunderstandings or to provide fake solutions and pressure to be adopted by all?
3. To go on negotiating transition and loss in spite of pain, anger, and helplessness or to become fragmented, confused and disoriented?
4. To listen, to see and to try to understand or to become emotionally deaf, blind or numb?
5. To struggle with uncertainty, human limitations and multiple points of view or to

become and remain addicted to a single viewpoint?

ACKNOWLEDGEMENTS

This work was made possible through a bequest from the Neil Wates Memorial Trust. Neil Wates spent his early working years with the London-based Wates building firm where he put into practice his special interest in the social responsibilities of business. Later, he explored environmentally sound farming techniques, supported various master craft and research projects and established a centre for meditation. His core philosophy was one of conscientious stewardship, responsive to the needs and potentials of people, the land and the environment.

A group of friends, relatives and colleagues had joined together in late 1985 to learn from the manner of Neil Wates' death. When they did so the focus which emerged was communication: the *communication* that took place—and that failed to take place—during his short illness and sudden death. It was decided to initiate this series of seminars to commemorate his life and the manner of his death. We thank the Trust for its generosity.

We would like also to thank Dr Patrick Pietroni, who jointly with Marilyn Pietroni, planned and directed the seminars, and Ms Anne Kilcoyne, who provided editorial advice and assistance on a monograph, on which some of this article is based.

REFERENCES

Bion W 1975 Selections from 'Experiences in groups'. In: Group Relations Reader 1. Coleman A D, Bexton H (eds). A K Rice Institute, Washington D. C.
Bion W 1978a The differentiation of the psychotic from the non-psychotic personality. In: Second thoughts. Heinemann, London
Bion W 1978b Language and schizophrenic thought, op. cit.
Bridger H 1978 Personal communication and unpublished paper on organisational change
Miller J, Rice A K 1975 Selections from 'Systems of organisation'. In: Group Relations Reader 1. Colman A D, Bexton H (eds). A K Rice Institute, Washington D. C.
Rice A K 1975 Selections from 'Learning for leadership'. In: Group Relations Reader 1. Coleman A D, Bexton H (eds). A K Rice Institute, Washington D. C.

CREATIVE COLLABORATION: INTERPROFESSIONAL LEARNING PRIORITIES IN PRIMARY HEALTH AND COMMUNITY CARE

Jill Spratley
Marilyn Pietroni

This is a shortened version of a report of a project undertaken by the Marylebone Centre Trust on behalf of CCETSW. The authors wish to thank CCETSW and Marylebone Centre Trust for the funding of this project.

INTRODUCTION

This report describes an action research project in the field of interprofessional training and education, developed and carried out in late 1992 by the Marylebone Centre Trust (MCT).

The aims were as follows:

1. To identify interprofessional learning priorities as seen by a wide range of contributors in professional development and training; policy; service organisation, management and delivery; carers' and users' networks.
2. To provide information concerning an approach to interprofessional learning developed by the Postgraduate Development Team at Marylebone Centre Trust (MCT).

A workshop method was used in which a range of workers were invited from the fields of primary health and community care to one of two workshops. Participants were asked to present for scrutiny current work projects which involved a high degree of collaboration across professional and agency boundaries. They were asked to identify what helped and what hindered collaboration, and to consider the implications for interprofessional training and education.

The key issues which emerged were recorded by a rapporteur, were later confirmed by the par-

Reproduced with kind permission from the Marylebone Centre Trust.

ticipants and were amended where necessary. The discussion and non-verbal behaviour were also noted by a non-participant observer, who identified notable areas of agreement, difference and conflict. The observers' findings were also fed back to participants to cross-check the data at the workshop. Follow-up sessions were held in which preliminary findings were presented to participants for their information and further review. Portfolios of work in process were also circulated as part of this model of collaborative research and the workshops as a whole were evaluated. This structured framework for the workshops enabled staff and participants to undertake specific roles and tasks, supported by the research management team. The project took place against a backcloth of great expansion in collaborative work and in interprofessional education and training.

The focus of the second aim was to confirm or modify an outline multiprofessional, post-qualifying curriculum at Masters level, developed by a team at MCT in the same year. This curriculum drew on reflective approaches to learning which included the use of observational study and small group work.

An interim report on the project presented to CCETSW by Jill Spratley (1992) described the proposed methods, the workshop participants, and the key issues to be addressed.

BACKGROUND TO INTER-PROFESSIONAL EDUCATION AND TRAINING

Developments in interprofessional practice, policy and organisation

The need for increased cooperation between the various agencies and professions which provide health and social care services was recognised a long time ago, perhaps most notably with the Report on the Enquiry into the Death of Maria Colwell (DHSS 1974). Of late, however, this need has emerged as a priority.

Since 1985 a number of key organisations have been established whose main aim is to foster collaboration and communication between professionals. These include the European Network for

Multiprofessional Education (1987); the joint CCETSW and ENB initiative in London and the South-East (1985); the umbrella organisation drawing the UK network together, known as the Centre for the Advancement of Interprofessional Education (CAIPE) (1987); the Marylebone Centre Trust (MCT) carrying out integrated practice, training and research (1988); the Centre for Interprofessional Studies in Nottingham (CIPS) (1989); Continuing Care at Home (Concah) (1990); and the Royal College of General Practitioners' (RCGP) Primary Care Alliance (1993) and Commission on Primary Care (1993). The aims, objectives and mission statements of all of these organisations highlight as watchwords the three Cs: communication, collaboration, and—much more difficult to achieve—cooperation. In addition, an annotated bibliography on Interprofessional Collaboration and Education has also been published by CAIPE (Toase 1991) and has been recently updated.

All this activity follows a pathway signposted some years earlier by a policy development group consisting of CCETSW, the then Council for Training in Health Visiting (CTHV) and the RCGP. In 1971 these three bodies circulated a joint letter to all course leaders recommending that 'regional arrangements be made for interdisciplinary meetings for discussion of common interests and problems ...' However, the difficulty of promoting collaborative training at that time was clearly indicated when only two groups responded. Undaunted, the policy development group continued its work. Two national meetings were held: in 1974 at the University of Nottingham and in 1975 at Cumberland Lodge. This relatively unknown strand in the history of interprofessional collaboration was reported by Flack (1976a, b) and reviewed recently by Thwaites (1993).

A study commissioned by CAIPE and carried out between 1987 and 1988 revealed 695 joint training initiatives, although over half were of a day's duration or less. A survey of the more substantial courses at Masters degree level was subsequently commissioned by the Journal of Interprofessional Care, launched by Marylebone Centre Trust in 1991. Undertaken by Janet Storrie, the survey revealed at least 15 higher education establishments offering higher degree courses in which interprofessional understanding and cooperation formed a significant focus. However, only two made these the main focus and only one of the programmes had started before 1990.

This massive expansion of interest had followed a series of government reports mainly concerned with child protection and published since the Maria Colwell Inquiry. These reports had brought the need for interprofessional cooperation to the top of the training and educational agenda (Jasmine Beckford (Brent 1985), Tyra Henry (Lambeth 1987), Kimberley Carlile (Greenwich 1987)). Subsequently, the Cleveland Inquiry (DHSS 1988) highlighted the issue of how individual professional decision-making and local agency policies determine communication and outcomes for better and for worse. The Department of Health's Working Together (1991) consolidated the findings of these inquiries.

Recognition of the need for better collaboration, however, spread far beyond the specialist field of child protection into other areas of specialist practice such as mental health, work with HIV/AIDS clients and elderly and disabled people. In fact, collaboration became a key issue in the direction of all health and community care services. Each profession was seeking to put its own house in order in this respect. When work tasks were re-examined it became obvious that, for services to be sensitive to the needs of users and to be genuinely influenced by their views, more cooperation was essential. It was also important to take seriously the related but often marginalised issues of user-participation and community development (Croft & Beresford 1992). The question of what part these issues should play in the overall stage of collaboration is, however, in practice a complex issue requiring specialist skills. Nevertheless, recent policy changes have ensured that such issues have moved from the margin to centre stage.

Changes in philosophy and legislation

Definitions of interprofessional collaboration have thus widened to reflect a more democratising philosophy, with reduced emphasis on professional hierarchies and their privileged areas of knowledge, information and skill. The idea of partnership between professions and agencies and with users and carers, whether in practice, training, or research, has increasingly found its way into many training strategy documents: those of health and local authorities, and in the mission statements of voluntary organisations and community trusts. A fundamental review of the role of professional knowledge and of the social hierarchy of professions and professionals is now taking place. This review has been developing in the individual professions over many years, notably in the Barclay Report (1982), Neighbourhood Nursing (Cumberlege 1986), and A New Kind of Doctor (Hart 1988).

These separate signposts were consolidated by three government reports which produced something like an overall map of the new integrative philosophies and practices: Community Care: an Agenda for Action (1988) (otherwise known as the Griffiths Report), Working for Patients (DoH 1989), and Caring for People (DHSS 1989).

Inevitably major legislative change soon followed. The Children Act 1989 centred the new partnership philosophy, and the NHS and Community Care Act 1990 charged all who were working in health and community care to work and plan together.

The reasons for increased pressure to work together were evident in all fields of practice, but the lack of professional management in social services and community health had also become a matter of serious concern. For the last 5 years management has therefore dominated training agendas and serious attempts are now being made to establish hard information from which priorities can be appropriately formulated. The high costs of inefficient services with poor information systems working in isolation from each other could not continue: poor communication was not only bad for the quality of services, it also affected the cost and quantity.

The NHS and Community Care Act 1990 brought about a fundamental re-organisation of resource and service management which extended the sphere of collaboration further still. Health and social care services were each structurally divided into purchasers and providers in an internal 'market' of care. This fundamental change meant that it was no longer possible to keep information about costs administratively separate from professional decision-making. As a result, the cost, volume and quality of services are now being linked at all levels of the health and social care systems. As an additional consequence, various forms of joint commissioning and joint service contracting have emerged, and the interprofessional training agenda, already greatly stretched, must now also include these forms of interagency collaboration. The purchaser/provider split has also, incidentally, put the development of information systems and their subsequent management on to the collaborative agenda. No longer can interprofessional and interagency collaboration be left to local inclination and habitual practices: it has become a matter of law, good management and technology.

These changes were no ordinary changes but expressed fundamental shifts in philosophy. They changed training priorities, brought new approaches to practice and generated new forms of organisation and management. They also increased conflict and ambiguity in the value-base of public health and welfare services. For example, Griffiths' proposal to increase the use of volunteers seemed likely to mitigate the excesses of professionalism and, at first sight, to increase cost-effectiveness as well; on the other hand and more cynically, it was widely viewed as a return to the values and practices of the nineteenth century and a means of providing dignified occupation for unemployed people. Another example is the increased emphasis on audit which has provided tighter linking between the volume, quality and cost of services. The results have made some feel that all that matters is counting and accounting: others see it as a chance to substantiate in hard terms the quality of the services they are providing and to strengthen their claims on the resource cake.

Competence is another issue which has risen to the top of the agenda as a result of changes in training policy. Hitherto, although nurse training had been substantially practice-based, most professional education had been based in educational institutions, often criticised for its remoteness from practice and from the priorities of employing agencies. The National Council for Vocational Qualifications, a government-led initiative, challenged this tradition by creating new, more generic and work-based learning pathways in health and social care. More flexible career paths should eventually result. Access to qualification and to professional education has already increased, notably for carers. Some have argued, however, that this change has been a covert way of securing cheap and tame labour without the high expenses and professional autonomy produced by college-based training. Nevertheless, a new national system for evaluating and accrediting work-based learning has been established. Whatever the cynics say, vocational education could revolutionise the relationship between practice, training and qualification, and produce a more truly integrated workforce which is used to seeing health and social care as one field. The issue of collaboration and learning could therefore, in the long term, be dramatically transformed.

In vocational education the emphasis is on the *connections* between fields of practice and knowledge right from the start, whereas professional education has usually been concerned to define fields of practice in which knowledge, roles, skills and identities are seen as unique. In the process of professional education participants are socialised into *separate* classes with a recognised place in the overall social structure.

These transformations in how we think about what we do in the fields of primary health and community care, and what approaches to learning are appropriate for that work, reflect deep social and philosophical changes. At the beginning of the twentieth century it was expected and accepted, fairly generally, that authority and dominance rested with the sciences; therefore areas of practice that had their roots in science, such as medicine, were automatically accorded high status. At the end of the century there exists a very different environment where uncertainty has been raised to the height of a scientific prin-

ciple. Philosophically our understanding of the world is that it is constructed by the particular viewpoint taken, itself determined by our cultural position and the language most available to us. Accordingly, all our perceptions and understandings are by definition prejudiced in favour of what is familiar. Within this new paradigm we recognise how difficult it is to know or properly understand what is outside our system, and that communication and development depend on our continual attempts to do so.

Finance for interprofessional education

Unfortunately, finance does not always follow integrative changes in educational philosophy and government policy. Thus the budgets available for postgraduate or post-qualifying training, whether or not it is of a collaborative nature, are somewhat fragmented between professions. GPs can access a Postgraduate Education Allowance (PGEA) conditional upon fulfilling an approved PGEA programme covering specific topic areas; this individual budget is additional to the budgets that underpin the GP regional training system (Meek & Pietroni 1991). The Vocational Training Scheme represents a key professional development resource in General Practice. In contrast, social work training at all levels is dependent upon the spending priorities of individual employers; training support funds are channelled from the Department of Health to employing agencies under specific client group headings such as child protection, learning difficulties and HIV/AIDS; however, a proportion of such funds are likely to be spent on collaborative aspects of this specialist work. Although post-qualifying training consortia in social work are currently being established, it is a very slow process and collaborative training is consequently still very low on the agendas of these consortia. The picture is slightly better for the community nursing disciplines; regional health authorities do provide grant support for selected training programmes, whether short or substantial, within and beyond the accredited systems of nurse training. The key issue here, however, is that nurses and social workers are bureau-profes-sionals who work to agency policies and agency training priorities in a much more specific way than the relatively autonomous GP. Thus, individual training allowances are not allocated at national level for social workers or nurses who wish to set their own training priorities within an overall approved training system.

Conceptual models

An excellent analysis of interprofessional and interagency training (Hey, Minty & Trowell 1991) draws on several different models of collaboration in practice:

1. Davidson (1983), who uses a typology based on degrees of collaboration:
   i. communication and consultation
   ii. cooperation
   iii. coordination
   iv. federation and teamwork
   v. merger.
2. Tibbit (1988), who builds on this typology to create a matrix by adding differentiations based on three organisational levels:
   i. service delivery
   ii. operational management
   iii. strategic planning.
3. Kane (1976), who analyses the knowledge, skills and attitudes required of members of interprofessional teams (Hey et al, p. 199).

Together with Huntington's study of social work and general practice (1981), which analyses the structural and cultural aspects of interprofessional collaboration, this history of past and present conceptual work in this field is impressive, although it is surprisingly under-used in practice and training settings.

In conclusion: from conflict to creativity

It has to be recognised that the history of inter-professional and interagency collaboration is, in practice, littered with disasters and discontents (Kilcoyne & Pietroni 1990). Partly, this is because the three key professions of medicine, nursing and social work have different histories and cultures, and are engaged in different tasks; their activities may interact, but their legislative frameworks, languages, values and emotional priorities are often quite different.

In the pages that follow it becomes clear, however, that the cynics and pessimists are not altogether right. Collaboration between agencies, professionals, carers and the users of services themselves gives to all concerned a sense of creativity that is missing when people work in isolation. Moreover, such collaboration goes some way towards recognising, and even creating, the kind of multi-perspective and multi-cultural practice that policy rhetoric can only signal.

THE WORKSHOPS

Preparation

The research project was designed as a collaborative inquiry using two consultative workshops which were structured to promote participative working. The workshops were held in early autumn 1992. They provided a forum in which interprofessional and interagency approaches to learning and working could be explored in some detail and during which there would be time for reflection.

The potential participants were identified through a mapping exercise which took account of local community health and social services, as well as networks in the voluntary sector, including carers and users. In order to examine a range of experience, representatives were invited from different organisational levels and different types of collaborative work.

A total of 128 invitations were despatched resulting in 64 replies (50%), and of these 40 individuals were seriously interested but unable to attend. A total of 24 participants were finally involved in the two workshops, with 15 attending workshop I, and nine attending workshop II. Members finally included representatives from Social Services, the Health Service, carer organisations, the voluntary sector, and educational institutions.

Significantly, all of the workshop presentations were offered spontaneously at the application stage, in response to a general invitation to incorporate participants' own material. Clearly this suggested that the participants were keen to talk about their work with interested others.

Feedback at the recruitment stage also suggested that the opportunity offered by the workshops for review and discussion of current work was very welcome. Unfortunately, factors such as workload and lack of replacement cover made it difficult to take up that opportunity. Interestingly, many people wrote or telephoned to explain these problems in some detail and asked if other opportunities would arise in the future.

Each workshop programme consisted of a one-day session, followed by a half-day follow-up meeting after a short period.

The questions

Throughout their presentations and discussions, participants were asked to keep in mind four key questions concerning interprofessional working and learning. The questions were:

1. What makes interprofessional collaboration work well?
2. What hinders interprofessional work?
3. What are the key issues or themes in interprofessional work?
4. What are the key interprofessional development needs and training priorities?

Staffing roles

An important aspect of the process management of the workshops was the inclusion of a staff support resource. Each small group was serviced by three staff members in specific roles: observer, facilitator and rapporteur. The facilitator and rapporteur fulfilled the functions of managing and recording the group work. The observer took a relatively non-participative role but prompted the small groups to reflect at the end of the first day on process issues witnessed during their work. Briefing notes were provided and briefing meetings held for those undertaking the staff roles. During the workshops, opportunities were created for brief periods of staff reflection in order to monitor and support the progress of the event.

The one-day event began with some brief input relating to the workshop aims, the programme structure, staff roles and the group work which formed the major part of the day's activities.

The presentations

The key events of the day were the brief presentations offered by participants, which formed the basis for group discussion. A wide range of topics were invited by the research team for these presentations, including interprofessional and interagency research, training, policy development, service management or organisation, service delivery, and users' or carers' experiences of collaborating with mixed teams on projects in any of these areas.

Seven of those attending workshop I and five of those attending workshop II provided presentations covering a range of topics and issues. The presentations are described in synopsis form. The key issues which emerged from the workshop discussions, as well as from observers of the process, are described.

Discussion and feedback arrangements

The plenary discussions which completed the first day of the programme included some preliminary feedback from staff who had been undertaking the role of observer during the group discussions.

The design of the workshops enabled the research team to analyse and structure the information and feedback from the first day, in order to present it in summary form to the workshop participants during the follow-up session.

The format for the follow-up session included structured feedback concerning the key issues which emerged from the group work, in addition to observation feedback, thus providing a second reflection cycle on the work previously undertaken.

Towards the end of the follow-up programme, information was provided on the reference point for the project, namely the interprofessional curriculum developed by the MCT, in order to examine this approach in the light of the workshop findings.

Following the workshop events, evaluation forms were sent to participants; the results indicated that participants valued the chance to discuss this complex work with others doing the same sort of thing. As part of the collaborative design, all participants and staff were also sent written interim feedback in Spring 1993 for comment. At that point, half the respondents asked for a further follow-up meeting. Owing to budget constraints it was not possible to organise a further follow-up at that time although it is hoped that this will be possible in the future.

Methodology

The two workshops were structured to follow an action and reflection cycle over one day with a second cycle on the follow-up day held a few weeks later.

Action in the first stage of the workshop was provided by the workshop presentations, vignettes of which are provided below.

Reflection was provided from four perspectives: small group discussion, the records of the rapporteurs and the feedback from the non-participative observers. This material was fed back and checked out with the small groups and later integrated by the rapporteurs into feedback for the large group discussion at the end of the first day.

The sources of data at the end of the first day of each workshop were therefore as follows:

- workshop presentations
- records from rapporteurs
- feedback from observers
- adjusted records from the plenary.

A spreadsheet format was developed to organise this material around the four research questions that shaped the collaborative enquiry.

It became evident at this stage, however, that the material was more detailed and often too subtle to fit into this simple structure. What emerged instead were some strong cross-cutting issues that arose in the course of collaborative work of different kinds. These issues were often dynamic and double-edged and deserved

attention in their own right. They were easily identifiable by following key words and phrases from the data sources. The data was therefore reorganised under these headings.

It was therefore not possible to produce clear-cut responses to the first three research questions.

The priorities in interprofessional learning were, however, emerging clearly but these were directly related to the conditions in the fields in which people worked, whether that was practice, training, research or management. It would have been artificial to separate the interprofessional learning priorities from these related issues. Interprofessional training and education can respond to needs generated by policy, management and organisation, and practice, but it cannot bear the full burden of this responsibility, some of which has to remain with the policy-makers, managers and practitioners themselves.

At the follow-up session, the research team therefore presented these cross-cutting issues alongside the interprofessional learning priorities to participants for further reflection. A more refined version was then produced and circulated to participants for final comment in writing. This concluded the second action and reflection cycle.

Workshop presentations

This section includes vignettes of the projects which were presented during the workshops. Discussion of the projects offered an important opportunity to experiment with a variety of different perspectives on the same piece of work. A constructive atmosphere emerged which indicated the potential of an interprofessional ethos that encourages individuals to work together across considerable differences.

Despite some of the problems described, the presentations demonstrate the 'art of the possible' in collaborative work across a range of agencies and disciplines at this time. Issues and challenges were identified and the vignettes describe some remarkable achievements. The range of projects included interprofessional and interagency practice with a variety of client groups, and collaborative training and research as follows:

Workshop 1 presentations

Presentation 1: Community mental health open referral system—an innovative form of service delivery

A description of a multidisciplinary early intervention service in the field of community mental health. The team includes an occupational therapist, social worker, community psychiatric nurse, psychologist and psychiatrist. A comparison is made between a more traditional model of referral where the GP is the gate-keeper, and the open referral system developed by the multidisciplinary team, designed to enhance ease of access and a more flexible service.

Presentation 2: A multidisciplinary approach to a homeless client group in a specified geographical patch of an NHS Trust

An account of an initiative led by a multidisciplinary Nursing Development Unit with some community outreach schemes. Liaison took place with GPs, social workers, housing provision groups and voluntary organisations. The aim of the project was to break down barriers surrounding different agencies and professional roles and, in so doing, to improve the provision of services to homeless people. The account identifies a number of key issues in the development of multidisciplinary work, including the need for shared interagency training and the introduction of new forms of skill-mix in appropriate areas.

Presentation 3: A primary care planning project in a District Health Authority

Against a background of policy changes, including the NHS and Community Care Act 1990, a review of community nursing in one District Health Authority identified a number of areas in which communication between local GPs and community nursing staff could be improved. This planning project examined aspects of current working practices across general practice and community nursing boundaries, with a view to facilitating improvements in communication and practice. The project exposed a lack of knowledge and understanding of different professional roles and considerable rivalry and prejudice. Changes were introduced to foster collaboration and produce a more user-centred approach.

Presentation 4: A multidisciplinary liaison group concerned with the needs of people with a dementing illness, and their carers, within a London Borough

This project describes the development of a conference organised by a substantial multidisciplinary and interagency liaison group which included carers. The conference was designed to raise awareness of the needs of people with dementia and their carers. It provided the opportunity for professionals to consult closely with carers concerning service provision, and facilitated continuing liaison between service planners, field workers and carers.

The outcomes from the event suggest that services can be improved by multiagency cooperation. The inclusion of carers as full members of the forum played a key part in promoting understanding of what users and carers need from the services. The experience of planning the conference confirmed previous findings (Wertheimer 1991) that much advance planning and careful funding is required to involve carers successfully.

Presentation 5: The development of shared learning in basic training for social workers, health visitors, district nurses, community psychiatric nurses, community mental handicap nurses, midwives and doctors

This shared learning initiative was developed within a University context, over a period of 10 years. The strategy was to make shared learning *integral* to courses, rather than an additional extra. Timetables and coordination presented particular challenges and required advance planning over several years. Outcomes included greater integration of different groups of students and teaching staff within the University and in practice settings. Shared interdisciplinary learning also deepened the understanding of, and respect for, different discipline roles.

Presentation 6: Interagency and interprofessional working between a community development project and a health centre

The essential element in this project was the development of collaboration between a health centre and a neighbouring community development project. Although such collaboration had been planned when both agencies were established, a pattern of isolated working practices had emerged. The community development project took the initiative to break this pattern in response to clearly identified needs articulated by users themselves. Challenges revolved primarily around the availability of resources, particularly in relation to the support of community-based workers, and in developing and maintaining liaison with Health Authority staff. Different cultures and styles of communication between the two agencies were also a key issue. Nonetheless, joint meetings continued to identify ways of establishing an agency partnership aimed at improving the health of the community in an integrated way.

Presentation 7: Meeting the needs of long-term house-bound people

This research project, based in the context of an inner-city group practice, was developed in order to identify the unmet needs of the long-term housebound population and their carers. An additional aim of the project was to promote a multiprofessional approach to the needs of users and carers. The study also evaluated the processes of the multiprofessional team, particularly in terms of how it related to effectiveness and the type of care offered (Koppel & Morris 1993).

Workshop 2 presentations

Presentation 1: Training within the primary health care team

This project describes an attempt to develop shared learning events on a monthly basis in a health centre in order to promote better team-working between GPs, practice nurses, community workers, receptionists and administrative staff. It proved difficult to accommodate radically different learning agendas at the same time as maintaining motivation and attendance.

Presentation 2: A multidisciplinary assessment service based in a health centre

For research purposes, using a collaborative inquiry approach, a short-term (2 years) assessment clinic was organised in a health centre. The assessment process was carried out in response to self-referral or GP referral of patients who often had chronic problems with their health and lifestyle, e.g. migraine, backache, diffuse pain, irritable bowel syndrome. The patients were seen individually over the period of one day by a range of therapists including an osteopath, homoeopath, massage therapist, counsellor and GP. Following this stage, all of those involved— GP, patient and therapists—met in order to discuss the meaning and management of the patient's presenting problem. The approach used took into account physical, mental, social and economic factors.

The project identifies a number of key issues arising from this process, including those relating to professional power and user empowerment, and the use of different models of assessment.

Presentation 3: Working with carers of people with learning difficulties: interprofessional collaboration in training

This project describes the development of a short course for a wide variety of lay and professional carers working with children and adults who have learning or developmental difficulties. The course was designed to provide support and offered time and opportunity to share the members' work experience. The course was largely experiential.

The members valued this way of learning and the regular and much-needed forum for discussion it provided. Over time it became possible for participants to look at the emotional impact of the work on themselves and gradually to focus on the interaction between themselves and their clients rather than simply on facts and procedures. The agencies in which the course members worked were an important focus of discussion as well, because little support or supervision was available in the workplace and the pressures from the work were considerable. It was as if the subtlety and complexity of the work were not recognised by the agencies. Rivalry between disciplines often, therefore, took over in the workplace. When looked at in a supportive environment on the course, workers were able instead to expose how vulnerable and frustrated they often felt.

Presentation 4: Including services for children and families in the community care joint planning process

This presentation explained what was happening in one local authority in relation to joint planning following major policy change in relation to community care and services for children.

Local authorities were required to develop Community Care Plans by the NHS and Community Care Act 1990. These plans covered services to elderly and disabled adults, people with learning difficulties, mental health clients and homeless people. Services to children were covered under separate legislation, the Children Act 1989, and separate social services policy and organisation existed in the social services department described.

As a result, in terms of policy, planning and implementation, two parallel, uncoordinated systems existed. In the community care services, change was rapid and fundamental. In the parts of the organisation providing services for children, there was a different ethos and approach, different working practices and different planning structures. Yet, in reality and taking a 'user-centred' view, families often had needs that crossed all of these boundaries. Also, the organisational structure included Joint Planning Teams (JPTs) for both sets of services. Representatives from other agency management systems sat on these JPTs. The presentation looked at the role of these

interagency Joint Planning Teams in the decision-making processes that influenced eventual joint commissioning of services.

Presentation 5: A multidisciplinary project in health promotion based in a health centre

The impetus for this project arose from health visitors linked to a health centre who wished to find new ways of promoting health and preventing disease, as well as providing information on benefits, housing and general welfare rights. Improving access to community services of all kinds was their key aim.

The presentation described their development of a health information desk and health promotion display, based in the health centre, and staffed by a rota of different professionals. A key aspect of the project was the wide range of information provided by the desk, and the wide variety of workers and agencies who worked and were otherwise linked together in a referral network. These included health visitors, district nurses, school nurses, benefits advisers, physiotherapists, speech therapists, interpreters, counsellors, housing officers, family planning workers and dieticians. Many unmet needs were identified and communication between all those involved was enhanced. Developments have included the spread of this idea to other health centres in the locality, as part of an integrated health and community care development.

CURRENT ISSUES AND THEMES IN INTERPROFESSIONAL COLLABORATION

Collaboration is not easy when organisational structures and professional histories militate against it. The workshop presentations summarised on pages 261–263 describe how participants achieved the 'art of the possible' in their own organisations. Feedback at the evaluation stage showed how much they valued this opportunity for reflecting together on their work, particularly in view of the scarcity of such opportunities in the workplace.

In this section, therefore, some current issues in interprofessional collaboration are identified as they emerged during the workshops. It had been intended to organise this material under the headings of the four questions originally asked but what emerged was far more specific than that structure allowed. The material has accordingly been gathered under the headings of a series of key issues and themes that were identified by the methodology described above.

The major issues and themes identified were:

1. Policy and organisational change in relation to basic professional roles.
2. The impact of basic professional education and training.
3. Difference is difficult/difference is creative.
4. Language, culture and values.
5. Collaboration with carers.
6. User-centredness.
7. Communication and negotiation.
8. Personality and collaboration.
9. Leadership.
10. Individuals working in groups.
11. Resourcing collaborative work.
12. The nature of ideas about collaboration.

Policy and organisational change in relation to basic professional roles

The strong forces for change working on all health and community care professionals and their employing organisations were much in evidence. These forces had done much to stir up existing structures and work patterns, sometimes for the better and sometimes for the worse. In particular, the pace and nature of change had created major insecurities about jobs, provider contracts and organisational survival which had greatly increased the anxiety from the usual hierarchical issues in multiprofessional teams and employer/employee relations. It was clear how little support many participants felt they had in order to meet these changes, because their organisations were often also under threat. Communication between policy makers and those working in the field was highlighted as

important if some dialogue concerning new developments in practice was to be maintained.

When the foundations of the working environment are disrupted and unhelpful in this way, it is difficult to unravel ordinary problems. Although multiprofessional teams and networks were clearly felt to be a very important booster to staff morale, and to the quality of practice in all fields, at this time of critical change teamwork often could not adequately sustain workers who were charged with assessing and supporting the health and welfare of others.

The critical policy changes of the last few years had not only produced new organisational structures, they had begun to challenge the definitions of basic professional roles and tasks. The issues here went beyond current controversies over skill-mix and job grading, and beyond the mere blurring of roles. The language and philosophy of recent policy guidance and legislation ('user-centred', 'seamlessness', 'partnership') had produced vigorous debates on the future direction of service developments and the specific role of each profession within these services.

At the centre of this re-think seemed to be a reformulation of the relationship between health and social care professionals. It was as if a search for appropriate organisational frameworks was taking place that would enable different tasks, skills and cultures to be brought into more creative collaboration. It seemed generally agreed that the community roots of much unhappiness and ill-health was based in poverty and deprivation. Although a significant number of the workshop presentations were drawn from primary health care settings, it was clear that here too the burden of change was in the direction of improved *social* care and of improved *community* liaison (e.g. Workshop 1, Presentations 3, 4, 6 and 7; Workshop 2, Presentations 1 and 5). The community-based projects with health or mental health dimensions were also moving away from a primarily medical model of diagnosis and treatment, towards a more integrated model. Practices included more holistic assessments (covering health and social aspects) and more integrated forms of care and service provision (e.g. Workshop 1, Presentations 1, 2, 4 and 6;

Workshop 2, Presentations 1 and 5). This tendency towards the integration of health and social care was also evident in the shared training programmes described (Workshop 1, Presentation 5; Workshop 2, Presentations 1 and 3), and in the research project (Workshop 1, Presentation 7).

Interestingly, the training programme which formed the reference point for this project proposed in its mission statement that primary health be recognised as a sub-set of community care, and that post-qualifying health and social care training be integrated right across the curriculum.

These developments seem to question whether the reformulation of professional categories, roles, and languages is in process.

The impact of basic professional education and training

The debate about the levels at which interprofessional training should take place was much in evidence. In positive terms, it was suggested that basic training provides security within a basic role and a professional identity. In turn, this foundation enhances people's capacity to make interprofessional links, frees them to be more receptive to the ideas and perspectives of others, and enables them to be less defensive about their own practice. In negative terms, it was pointed out that basic training establishes such different cultures about decision-making and priority-setting, and such different attitudes towards collaboration, that much of the focus of post-qualifying and continuing education must inevitably be on undoing what has gone before.

Doctors

During one of the periods of workshop discussion these issues were looked at in some detail. Doctors described how they are trained during medical school and their years of 'house jobs' in teaching hospitals to become autonomous professionals. They learn to shoulder solitary responsibility and to arrive at clear priorities when prioritising ('triaging') in emergencies. They are trained into making difficult decisions

on their own. Coincidentally, this heightens their sense of the preciousness of resources: knowledge, skill and, particularly, time. They are also presented with the model of hospital consultant and ward round as their paradigm of leadership and of relations between the individual and the group or team. Later, in their professional career, these old habits die hard and make interprofessional collaboration, and the complex and sometimes consensual decision-making sometimes required, difficult. This is especially so if, in the course of interagency collaboration, prioritising is less than rigorous, and decisions are left wholly unclear.

Nurses

The nursing disciplines have traditionally been trained within a hospital setting to complement the medical model. Recent changes in nursing roles and attitudes have been brought about, however, by new management systems, the drive toward graduate status and the introduction of a very different basic training model with Project 2000. Social changes have also brought greater awareness of gender issues which had made the power-relation between doctors and nurses a key training issue. There is also now a drive at advanced levels to establish the more autonomous grade of nurse-practitioner, but there is far from united support for this change and at basic levels nurses are trained to work efficiently to clear professional guidelines within a hierarchical and often bureaucratic framework. Their basic models for collaboration, decision-making and priority-setting are influenced accordingly.

Social workers

Social workers have a very different basic training from that of doctors and nurses, centred on statutory responses to the conflicting needs of deprived, disabled and under-privileged groups in society. Their training usually takes place in the community, often in a range of different settings. The focus is on social care and the priorities are set by the political and statutory framework of social services, and the resources allocated to it. Great emphasis is given to values that underpin services of all kinds, and particularly to equality of opportunity. The knowledge base of social work, though now tied more closely to evaluative research, does not have its roots in the hard sciences, and its status has always been that of a semi-profession. Indeed, professionals and professionalism have sometimes been regarded with suspicion in social work because of their place within the same class and privilege structures that disadvantage social services clients.

The statutory and bureaucratic structures that frame social services also mean that social workers are trained to function as bureau-professionals who make decisions and set priorities according to local and central policy and in consultation with others, usually within a many-tiered line-management system. The contrast with models of authority, autonomy and hierarchy generated by training for the health care professions could hardly be greater.

Difference is difficult/difference is creative

Workshop members seemed very aware of their individual differences and their different professional agendas both within the workshops and at work. Such differences were recognised both as a potential source of difficulty requiring acknowledgement and sensitivity, and as an important focus of work. Friction was considered to be a healthy sign of life and of active communication across real differences.

One of the risks of collaboration in the light of these differences was felt to be the danger of turning different professional knowledge, skills and identities into some kind of interprofessional 'porridge'. The ways in which the Seebohm recommendations for generic social services were implemented and the impact of these recommendations were quoted several times as a warning example. Such issues again raised the question of skill-mix: should flexible, multi-skilled workers be developed to reconcile existing interprofessional differences within new roles? The allied issues of whether common core

skills, knowledge and attitudes were needed by all primary health and community care workers, and at what stage they should be acquired, were also frequently raised.

Different organisational structures and practices, particularly those surrounding child care and mental health were felt to be something of a puzzle. It was a further puzzle, particularly to the health care professionals present, that the term 'community care' in some social services departments was taken to exclude child care and mental health. On the one hand, these differences broke up the life-cycle approach to practice, and continuity of care, and were a barrier to collaboration across client groups; on the other, these same differences represented hard-won specialist expertise that was threatened by collaboration. There was clearly no easy solution here.

One of the key differences between disciplines that surfaced repeatedly in discussions about work roles and tasks was that of language, which seemed fundamental enough to be addressed under a heading in its own right.

Language, culture and values

It became clear during the workshops that language is a key issue when developing interprofessional training, practice or research. Differing perceptions and descriptions of work tasks reflect frameworks of language and meaning developed early on in basic professional training. These frameworks have often been reinforced later by restrictive approaches within agencies and professions to joint working and training. Indeed, the individualistic nature of some professional activities generates anxiety about stepping outside the familiar. The projects described represent a significant move away from this history.

Different professional language systems can be seen as the exchange currencies of collaborative work. Workshop participants described how genuine misunderstandings arise across professional and agency boundaries because the same words have different meanings in different contexts or sub-systems. For example, 'community care' itself is a problematic term, the meaning of which varies not only between professions, but also between agencies. In one agency, it means the care of elderly, disabled and sick people, but excludes other care groups; in another it is an inclusive term; in primary health the meaning may be different again. To the lay person, 'community care' may sound like an inclusive term. In fact, it is, of course, selective. Some local authorities use the term to include elderly, sick and disabled people only, thus excluding mental health services as well as child care from their in-house definition. The local and national meanings of community care are therefore far from user-centred; they are constructed within bureaucratic and legislative languages that can mystify not only users and their families but also professionals from another part of the overall system where the local meanings-in-use are different.

These differences of meaning can befuddle collaborative work and take time to unravel. During the workshops many examples arose in relation to the work being presented, and some misunderstandings occurred.

The practical use of language is as important as the terminology itself, and is clearly derived from different professional cultures and their different value-bases. For example, the use of the terms 'mentally handicapped', 'learning difficulty', or 'learning disability' varies within and between professional groups. There are also variations as to whether work with mentally handicapped people and work with those with mental health problems belong in the same category or specialty. When professional groups behave as if a consensus is widely shared about these issues, and as if 'politically correct' terminology and categorisations are fully accepted across the board, then problems develop between the different groups when these assumptions prove to be misplaced. Collaborative work, it was pointed out, can run aground on the pride associated with occupying the high moral ground, just as easily as it can on the prejudice associated with ignorance, or with protecting the status quo.

Language, and the professional cultures and values within it were considered by participants to be some of the most important issues in inter-

professional work. It was felt that working and learning together could produce new shared languages, a common-enough culture and negotiated values, but that this 'shaking-down' process would take time. If time is not taken then the quality of the work or learning is likely to be blocked or compromised and stress, then related to anti-task, defensive behaviour, is more likely.

Collaboration with carers

The definition of the collaborative team or network had been extended by several of the projects presented to include carers as well as professionally trained workers (Workshop 1, Presentations 2, 4 and 7; Workshop 2, Presentations 3 and 5). One of the most innovative pieces of work presented was, in fact, carried out by a specially appointed carers' development worker (Workshop 1, Presentation 4). The redefinition of the multidisciplinary network required very intricate planning and confirmed previous project work in this area carried out by The King's Fund (Wertheimer 1991). Both projects indicate the need for particular attention to be paid at the planning stage to funding carers' time, providing transport and arranging potential respite cover. This lengthens the planning stage considerably but is well worth it in terms of the increased understanding and quality of collaboration produced between carers and professionals.

Collaboration with carers was felt to be a complex task, especially, for example, where carer and user were in competition with each other for professional time or attention, or where the needs of carer and professional conflicted over medication or respite care. Creating a representative carer voice in local policy and planning groups could also be a delicate issue, with a tendency for those who were the most vocal or organised to take up central roles. Those in greatest need might have no way of making their voices heard except through a census or locality profiling. A great deal of community development work was necessary, it was felt, to follow up on this basic information and make collaboration with carers the rule rather than the exception.

Here, again, are implications for interprofessional training. The reference point project provides one training solution where carer organisers, support workers, and volunteer organisers train alongside other health and social care professionals as integral members of a shared learning group.

User-centredness

Most, if not all, of the projects presented were actively user-centred in a way that went far beyond rhetoric. Workshop 1, Presentation 1 offered direct and open access to services for mental health users in place of the traditional GP referral model. These innovations had significantly increased access and had also changed the nature of the services offered. Workshop 1, Presentation 2 took a similar open access approach to homeless users. Again, the watchwords were 'flexibility' and 'choice'. The coordinating worker was of central importance in working towards a more flexible approach. The primary care planning project (Workshop 1, Presentation 3) was also concerned to develop connections between professionals who were organised, managed and trained differently but provided complementary services. Primary care teams must link up if the user is not to fall between two or more stools. So the story continued in all the projects described, including Workshop 2, Presentation 4, where the bureaucratic and statutory separation of services for children and community care services was described in graphic terms.

User-centredness was nevertheless felt to be a complex issue. Similar arguments apply to those outlined above with regard to carers: each user is an individual with unique needs not easily represented by user-groups; user-groups are not unified, and whereas policy may be influenced by them, there are no guarantees that practice or resources will follow. The Patient's and Citizens' Charters have raised the profile of the user, as well as raising users' hopes for more say in a better service. However, professionals are weary of doing a difficult job in the full glare of public criticism, and some professionals felt exploited by demands to meet

ever-increasing need with ever fewer resources in a context of ever more complex change. Within this climate, it was proposed by workshop participants that user and carer organisations must share the responsibility for promoting good collaboration with professionals along a 'two-way street'.

Some also felt that the recent emphasis on users and carers was not merely a matter of good practice and productive social change. It was also seen as a cost-cutting exercise that enabled 'divide and rule' managerial processes to occur. It was therefore felt to be a means of reducing hard-won professional expertise and the power and effectiveness of the professionals. Some felt that whilst change was necessary, the pendulum could swing too far.

Communication and negotiation

The complexity of interprofessional and interagency collaboration places a large burden on communication skills. Participants emphasised how important it was, therefore, for shared learning to take place around real examples that are capable of generating a new and genuine understanding of the intricacies of the different perspectives involved. This takes time and the multidisciplinary communication involved is extremely complex (e.g. Workshop 1, Presentation 5), because ignorance and stereotyping have to be addressed as well as the substantive practice issues.

Similarly, building collaborative practice or policy at a local level is time-consuming and requires a high degree of motivation and skilled communication if the inevitable human, professional and bureaucratic impediments are to be overcome (e.g. Workshop 1, Presentations 3, 4, 6 and 7; Workshop 2, Presentation 2). Here, planning presents a real challenge and it is necessary to use and sustain different kinds of communication and negotiation. Those involved, and especially those in leadership roles, have to be able to tolerate and work with disparate or opposed views, and radically different constructions of what the problems and potential solutions really are. They have to be able to mediate between these different perspectives with a high degree of diplomatic skill, as well as with pragmatism and with power. A capacity to use both written and oral, and informal and formal styles of communication was felt to be essential in bridging the inevitable gaps between viewpoints. Indeed, a personal, flexible style might be seen as part of a repertoire of communication skills which are a necessary part of getting to grips with the differences between individuals and professional groups.

Time for communication and a safe space for reflecting on the issues and difficulties of collaborative work is in short supply in the workplace. Indeed, the workshops were valued because they provided the opportunity for this to take place. The anxiety generated by collaborative work is often considerable (whatever the precise nature of the work), and that anxiety is responded to more defensively if time for digesting complex experience is not available. Communication problems are then more likely to ensue and the quality of practice is likely to suffer. There are implications here for managers, trainers and practitioners.

Personality and collaboration

An interesting focus which emerged quite clearly from both workshops was the important part that individual personality plays in helping or hindering collaborative work. When all that is familiar is in the process of change, it seems that personalities matter much more. Bureaucratic and professional constraints can be, and often are, organisationally defensive, sustained by the anxiety and pressure of the work itself and by human rigidity (Menzies 1960). Where professionals and agencies have to collaborate, however, these human and organisational rigidities are far from sustaining. Time and again workshop participants used the word 'flexible', and phrases like 'flexible human response', or 'it was no good being rigid', whereas in the past the blame for collaborative difficulties might have been laid at the door of a particular profession, organisation, or even client.

There was a recognition of the central importance of individual personality, particularly

where someone was on a boundary-crossing, or in a boundary-maintaining role. Collaborative work, it was said, requires flexible personalities who can 'see round corners' to 'get things done' and 'make the right connections'; yet they must remain true to their professional identity, their agency, and to the key work tasks. Personalities could 'make or break the collaborative tasks'. This was regarded as a key issue and formed an important basis for discussion on the follow-up day. It also has implications for training and professional ideologies.

Leadership

One of the most interesting issues to emerge as a key theme in the collaborative projects was leadership. Many felt that in order for the complexity of interagency work to be managed, and the gaps and conflicts between different professional viewpoints, or practices, not only to be bridged, but also to be creatively exploited, skilled leadership was essential. Even where this was not made explicit, the discussion of the work made it clear that this was indeed the case. Different styles of leadership were both modelled and described in the workshop, and clearly affected the success of the projects and the experience of all concerned with them. A capacity to move between different leadership styles seemed to be particularly necessary to the progress and outcome of the more complex projects, although it probably applied across the board. Opinions varied concerning the extent to which single discipline leaders help or hinder the collaborative process. However, it was suggested that a multiprofessional team needs different types of leadership at different stages.

Creativity can be maximised and sustained, it was felt, by skilled and artful leadership. Learning for leadership in interprofessional work seems therefore to be a key issue, whether the work is carried out by a front-line practice team, an interagency network, or a policy or training group. The creative use of ideas and differences will contribute to the resources which, in turn, will benefit users and improve the quality of services.

Individuals working in groups

Some very basic issues arose concerning the way that individuals and professional groups conduct themselves in the course of interprofessional collaboration. In practice settings, for example, there were competitive problems about the 'ownership' of clients and patients, and the control over decision-making. Similar issues arose in the course of collaborative research and training. In all three settings—practice, training and research—professionals acknowledged that they 'needed to be needed' and yet often felt they had insufficient expertise for the complex tasks that confronted them in their daily work. They were often struggling with a sense of impotence and frustration generated by different aspects of the work itself: people in great need, people demanding what was not possible or sometimes not available, and, of course, a serious lack of resources.

These struggles to 'contain the uncontainable' and 'cope with the impossible' seemed to feed professional rivalry at the very same time as stimulating a greater need for collaboration and interdependence. Thus, if particular professional groups absented themselves from interprofessional team meetings, their absence was perceived as a disappointing, powerful and intrusive factor to the sometimes fragile working of the team or group. In addition, conflict within groups was sometimes projected on to 'outside forces' such as other agencies and institutions. On closer examination during the reflective part of the workshop, the roots of these difficulties were found to be related not only to different professional roles, tasks and defences but also to patterns of collaboration established in basic training as described above.

Resourcing collaborative work

Inevitably, resources were a major issue in nearly all of the workshop presentations.

Time appeared to be the most important resource of all: time for planning and doing the work; for thinking about the work; and then for developing or improving it. Human resources could only be developed and utilised fully if time permitted that cycle to take place. Without time, stress levels increased, and the quality of communication, and hence of the work itself, diminished.

Funding collaborative work is a highly technical issue because sources of funding for practice, training and research are fragmented across either the professional groups, or different areas of specialist practice, such as child protection, mental health, HIV/AIDS, or work with elderly people. Specific funding issues are raised where projects include carers and users (see Workshop 1, Presentation 4), where transport costs and substitute care must be provided and extra induction, debriefing and follow-up times are needed.

Several vignettes described how a commitment to support collaboration by sanctioning time and finance at management level is necessary for interprofessional and interagency projects to succeed. There was more than one instance (e.g. Workshop 1, Presentations 3 and 6; Workshop 2, Presentation 1) of the management of one discipline cutting across collaborative work, because it was considered to be a loss of resources to the primary task of that discipline, or because the line managers were frightened of losing control of their own staff. This finding reinforces the findings of Manchester workshops of the 1970s (Flack 1976). Some argued that the first step in every collaborative project should be to establish the commitment and collaboration within the various management systems implicated.

One further interesting issue about resources was the importance of central or charitable sources of funding to stimulate new projects and offset long-standing separatist patterns of local care. The devolution of budgets to localities is therefore a mixed blessing, since existing local rivalries may well be simply perpetuated by the regular rush for cash in the internal market. If, however, the terms of grants and pump-priming monies clearly require interagency collaboration this tendency could be offset.

The nature of ideas about collaboration

The idea of working together seems to have been a

very important antidote to a historical legacy of professional and agency demarcation. Clearly those who attended the workshops were enthusiasts, but the effort and hard work that had gone into making interagency collaboration possible, usually over several years, was exceptional. Often there seemed to have been quite high expectations of what such collaboration might produce. Surprisingly, the evidence of the projects described suggested that these high hopes were often fulfilled.

Participants stated that working together made more sense of their difficult and sometimes unrewarding work, and produced better outcomes. The sheer difficulty of some aspects of work in primary health and community care had made people feel progressively de-skilled when working solely within their own professional and organisational frameworks. They said they needed the broader, more integrative approach, because it fitted more accurately the problems with which they were faced and made them feel more supported and effective. Their experience thus confirmed the views of writers such as Schön (1987), Pietroni (1992), and Hornby (1993), and supported the direction of other initiatives designed to foster collaboration.

In the course of the workshop discussion, references to the more sinister meaning of collaboration also arose. Why, it was asked, should such a good idea, so deeply rooted in good practice, only *now* be taken up with such vigour and placed at the centre of policy? And why should colleagues from other professions, particularly senior managers with backgrounds outside community care or primary health, be embracing a field they had hitherto neglected? Although people clearly would have liked to believe that policy was actually supporting good practice, the storm of policy change and its paramount focus on saving costs and increasing efficiency, made them suspicious.

Uncertainty about the policy motives for increased collaboration was not the only impediment to collaboration, however. It was pointed out that mistaken perceptions concerning the roles, knowledge-base and professional skills of others often hindered the extent to which collaboration could be thought about constructively and then turned into practice. This was particularly found to be so in the early stages of the district-wide research and planning project (Workshop 1, Presentation 3) which sought to promote a multiprofessional approach to primary health care teams. In addition, it was stated that liaison between community and primary care was often difficult as a result of different agendas, cultures and working practices. Skilful management is required to make it work.

SUMMARY OF KEY ISSUES AND INTERPROFESSIONAL LEARNING PRIORITIES

In this section, whilst the primary focus concerns the implications for interprofessional learning priorities, a number of issues relating to practice, management and organisation and policy are also presented. Such issues emerged from the workshop discussions as an important part of the *context* of interprofessional activity.

Practice issues

1. An integrated approach to practice more accurately fits users' needs, and can sustain and raise the morale of staff.
2. Interprofessional rivalry is stimulated by the sense of frustration and impotence which comes from practice in a field in which there are often no solutions.
3. Carers' representatives and carers' development workers are vital contributors to multi-disciplinary teams and networks.
4. Direct self-referral to some services improves access, influences the nature of the service offered and is likely to meet users' needs more effectively; inappropriate gate-keeping is to be avoided.
5. Flexibility is essential in administrative and professional roles and tasks to facilitate collaboration across complex agency boundaries.

Management and organisational issues

1. Individual agency management systems need to make a clear time, space and funding commitment to fostering interagency work.
2. The development of interagency management systems is likely to enhance the establishment of formal collaborative structures at all levels.
3. Managers at local, regional and central level need good access to information concerning evaluated, innovative projects involving collaborative work in order to guide policy and resource priorities.
4. Carers' development workers and care coordinators contribute significantly to the sensitivity of services to meet the needs of carers and users.
5. Stress management training for staff is a high priority.
6. Support systems for staff are critical at times of great change.
7. A common language across health and social care is needed to facilitate collaboration across health and social care. Terminologies in use in different specialties such as child care, mental health and work with elderly people, as well as in the different agencies, are confusing.

Policy issues

1. The high profile given to collaborative work has been well received, although some practitioners and middle managers have anxiety about recent policy changes and the vulnerability of the welfare state.
2. Rapid and fundamental policy change has tended to divert energy and attention from the collaborative practice agenda towards personal, professional and organisational survival.
3. Skilful, flexible leadership is of utmost importance in developing collaborative initiatives.
4. Collaborative research and development, though a complex activity, enhances interagency understanding and fosters common knowledge and language.

5. A more integrated language is needed to foster collaboration and cooperation between health and social care.
6. Public education is needed concerning what is a responsible use of health and social care services to ensure that services are used appropriately and go to those with greatest need.
7. Mechanisms for funding more collaborative work are needed, including training, research and practice, if fragmentation of resources and effort is to be avoided.

Interprofessonal learning priorities

There are key implications arising from the *culture, organisation* and *management* of interprofessional learning, as well as from the development of appropriate *skills, knowledge* and *attitudes.*

In terms of the culture, organisation and management of interprofessional learning it is important to:

1. Address through shared learning the mistaken perceptions and professional stereotypes that impede interprofessional work.
2. Provide an understanding of the languages, cultures and values of the different professions so that the quality of collaborative work can be improved.
3. Give greater priority to the specific profiles and development needs of individual practitioners and managers since individuals can make or break collaborative working.
4. Stimulate the capacity for managing, and making the most of differences of all kinds, and particularly for working at understanding basic professional differences of all kinds which stem from basic training, in relation to core values and to models of authority, leadership and decision-making and collaboration.
5. Create a definition of collaborative work in which collaboration with carers' representatives is the rule rather than the exception, and in which the intricate nature of that collaboration is understood, including the often different perspectives of users themselves.
6. Promote shared learning around real practice

problems since, though time consuming, this generates understanding, shared language and new conceptualisations, all of which facilitate collaboration.

7. Allow time and a safe space for digesting the stress and anxiety of practice and for thinking about interprofessional and interagency collaboration.

8. Develop a learning culture in which evaluation, reflection and feedback are key elements since interprofessional differences can be addressed and digested in the course of the cyclical patterns of action and learning that result.

9. Provide training opportunities which include a range of workers from different agencies and different organisational levels to promote multi-perspective thinking.

10. Earmark funds, time and adequate room-space for interprofessional and interagency training.

11. Take account of differing professional, agency and course timetables in long-term planning for shared learning.

12. Make available good examples of interprofessional and interagency collaboration in order to demonstrate 'the art of the possible'.

13. Develop a broad range of teaching methods, with particular emphasis on experiential learning, since this allows the complexity of interprofessional and interagency collaboration to be explored and understood.

14. Facilitate the development of teams and networks by sharing real work experiences in a non-judgemental environment which enables those involved to identify and explore shared preoccupations and significant differences.

In terms of the development of *skills, knowledge* and *attitudes* for interprofessional collaboration it is necessary to:

1. Develop flexibility and creative thinking in individual professionals who have to work in a context of continual change and uncertainty.

2. Develop wide-ranging skills in communication, both written and oral, formal and informal, since a flexible personal style of communication is a great asset to collaborative work.

3. Give priority to stress management skills.

4. Increase knowledge, understanding and skills with regard to working in small and large groups and extended networks and functioning as part of a team.

5. Develop the capacity for leadership through an appropriate knowledge base and a range of leadership skills which are suited to complex multi-agency teams and networks.

6. Provide senior managers (RHA, DHA, FHSA, Senior SSD staff) with access to learning opportunities which include skills relating to interprofessional and interagency collaboration across sectors and systems, as well as communication and groupwork skills.

7. Provide those involved in interprofessional education and training with opportunities for personal and professional development and continuous updating.

ACKNOWLEDGEMENTS FOR NETWORKING AND TEAMWORK

This project has been a collaborative endeavour. The authors wish to thank particularly those who presented their own work for scrutiny in the workshops and those who contributed to the discussion. Without them this publication would not have been possible. Particular thanks are also due to the team and staff at Marylebone Centre Trust, who helped to organise and provide administrative support for the project, notably: Sally Kneeshaw who did much of the original work concerning networks in order to establish a suitable membership; Sheelagh Taylor for her meticulous typing of the manuscript; and Moira Jenkins and Carol Pyper for administration.

The two workshop staff teams contributed to preparatory thinking, and provided skilled help on the day. They included: Joan Browne, Peter Davies, Angela Foster, Jan Hatch, Sally Kneeshaw, Richard McLaren, David Peters, Margaret Thwaites, Sybilla de Uray-Ura, Vivien Webber.

Marylebone Centre Trust relies heavily on volunteer help in the library, with publications and with other day-to-day work. From this team we wish to thank Bunny Hoover for help with organisation and Reg Mares for help with mailing. Here also, Maggie Linford and Hermione Raven worked on the final manuscript with remarkable good humour.

Finally, we wish to thank Simon Biggs and Mary Winner, our CCETSW project officers, who made the project possible and provided advice when needed.

Although the project has been very much a collaborative endeavour, this publication contains comment, analysis and interpretation for which the authors alone are responsible.

REFERENCES

Andrews J 1993 Joint training for doctors and staff (news item) Doctor, 16.9.93

Areskog N-H 1989 Man—society, multiprofessional integrated study programme Faculty of Health Sciences, Linköping University, Sweden

Areskog N-H 1993 Interprofessional and multiprofessional education in Europe, Nicosia Conference WHO, Conference presentation. European Network for Development of Multiprofessional Education in Health Sciences (EMPE) Conference, Kracow, Poland, Sept. 1993

Barclay P 1982 Social workers: their role & tasks. NISW Bedford Square Press, London

Barker I (ed) 1989 Multidisciplinary teamwork; models of good practice. Central Council for Education & Training in Social Work, London

Bennett P, Dawar A, Dick A 1972 Interprofessional cooperation, Journal of Royal College of General Practitioners, 22, 603

Bines H, Watson D 1992 Developing professional education. The Society for Research into Higher Education and Open University Press

Brent: London Borough of 1985 A child in trust. Report of the Panel of Inquiry into the circumstances surrounding the death of Jasmine Beckford. London

Brill N I 1976 Teamwork: working together in human services. J B Lippincott, Philadelphia

Children Act 1988. HMSO, London

Croft S, Beresford P 1989 User involvement, citizenship and social policy. Critical Social Policy, vol. 9, no. 2, Autumn

Croft S, Beresford P 1992 The politics of participation. Critical Social Policy, vol. 12, no. 2, Autumn

Crombie D L 1984 Social class and health status: inequality and difference. RCGP Occasional paper 25

Cumberlege J 1986 Neighbourhood nursing—A focus for care. Report of the Community Nursing Review. HMSO, London

Dartington T 1986 The limits of altruism—elderly mentally infirm people as a test case for collaboration. The King's Fund, London

Davidson S 1983 Planning and coordination of social services in multiorganisational contexts. Social Services Review,

vol. 50, no. 1, 117–137

DHSS 1974 Report of the Committee of Inquiry into the care and supervision provided in relation to Maria Colwell. HMSO, London

DHSS 1988 Report of the Inquiry into child abuse in Cleveland 1987 (Chair: Justice Butler-Sloss). HMSO Cmd 412, London

DHSS 1989 Caring for people: community care in the next decade and beyond. HMSO, London

DoH 1989 Working for patients. The Health Service caring for the 1990s. HMSO, London

DoH 1991a Working together—under the Children Act 1989. HMSO, London

DoH 1991b The health of the nation, A consultative document for health in England. HMSO, London

Dingwall R 1975 Health visiting and social work—what are the boundaries? Health & Social Services Journal, 85, 2608–2609

Flack G 1976a Team training—to bring the professionals to the people, Health & Social Services Journal, Dec. 10

Flack G 1976b Looking for dividends from the cooperative movement: Report on a multidisciplinary seminar. Health & Social Services Journal, Mar. 11

Flack G 1979 Education for cooperation in health and social work—papers from Symposium on interprofessional learning, University of Nottingham, July 1979. RCGP, London. Occasional paper 14

Goodlad S (ed) 1984 Education for professions, Quis Custodiet. Guildford, Surrey, SRHE & NFER–Nelson

Greenwich, London Borough of 1987 A child in mind. Report of the Commission of Inquiry into the circumstances surrounding the death of Kimberley Carlile. London

Gregson B A, Cartlidge A, Bond J 1991 Interprofessional collaboration in primary health care organisations. RCGP, London. Occasional paper, 52

Griffiths Sir Roy 1988 Community care: agenda for action. HMSO, London

Hart J T 1988 A new kind of doctor: the general practitioner's part in the health of the community. Merlin Press, London

Henkel M 1991 Some notes on 'Changing ideas about knowledge and education', Brunel University

Hey A, Minty B, Trowell J 1991 Interprofessional & interagency work: theory, practice and training for the nineties, ch 11. In: Pietroni M (ed) Right or privilege? CCETSW, London

Hornby S 1993 Collaborative care—interprofessional, interagency and interpersonal. Blackwell Scientific Publications, Oxford

Hull M 1992 Report on inter/multidisciplinary training developments in the Learning Difficulties programme (1986–1991) with particular reference to CCETSW London & South East Region, Internal Report

Huntington J 1981 Social work and general medical practice. George Allen & Unwin, London

Jones R V H 1986 Working together—learning together. RCGP, London. Occasional paper 33

Kane R 1976 Interprofessional teamwork. Syracuse University School of Social Work, New York

Kilcoyne A, Pietroni P 1990 The history of the primary health care team. Article in Members Reference Book. RCGP, 307–311

Koppel I V, Morris B 1993 Meeting the needs of the long-term housebound. Grove Health Centre, London

Lambeth, London Borough of 1987 Report of the Public

Inquiry into the death of Tyra Henry. London

Leathard A 1992 Interprofessional developments at South Bank Polytechnic London. Journal of Interprofessional Care, vol. 6, no. 1, 17–24

Lonsdale A, Webb A, Briggs T L 1980 Teamwork in the personal social services and health care. Croom Helm, London

Marten R, Mond N C 1971 General practitioners and the social services departments. Jnl RCGP, 21, no. 103, 101–104

Meek H, Pietroni M 1991 Other models of post-qualifying training 1—general practice, ch 6. In Pietroni M (ed) Right or privilege. CCETSW, London, pp 56–64

Mental Health Act 1983. HMSO, London

Menzies I E P 1960 A case study in the functioning of social systems as a defence against anxiety. Human Relations, 13, 95–121

National Health Service and Community Care Act 1990. HMSO, London

Pietroni P C 1992 Towards reflective practice—the languages of health and social care, JIPC, vol. 6, no. 1, 7–16

Royal College of General Practitioners Working Party 1972 The future general practitioner: learning and teaching: BMJ

Royal College of General Practitioners Working Party 1990 Primary care of people with mental handicap. RCGP, London. Occasional paper 47

Schön D 1983 The reflective practitioner. How practitioners think in action. Harper Collins

Schön D 1987 Educating the reflective practitioner. Jossey-Bass, San Francisco

Schön D 1992 The crisis of professional knowledge and the pursuit of an epistemology of practice. JIPC, vol. 6, no. 1.

Shakespeare H, Tucker W, Northover J 1989 Manpower planning advisory group. Report of a national survey on interprofessional education in primary health care. Centre for the Advancement of Interprofessional Education (CAIPE)

Spratley J 1989 Disease prevention and health promotion in primary health care. Team workshops organised by the Health Education Authority. Evaluation report, Health Education Authority, London

Spratley J 1992 Community care—towards a model of interprofessional learning for advanced practice. Research project—Interim Report. Marylebone Centre Trust, London

Stallibrass A 1989 Being me and also us—lessons from the Peckham Experiment. Scottish Academic Press, Edinburgh

Stevens A 1992 Joint & shared training: Community Care issues. CCETSW, Internal Discussion Paper

Stevens A, Gabbey J 1991 Needs assessment health trends. vol. 23, no. 1, 20–23

Storrie J 1992 Mastering interprofessionalism—an inquiry into the development of Masters programmes with an interprofessional focus. JIPC, vol. 6, no. 3, 253–259

Taylor R C, Ford E G 1983 The elderly at risk. Jnl RCGP, 33, 699–705

Thwaites M 1993 Interprofessional education and training. CAIPE Bulletin, No. 6, Summer

Tibbit R 1988 Health and personal Social Services in the United Kingdom: interorganisational behaviour and service development. In: Williamson A, Room G (eds) Health and welfare state in Britain. Heinemann, London

Tiivas A 1991 Report to Hammersmith and Fulham, ACPC re multidisciplinary training 1991. Internal report

Toase M (ed) 1991 Interprofessional collaboration and education—an annotated bibliography. Centre for the Advancement of Interprofessional Education in Primary Health and Community Care (CAIPE), London

Tsouros A D (ed) 1990 Healthy cities project. A project becomes a movement. Review of progress, 1987–1990. World Health Organization

Wertheimer A 1991 A chance to speak out—consulting service users and carers about community care. The King's Fund, London

Whittington C 1962 Teaching and assessing social workers for organisational and interprofessional practice. CCETSW/King's College Project: Stage I, CCETSW

Whittington C, Bell L, Holland R 1993 Summary papers on learning for organisational and interprofessional competence in social work. CCETSW/King's College Project: Stage II, CCETSW.

Woodhouse D, Penegelly P 1991 Anxiety and the dynamics of collaboration, Aberdeen University Press

WHO 1986 Health for all by the year 2000. Charter for Action. Faculty of Community Medicine, London

WHO 1900 Healthy cities. Second Inter-Regional Healthy Cities Conference, Montpelier 8–11 October

Index

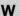